Management of Prader-Willi Syndrome

Louise R. Greenswag Randell C. Alexander
Editors

Management of Prader-Willi Syndrome

Under the Sponsorship of The Prader-Willi Syndrome Association

Springer-Verlag New York Berlin Heidelberg
London Paris Tokyo

Louise R. Greenswag, R.N., PH.D.
Adjunct Professor, College of Nursing
Program Consultant for Prader-Willi Syndrome
Iowa Child Health Specialty Clinics
University Hospital School
The University of Iowa Hospitals and Clinics
Iowa City, Iowa 52242, USA

Randell C. Alexander, M.D., PH.D.
University Hospital School
The University of Iowa Hospitals and Clinics
Iowa City, Iowa 52242, USA

Library of Congress Cataloging-in-Publication Data
Management of Prader-Willi syndrome / edited by Louise R. Greenswag, Randell C. Alexander.
p. cm.
Bibliography: p.
Includes index.
1. Prader-Willi syndrome. I. Greenswag, Louise R. II. Alexander, Randell C.
RJ520.P7M36 1988
618.92'0043—dc19 87-37640

Typeset by Asco Trade Typesetting Ltd., Hong Kong.
Printed and bound by Edwards Brothers, Ann Arbor, Michigan.
Printed in the United States of America.

9 8 7 6 5 4 3 2 1

ISBN 0-387-96687-0 Springer-Verlag New York Berlin Heidelberg
ISBN 3-540-96687-0 Springer-Verlag Berlin Heidelberg New York

To children with Prader-Willi syndrome and their families,
and to
Sidney Greenswag and Carol Alexander
for their encouragement and patience.

Foreword

I have had a major interest in Prader-Willi syndrome (PWS) for over 30 years and, having dealt with many patients, have reached the conclusion that PWS is one of the two most grave ailments I have encountered—the other being Huntington's Disease (HD). Anyone who has witnessed the mood swings and the relentless, progressive, intellectual, and physical deterioration associated with HD would agree beyond a doubt that it is a devastating condition. PWS is an equally devastating birth defect that characteristically presents major problems from birth. The enormous difficulties associated with the first phase of PWS cause frustration and guilt in mothers who perceive themselves as inept at feeding and nurturing their affected child. This guilt intensifies during the second phase, as PWS children constantly appear plagued by a relentless hunger that dominates their lives. The presence of this insatiable urge to eat, which is beyond the control of the patient, his family, or physician, becomes the primary focus for the child and inhibits all other activities and interests. In addition to the issue of satiety, a PWS child faces a life of sexual incompetence. Reactions to these problems are further aggravated by hypothalamic dysregulation, which seems to affect temperament. It is not surprising, therefore, that emotional incontinence increases in severity and frequency as the PWS child grows older. Parents, usually unable to manage diets, food-seeking activities, and bizarre behavior, become distraught and emotionally drained. Family systems deteriorate and life becomes hell for all concerned. In my experience, parents of PWS children come to the physician's office in great distress and total despair more often than parents of children with any other birth defect. They speak of their helplessness, the sacrifices of other family members, their love for their affected child, and their concerns about the future. One common theme is the reluctance of many parents to consider alternative living arrangements. This may reflect attempts at denial that a problem exists with which they cannot cope. Fortunately, effective management, even for the most severe cases, is a realistic possibility, particularly after parents are finally able to accept the fact that the family home is not the best place for the affected adolescent or adult.

It has taken years to recognize that solutions to the multifaceted problems of PWS require the expertise of many specialists—pediatricians, neurologists, endocrinologists, nutritionists, psychologists, nurses, special education consultants, speech therapists, physiotherapists, and occupational therapists—all play important, collaborative roles in the lives of PWS individuals and their families.

This book is the result of the realization of its editors that a cooperative effort is needed to ensure appropriate interventions. They were able to assemble an array of experts, each of whom presents suggestions for how a specific discipline can best help. The book gives useful directions to all of those involved in the care of children and adults with PWS, not least to the parents. It may not only help to provide a sophisticated treatment program for PWS, but it may also encourage specialists to collaborate to help the PWS individuals and their families to carry their lot.

Iowa City, Iowa HANS ZELLWEGER, M.D.

Preface

Ten years after Hans Zellweger started a registry of newborns with the characteristic of hypotonia (floppy babies), Prader-Willi syndrome was described as a subset of that group. During the next 20 years, a modest number of new cases was added to the literature, but no success was achieved in creating an awareness among the medical community that this unusual disorder existed. For the few families that had been given the diagnosis, there was little else to offer.

This was the situation in 1975, nearly 30 years after Dr. Zellweger's initial efforts, when Gene and Fausta Deterling were told that their newborn son, Curtis, had the condition. To be told that physicians knew little about the problem and even less about what to do, either for those with the affliction or for their families, became an unacceptable obstacle. The Deterling's efforts stimulated the formation of the Prader-Willi Syndrome Association. This association has become more than just a parent support group and now focuses not only on Prader-Willi persons, but on assisting their families, informing concerned professionals, and educating the public.

Louise R. Greenswag and Randell C. Alexander bring further insight and expanded recognition of the multifacted characteristics of Prader-Willi syndrome. They accomplish this not merely by description but, most importantly, by gathering together experiences gained during the past decade. Does one dare to hope that the years to come will continue to be as fruitful, perhaps with the development of genetically engineered treatments for this type of disorder?

Portola Valley, California

DELFIN J. BELTRAN, M.D.

Acknowledgments

A great many people have made valuable contributions directly and indirectly to the development of this volume. First and foremost, our debt to the Prader-Willi Syndrome Association (PWSA) is deep and lasting. This book exists because this remarkable organization of parents and professionals shared our vision. We are grateful to the PWSA Board of Directors for their willingness to contribute generous financial support in the preparation and publication of the text and for their intellectual and personal encouragement. Special thanks are due to Marge Wett, Executive Director of PWSA, who spent innumerable hours reviewing content and provided extensive assistance and valuable feedback.

We wish to acknowledge the authors of each chapter who graciously and without remuneration took the time to contribute their expertise despite heavy professional and personal commitments.

We are especially indebted to M. Joan Soucek for her technical assistance "par excellence," for her patience, endurance, and perseverance during every step in the preparation and refinement of the manuscript. Appreciation is extended to The University of Iowa Hospitals and Clinics—the Department of Medical Genetics and the Department of Pediatrics, Division of Developmental Disabilities—and particularly to Janice L. Held for her technical assistance and to Richard T. Huber for his outstanding graphic art.

Credit is due to the people at Springer-Verlag, who offered numerous important suggestions for additions and revisions.

Very special thanks are extended to Dr. Hans Zellweger and Dr. James Hanson. Their personal commitment, in addition to their contributions to the text, gave us an extra measure of inspiration. They served as both teachers and friends.

We are primarily indebted to the children born with this unusual birth defect and to their families who allowed us access to their struggles and brought us to a deeper understanding of the condition known as Prader-Willi syndrome.

LOUISE R. GREENSWAG, R.N., PH.D.
RANDELL C. ALEXANDER, M.D., PH.D.

Contents

Contributors

RANDELL C. ALEXANDER, M.D., PH.D. Department of Pediatrics, University Hospital School, The University of Iowa Hospitals and Clinics, Iowa City, Iowa 52242

DELFIN J. BELTRAN, M.D. President, Prader-Willi Syndrome Association, Portola Valley, California 94025

WILLIAM D. BLEVINS, M.ED. Director, Residential Services, Rehabilitative Services Program, The Woods Schools and Residential Treatment Center, Langhorne, Pennsylvania 19047

TRUE CARR, O.T.R. Senior Occupational Therapist, University Hospital School, The University of Iowa Hospitals and Clinics, Iowa City, Iowa 52242

SUZANNE B. CASSIDY, M.D. Director, Division of Human Genetics; Associate Professor, Department of Pediatrics, University of Connecticut Health Center, Farmington, Connecticut 06032

RHETT ELEAZER, ESQ. Board Member, Prader-Willi Syndrome Association; Eleazer and Sautter, Attorneys and Counselors at Law, Columbia, South Carolina 29201

GERALD ENTE, M.D., F.A.A.P. Clinical Director of Neonatology, Nassau County Medical Center, East Meadow, New York 11554

JERI J. GOLDMAN, PH.D. Director, Clinical Services, Rehabilitative Services Program, The Woods Schools and Residential Treatment Center, Langhorne, Pennsylvania 19047

LOUISE R. GREENSWAG, R.N., PH.D. Adjunct Professor, College of Nursing; Progam Consultant for Prader-Willi Syndrome, Iowa Child Health Specialty Clinics, University Hospital School, The University of Iowa Hospitals and Clinics, Iowa City, Iowa 52242

JAMES W. HANSON, M.D. Division of Medical Genetics, Department of Pediatrics, The University of Iowa Hospitals and Clinics, Iowa City, Iowa 52242

VANJA A. HOLM, M.D. Department of Pediatrics, Child Development and Mental Retardation Center, The University of Washington, Seattle, Washington 98195

JAMES TIMOTHY INWOOD, B.S. Behavior Modification Specialist, Department of Mental Retardation—Region 4, Norwalk, Connecticut 06850

MARSHA H. LUPI, ED.D. Department of Special Education, Hunter College, New York, New York 10021

MARY ALICE DUESTERHAUS MINOR, M.S. Department of Physical Therapy, College of Allied Health Professions, University of Kentucky, Lexington, Kentucky 40536

WILLIAM MITCHELL, ED.D. Psychologist, Learning Disabilities Program, Boston Children's Hospital, Boston, Massachusetts 02115

JOYCE A. MUNSON-DAVIS, M.A. Speech-Language Pathologist, University Hospital School, The University of Iowa Hospitals and Clinics, Iowa City, Iowa 52242

RALPH NEWBERT, ED.D. Labor Law Project Coordinator, Labor Law Bureau, University of Maine, Orono, Maine 04469

ARTHUR J. NOWAK, D.M.D. Departments of Pediatric Dentistry and Pediatrics, Colleges of Dentistry and Medicine, The University of Iowa, Iowa City, Iowa 52242

JAMES F. PORTER, M.S.W. Social Services, Division of Developmental Disabilities, University Hospital School, The University of Iowa Hospitals and Clinics, Iowa City, Iowa 52242

KAREN RUBIN, M.D. Assistant Professor, Division of Pediatric Endocrinology, Department of Pediatrics; Joint appointment—OB-GYN, The University of Connecticut Health Center, Farmington, Connecticut 06032

JACK SHERMAN, M.D., F.A.A.P. Director, Pediatric Clinical Genetics, Nassau County Medical Center, East Meadow, New York 11554

DIANE D. STADLER, M.S. Nutritionist, Division of Developmental Disabilities, University Hospital School, The University of Iowa Hospitals and Clinics, Iowa City, Iowa 52242

STEPHEN SULZBACHER, PH.D. Associate Professor of Psychiatry and Behavioral Science and Pediatrics, Children's Hospital and Medical Center, The University of Washington, Seattle, Washington 98105

DOROTHY G. THOMPSON, Residential and Program Development Consultant for Prader-Willi Syndrome, 5505 12th Avenue South, Minneapolis, Minnesota 55417

ELIZABETH J. THOMSON, R.N., M.S. Clinical Coordinator, Regional Genetics Consultation Service, Department of Pediatrics, The University of Iowa Hospitals and Clinics, Iowa City, Iowa 52242

JANALEE TOMASESKI-HEINEMANN, M.S.W. Social Services, Children's Hospital at Washington University Medical Center, St. Louis, Missouri, 63110

MARJORIE A. WETT, Executive Director, Prader-Willi Syndrome Association, Edina, Minnesota 55436

HANS ZELLWEGER, M.D. Professor Emeritus, Division of Medical Genetics, Department of Pediatrics, The University of Iowa Hospitals and Clinics, Iowa City, Iowa 52242

Introduction

K is capable of gaining several pounds in one week and must be under constant supervision to control her weight. If my husband or I die and V [her sister] either dies or marries someone who can't handle her, who will look after her? Her other brother and sisters cannot be depended upon as their spouses object. K has a beau who wants to marry her. He is mildly retarded and attends a workshop. No one seems able to answer my questions about whether they can marry and still be state supported. . . they cannot reproduce so that is not a problem. V says she will not take care of her [K]. I can't seem to get a PWS organization going. If she is not in a PWS home of some kind, she will kill herself with her fork. . . .

Providing services to the Prader-Willi syndrome (PWS) population at The University of Iowa led us to the realization that information about case management of the syndrome has been limited in scope, fragmented, and that continuing professional help has been slow to develop. Similar experiences reported by colleagues in other major centers convinced us that a comprehensive resource, offering a blend of knowledge and common-sense guidelines, was needed.

To this end, we have brought together the contributions of professionals with considerable expertise in diagnosis and management of PWS. Clinical, social, family, and community issues are explored and management strategies identified. To sharpen the perceptions of the reader to the "human dimensions" of PWS, selected personal experiences of parents are integrated throughout the text.

Designed for clarity and conciseness in communicating ideas, this text nonetheless represents a diversity of approaches to management, and the diversity itself is reflected in the format. In some chapters, contributions are more personalized than in others. Although there may not be an equal representation of disciplines, and writing styles may vary, each chapter is significant and represents contributions far beyond the capability of a single author. *Management of Prader-Willi Syndrome* is a "how-to" book. It addresses the everyday concerns of PWS individuals and their families. The text initially presents historical, medical, and genetic information to orient the reader. The major portion deals with pragmatic guidelines, rather than research and diagnosis, and is directed to health and educational specialists in academic, clinical, and community settings, who are members of a team or independent practitioners. Our goal is to reach professionals, parents, extended family and friends, and anyone else interested in learning about Prader-Willi syndrome.

In the discussion and planning stages of this book, many aspects of PWS were examined. It was apparent that serious attention needed to be given to emotional and social problems, as well as to physical aspects. As the manuscript progressed, several issues came into focus.

Individuals with PWS are usually diagnosed at major genetic centers and followed in outpatient clinics. Because academics have become better educated about the syndrome, neonatal and pre-obesity diagnosis is now on the increase. These academic centers remain a resource for primary practitioners.

Although PWS must be considered within the context of other developmental disabilities, the nature of this condition requires a unique approach to services. This is by no means an effort to diminish the needs of other handicapping conditions, but rather an attempt to address problems specific to PWS. Clearly, PWS is an eating rather than a weight disorder. Service providers must be aware that the overpowering hunger drive that these individuals experience is a physiological fact of life. Unlike those with exogenous obesity, the PWS person *never* feels full. Left alone, children with this syndrome will literally eat themselves to death. With few exceptions, which start early in life, the typical case begins to search compulsively for food much as a drug addict seeks out heroin. But unlike the withdrawal of an addictive drug, total withdrawal of food is fatal. The presence of this lack of satiety is compounded by the fact that most affected individuals lack the cognitive capacity to comply with unsupervised food intake regimes.

Early intervention before initial weight gain is critical. In many instances, services focus primarily on weight reduction because parents tend to seek help only *after* their child has become grossly obese. Unfortunately, some parents and professionals expect that weight loss will enhance the child's development, reduce inappropriate behaviors, and improve family life.

More recently, cases of PWS have been identified during the pre-obesity stage of the syndrome, and strict nutritional management has prevented marked weight gain. However, the absence of obesity in older children and adults does not preclude the presence of the syndrome.

Although supervision of food intake is a major component of case management, the social dimensions of PWS require equal consideration as PWS individuals develop considerable emotional lability over time. These children, usually affable in early childhood, demonstrate bizarre and inappropriate behaviors as they grow older.

Children who previously died young due to complications of obesity now face unique problems as developmentally disabled adults. Additional services are required to meet the appropriate residential, psycho-social, and vocational needs of this population. Thus a variety of primary providers are involved in delivery of direct services. For purposes of clarity, the text has been divided into five main parts:

I Physiological and Genetics Considerations: Chapter 1 presents an overview of Prader-Willi syndrome, its history, etiology, and clinical characteristics. Differential diagnosis in PWS is identified in Chapter 2. Chapter 3 considers endocrinological management, and the significance of genetic counseling is addressed in Chapter 4.

II A Case Presentation: The ongoing efforts of devoted and persevering parents, whose daughter remained undiagnosed until she was 26 years of age, are described sensitively in Chapter 5.

III The Interdisciplinary Process: Chapter 6 discusses the team approach to management. Chapters 7–15 describe case management in the fields of medicine, nursing, dentistry, nutrition, psychology, speech and language, education, physical and occupational therapies, vocational training, and social services.

IV The Socialization Process: Chapter 16 presents a format for teaching direct-care staff how to help clients with PWS develop interpersonal skills. Chapter 17 offers information about psychosexuality in individuals with PWS. Chapter 18 describes the personal experiences and feelings of the parents of a boy with PWS.

V Delivery of Services: Chapters 19 and 20 include selected topics about the advocacy and residential facilities, all of which have implications for parents and community service providers. Chapter 21 addresses the establishment of the national Prader-Willi Syndrome Association and examines its expanding role as a resource of support and information.

The final sections of the text consist of a glossary of terms, a selected reading list, and appendices. A list of references follows each chapter, and tables, diagrams and photographs are used throughout the book to illustrate and emphasize the material.

We believe that direct services to individuals with PWS and their families have "come of age." We hope that the descriptions and prescriptions chronicled here will provide a cornerstone for effective care.

LOUISE R. GREENSWAG, R.N., PH.D.
RANDELL C. ALEXANDER, M.D., PH.D.

Part I Physiological and Genetics Considerations

This baby was several weeks overdue when born. It was a difficult forced labor with I.V. medicines and breaking the water. I was kept medicated for days and never knew what was happening. I was told nothing [in the hospital] and very little when I went home. We left the baby there for a few days. He had difficulty nursing and seldom cried. He was a funny kind of dusky color and cried weakly. We were told at the clinic we took him to when he was about 3 years old that it was "hypothalmus" [sic]. It was a nightmare not knowing the problem or what to do.

We wish we knew for sure if it [PWS] is in our genes. We worry about our normal son. Can he have a PW child?

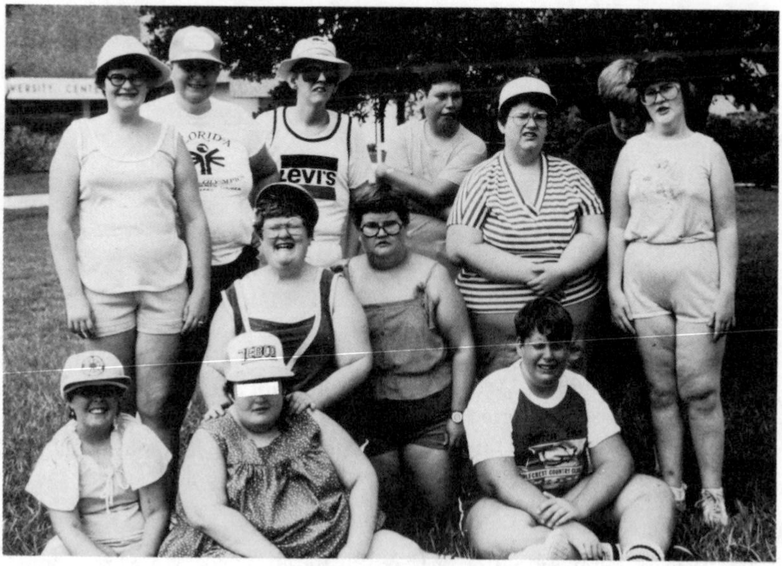

Prader-Willi Summer Camp 1980

1
Overview

RANDELL C. ALEXANDER and JAMES W. HANSON

Prader-Willi syndrome (PWS) is a recognizable pattern of altered growth and development, the etiology and pathogenesis of which remain unclear. Affected persons face life as potentially overweight, short, sexually immature, developmentally delayed individuals with poor gross motor skills. Usually at least mildly retarded, stubborn, egocentric, and emotionally labile, they rarely develop the ability to cope with their insatiable hunger and require environmental restrictions to prevent life-threatening obesity. Although individuals with PWS and their families face many of the same problems as others who are developmentally disabled, the unique characteristics of the syndrome—cognitive impairment and gross obesity due to uncontrollable hunger—require special care and services.

Although PWS is not a common disorder, it is not rare. Estimates of the incidence of PWS vary between 1:10,000 and 1:25,000, placing this disorder among the more frequent of the recognized malformation syndromes. According to the Prader-Willi Syndrome Association, over 3,000 cases of PWS have been identified throughout the world. More than 1,000 subjects have been described in more than 160 reports; of these, 90% are case descriptions (Bray et al., 1983). Males and females are equally affected, and PWS has not been shown to be associated with specific racial/ethnic groups, socioeconomic classes, or geographic regions.

However, PWS is an important condition for other than reasons of frequency or the complexity of management issues. This unique disorder manifests abnormalities of growth, learning, and physical development that may provide a window to understanding larger issues, including eating disorders and weight control, the neurophysiology of behavior, and the genetic control of morphogenesis.

History

In 1956, Prader, Labhart, and Willi published the first report of PWS. Although primarily interested in endocrinology, these authors reported an unusual pattern of other abnormalities: diminished fetal activity, profound poor muscle tone (hypotonia), feeding problems in infancy, underdeveloped sex organs (hypogonadism and hypogenitalism), short stature and retarded bone age, small hands and feet, delayed developmental milestones, characteristic facies, cognitive impairment, onset of gross obesity in early childhood due to insatiable hunger, and a tendency to develop diabetes in adolescence. A second report followed that same year (Prader, Labhart, Willi, & Fanconi, 1956). By 1961 fourteen cases had been studied in Switzerland (Prader & Willi, 1961) and six in England (Laurance, 1961). Prader and Willi published a follow-up of their original nine cases and added diabetes mellitus and mental retardation to the clinical picture in 1963.

Landmark studies include follow-up accounts of earlier cases by Gabilan and Royer (1968), Zellweger and Schneider (1968), and Dunn (1968). These reports indicated orthopedic, dental, and developmental characteristics that may assist in differential diagnosis and strongly suggest that the PWS syndrome has two clearly identifiable phases (see Chapter 2). Hall and Smith (1972) gave a detailed account of 32 PWS patients that not only supported earlier diagnostic criteria, but also described behavior and personality problems that appeared to increase with age. Medical problems associated with PWS have been discussed by Kriz and Clonniger (1981), Holm and Laurnen (1981), and Bray et al. (1983) (see Chapter 7).

A compendium of current findings that had been presented to the 1979 national conference of the Prader-Willi Syndrome Association was published (Holm, Sulzbacher, & Pipes, 1981) and Cassidy wrote a comprehensive monograph in 1984. A study of 232 individuals with PWS, age 16 and over, indicated that with appropriate nutritional control, the life expectancy of the population has been extended; that emotional lability increases with age and independent of the presence of obesity; that psychosocial adaptation to adulthood requires special management; and that the presence of PWS has a profound impact on family life (Greenswag, 1987).

Natural History and Clinical Manifestations

The characteristics that constitute Prader-Willi syndrome may be regarded as falling into three major categories:

1. Structural (morphological)
    a. Facial features
    b. A central pattern of fat distribution disproportionately seen on the trunk, hips, and thighs
    c. Eye difficulties such as myopia and strabismus
    d. Short stature
    e. Hypogonadism
2. Functional (or regulatory)

a. Decreased motor skills, particularly gross motor skills and speech
b. Hypotonia
c. An apparently high pain threshold
d. Skin scratching and picking, which may be related to the high pain threshold but which are not explained entirely by this mechanism
e. Thermoregulation problems (low body tempature is sometimes seen)
f. Hyperphagia (a seemingly insatiable appetite)
g. Higher vomiting threshold
h. Disturbances in sleep/respiratory functioning such as sleep apnea, or problems with falling asleep during the day
i. Decreased activity level, with concomitant requirement of considerably fewer calories
j. Limited sex hormone production

3. Cognitive
a. Low intelligence; most cases are at least mildly retarded, and some individuals who have higher IQ scores nevertheless function at considerably lower levels
b. Language problems
c. Behavior problems (such as stubbornness and lability)

Other characteristics seen in PWS are most likely secondary effects of more fundamental features. These include:

Poor dentition: Lowered cognitive ability, unauthorized snacking, changes in saliva, and possible rumination may contribute to this finding.
Scoliosis: This is very likely a result of generalized hypotonia.
Undescended testes (and inguinal hernias): Deficiency in sex hormones may alter the physical development of these structures.
Diabetes: This appears to be weight related, and is most commonly adult-onset (Type II).

The diagnostic picture of an individual with PWS appears to change as the child matures (Hoefnagel, Costello, & Hatoum, 1967), and only recently have minimum diagnostic criteria been established (Holm, 1981). Zellweger (1969) divided the syndrome into two phases, the first of which occurs in the pre- and neonatal period and early infancy.

Compared with a normal fetus, the PWS child is less active in utero, is more likely to be delivered in a breech or shoulder position, and may have an excessive amount of amniotic fluid (Hall & Smith, 1972). The diminished fetal activity and high breech presentation suggest that profound hypotonia may be present early in fetal life. The neonatal phase is marked by below-average weight, poor suck, reflexes that are difficult to elicit, extreme hypotonia, apathy, small genitalia (more noticeable in males), and skeletal anomalies of the head (Zellweger, 1984). Sometimes the severe lack of muscle tone (amyotonia) will "mimic flaccid paralysis" (Zellweger,

1981). Because of poor muscle tone, these babies have little facial expression and a weak cry, and may present feeding problems for weeks or months, necessitating special feeding techniques. Some infants may be labeled as having "failure to thrive" and may be mistakenly diagnosed as having some form of congenital hypotonia or muscular dystrophy. The hypotonia eventually resolves itself to the point where the infant can feed by himself or herself, although suck remains weak and feeding times are prolonged. Another consequence of the hypotonia is that motor development is also delayed beyond even that expected as a result of limited mental ability. However, some time after the first year of life, muscle tone improves to the point where the child begins to function in a fairly normal fashion.

Unfortunately, within the first 2 to 3 years of life, the first phase of PWS is insidiously replaced by a second phase, when an uncontrollable hunger drive causes children to gorge themselves and become grossly obese (Zellweger, 1981). Although the insatiable hunger drive *may* be present earlier (in the first phase), it is masked by the hypotonia. It is important to note that children with PWS are not merely overeaters; they are compulsively obsessed with food, demonstrate bizarre food-seeking behaviors, and during their early years may eat nonfood items. Unable to satisfy their ravenous hunger, their life is "one endless meal" (See, 1976). Early in the second phase, relieved parents, who initially struggled with earlier feeding problems, are delighted when their children appear eager to eat. However, all too quickly these toddlers bloom into poorly coordinated, grossly overweight, impulsive, and temperamental children with whom families must learn to cope.

The body fat of individuals with PWS characteristically is distributed in the adipose tissue of the trunk and thighs while the lower arms and legs remain lean; the hands and feet are unusually small (Holm, 1981; Nugent & Holm, 1981). On growth curve records, bone age is significantly delayed; when the epiphyses fuse, final stature is small (Dunn, 1968; Nugent & Holm, 1981). When the physiological hunger drive is left unmanaged, gross obesity and death result (Zellweger, 1981). Although PWS children are initially friendly and affectionate, their behaviors appear to deteriorate as they mature (Cassidy, 1984). Their emotional lability is characterized by placid affability and sudden, severe, unpredictable, uncontrollable outbursts of anger, hindering psychosocial adaptation (Greenswag, 1987).

Etiology and Pathogenesis

Despite over 30 years of investigation, the etiology and pathogenesis of PWS remain poorly understood. A host of causal hypotheses, including monogenic, polygenic, cytogenetic, and teratogenic etiologies, have been advanced (e.g., Holm, Sulzbacher, & Pipes, 1981), but none appear entirely satisfactory.

Although the vast majority of cases of PWS occur as sporadic events in families, several familial recurrences have been documented. An early report by Gabilan and Royer (1968) detailed two cases in the same family (a brother and sister) and another case from related parents. More recently, there have been additional reports of PWS in siblings (Bolanos, Lopez-Amor, Vasquez, Lisker, & Morato, 1974; Cohen, Hall, Smith, Graham, & Lampert, 1973; Endo, Tasaka, Matsuura, & Matsuda, 1976). Hall and Smith (1972) reported an instance of affected first cousins and Jancar (1971) reported two brothers, one of whom had a normal twin sister; as did Evans (1969). Brissenden and Levy (1973) and Ikeda, Asaka, Inouye, Kaihara, & Kinoshita (1973) reported instances of monozygotic twins. DeFraites, Thurmon, and Farhadian (1974) identified one family with five cases of PWS and believed the syndrome arose as an autosomal recessive trait. Lubinsky et al. (1987) described a family of four siblings (two female, two male) with PWS and no normal children. Diagnosis was made clinically on the basis of history, physical findings, and behavior in three of the children (the other had died at 10 months with a similar history). No chromosomal abnormality was identified in either the siblings or their parents. These recurrences within families have been cited as evidence of a genetic, possibly autosomal recessive etiology. However, this seems difficult to reconcile with the recurrence risk of 1.6% suggested by Clarren and Smith (1977).

A more appealing proposal advanced by Ledbetter and coworkers (1981) related PWS to a specific cytogenetic deletion in the long arm of chromosome 15. Unfortunately, not all PWS individuals display this abnormality, even when studied using advanced DNA molecular technology. Furthermore, some individuals with an apparently similar deletion have been identified who lack many of the characteristic stigmata of PWS (Greenberg & Ledbetter, 1988).

When PWS individuals with a known chromosomal deletion have been compared with those with apparently normal chromosomes, no compelling phenotypic differences have yet been noted (Greenswag, 1987). It may be that a very small and as yet undetectable chromosomal deletion in the same location may exist for affected individuals with apparently "normal" chromosomes. There is also a possibility of mosaicism in those in whom the chromosomal deletion has not been found.

It should also be kept in mind that PWS may well be etiologically heterogeneous. It is possible that a variety of different genetic and/or environmental agents may adversely affect either a single anatomical region or biochemical pathway in the developing fetus, leading to a common phenotype at birth (see Figure 1.1). This possibility requires serious investigation because it could have substantial implications, not only for the care and counseling of affected individuals and families, but also for prevention. Furthermore, it could profoundly affect our understanding of this condition, its frequency, and its variability.

If PWS is, as has been suggested (Hanson, 1981), in fact a "sequence" (a

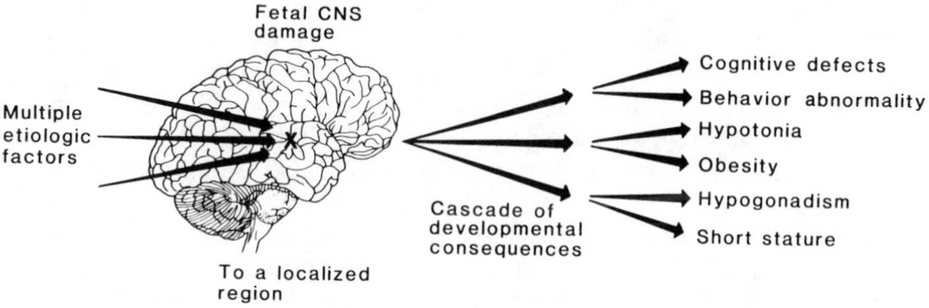

FIGURE 1.1. Pathogenetic model of PWS: Sequence.

pattern of altered growth, development, and function stemming from a single localized area of damage in the fetus) arising in the central nervous system, it could be predicted that a host of factors, both genetic and environmental, might cause this disorder. A few genetic problems (monogenic or cytogenetic) occurring in a portion of families could explain the low recurrence risk overall, with a few exceptional families presenting with unusual recurrence patterns. Furthermore, this model of causation would predict wide variability in phenotypic outcome based upon the exact location, extent, and timing of the proposed defect in fetal nervous system morphogenesis. One might expect that within the familial cases this variability would be substantially less than among sporadic cases. However, this could be difficult to demonstrate since the definition of a case would require modification. The family reported by Clarren and Smith (1977) may illustrate this problem.

On the other hand, PWS may be regarded as a true malformation syndrome. This implies a more restricted (and very probably genetic) group of causal factors that each affect a single (or few) biochemical or developmental process(es) in a group of tissues leading to the observed range of phenotypic consequences (pleiotropy) (see Figure 1.2). This model suggests a more restricted case definition, but also allows for some variability both between and within families. Although a few families with monogenic disorders concealed within the larger population of PWS could explain the observed recurrence patterns, cytogenetic rearrangements (at either the microscopic or molecular level) afford a more robust explanation. Deletions and other unbalanced rearrangements of a chromosome could well affect more than a single genetic locus ("contiguous gene disorders"), producing variable consequences. Indeed, "balanced" chromosomal rearrangements in a parent (inversions, translocations, etc.) might account for occasional recurrences in a few families. An alternative explanation for occasional recurrences among children of apparently normal couples is gonadal mosaicism.

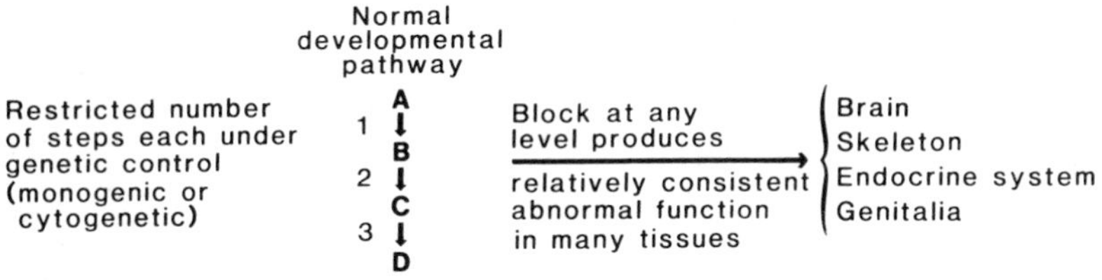

FIGURE 1.2. Pathogenetic model of PWS: Syndrome.

Answers as to which, if any, of these alternate explanations of PWS may be correct await clarification. It seems likely that such answers may be of substantial interest for such diverse areas of medical science as endocrinology, weight control, neurophysiology, psychology, and morphogenesis. The early results of the recent expansion of research activities from simple phenotype/function correlations to the utilization of molecular genetic techniques to help delineate basic developmental processes suggest that the wait for these answers may not be long.

Although the cause of PWS may not be clear-cut, the observed abnormalities may result from a localized primary disturbance in the development of the brain above the spinal cord, such as a defect in the hypothalmic-pituitary axis (Gorlin, Pindborg, & Cohen, 1976; Hanson, 1981). Afifi and Zellweger (1969) and Tze, Dunn, and Rothstein (1981) also suggested the presence of a fat metabolism defect. Schwartz, Brunzell, and Bierman (1979) believes that the level of the lipoprotein lipase enzyme may be one of the critical mechanisms by which the brain regulates the number, size, and metabolism of fat cells in the body, and suggested a biochemical explanation for the presence of PWS.

The number of alterations in the body's homeostatic mechanisms (regulatory functions) in PWS implicates the hypothalmus as the probable site of major dysfunction in the brain. For example, both the satiety and the feeding centers are located in the hypothalmus, and appetite disturbance may be a function of overactivity or underactivity of one of these centers or a problem in the balance between the two. The hypothalmus also helps to regulate production of growth and sex hormones. Sleep, breathing, and body temperature may also be affected, either in this area or in adjacent brain structures. Additionally, the hypothalmus and adjoining areas are also responsible for activity levels and the propensity for vomiting. To date, neither computed tomography scans of the brain nor autopsy results have yielded any specific defect or abnormality. It is possible that flaws exist in specific types or balances of neurotransmitters regulating brain cell-to-cell communication.

Finally, other abnormalities seem to reflect problems with areas of the brain that are either more diffuse or less clearly understood. Intelligence, behavior problems, and speech and language skills (cognitive functions) may represent somewhat more global differences in brain functioning. Future research may establish an underlying biochemical defect or microstructural abnormality in the brain that would account for the characteristic symptoms.

Management

Case management begins with the recognition by the parents and extended family that PWS is present. Care providers must understand that the syndrome will not disappear and cannot be corrected, and that intervention means the management of symptoms.

The child with PWS and his or her family undergo significant developmental changes with time. Although professionals working with a family naturally focus on their own discipline, they must be cognizant of the impact of the condition on other spheres of both the child's and family's existence. Even in cases when diagnosis is made early and excessive weight gain is avoided, extensive interdisciplinary interventions are essential. As is true for all low-incidence handicapping conditions, the relative lack of professional experience with such cases makes it imperative that the considerable knowledge of parents be incorporated into the management strategies. Specific interventions emphasize genetic counseling, prevention of obesity, behavior modification including environmental controls, planned physical activity, recognition of special educational and vocational needs, and psychotherapeutic guidance for the PWS person and those who have the responsibility of planning for his or her future.

It is very difficult to discourage food foraging habits since the insatiable hunger drive does not diminish. Effective nutritional programs take considerable time, planning, and commitment, and require accurate baseline data, education of the care providers, environmental control, and frequent monitoring of growth curves and caloric intake. More recently, affected individuals are being diagnosed early enough to avoid initial weight gain. However, the effect of early diagnosis on subsequent weight and behavior management is as yet unknown.

Individuals with PWS have special educational needs, the planning for which should take into account their cognitive limitations. In this respect, their parents share concerns similar to those of parents of children with other handicapping conditions.

As indicated earlier, behavioral problems appear to intensify with age, regardless of nutritional control. Prader and Willi (1963) reported their cases as good-natured children with silly, contented facial expressions. Others described younger children as placid, affectionate, and outgoing (Cassidy, 1984; Hanson, 1981). Zellweger and Schneider (1968) suggested that definitive behavioral changes take place between the ages of 3 and 5 as the universal symptom of insatiable hunger emerges. Stubbornness and hyperactivity replace affability; repetitive and incessant chattering, verbal aggressiveness, and self-assaultive acts are observed; erratic, unpredictable rages increase; signs of depression and, in rare instances, psychotic episodes may occur (Hall & Smith, 1972; Zellweger, 1984). Constant efforts to satisfy hunger seem to result in aggressive and bizarre food-seeking activities such as foraging, hoarding, and gorging (Byrt, 1969a, 1969b; Dunn, Tze, Alisharan, & Schulzer, 1981; Marshall et al., 1981). Older children and adolescents frequently appear to develop serious personality problems ranging from being secretive and manipulative to being dull, lethargic, and indifferent (Hall & Smith, 1972; Kollrack & Wolff, 1966). When normal secondary sex characteristics fail to develop in adolescence, feelings of loneliness and isolation increase.

Greenswag (1984) indicated that emotional instability is a predictable problem that limits psychosocial adaptation in adolescence and adulthood; it functions independently of weight and complicates case management. For the older person with PWS, lack of social experience and interpersonal relationships seem to worsen as a result of poor physical skills and increased antisocial behaviors. Although the danger of pregnancy does not exist, concerns about sexuality and the capacity for independent living increase during the teen years. When PWS children finish their schooling, responsibility for social stimulation falls on the family. Parents/care providers face a future of restricted family life (locked food) and intolerable behaviors even though some adolescents and adults have begun to participate in sheltered workshop programs. Future planning, wills, and residential placement in the least restrictive environment have become important concerns.

Future Trends

When a new syndrome is first described, its distinctive characteristics are likely to represent those severely affected cases that appear to belong together and present homogeneously. PWS, as delineated over 30 years ago by Prader, Willi, and Labhart, constitutes the "classic" case description.

With the gradual accumulation of additional cases, variants of the classic syndrome are being noted, and more subtle, common features identified. Although the discovery of a genetic marker further expands the identification of atypical cases, the specific deletion in the 15th chromosome is not seen in all cases diagnosed as having PWS. Conversely, an increasing number of individuals have been identified who have the chromosomal deletion but who have fewer classic characteristics. A significant portion of current research about PWS focuses on potential chromosomal abnormalities.

Based upon a significant increase in the number of less-classic variants, a third phase of syndrome identification is being developed that readdresses dental, homeostatic, behavioral, cognitive, and nutritional issues. For example, it has been recently shown that children with PWS may indeed vomit, contrary to earlier opinions, although apparently at a reduced level (Alexander, Greenswag, & Nowak, 1987). In the same study, rumination was found to be a minor characteristic of the syndrome. Exploring significant features and clarifying subgroupings may enhance case management.

Research continues to be directed toward fundamental understanding of the genetic, metabolic, and physical manifestations of PWS with the goal of developing interventions to correct or ameliorate this condition. Only in the coming decades will the natural history of individuals who are managed sufficiently to avoid obesity and its complications be known.

In addition to major medical and weight management concerns, the psychosocial aspects of the syndrome need considerable study. Little is known about the nonmedical aspects of this birth defect, either its psychosocial significance on the PWS person or its impact on his or her significant others. After diagnosis, what does the future hold for these individuals? Certainly, the functional, emotional, and social patterns of a large group of individuals with PWS need to be investigated in order to enhance their capacity to contribute as productive members of society. In this undertaking, the National Prader-Willi Syndrome Association, a group of parents and professionals dedicated to ongoing research and support of the children and their families, will play a most significant role (see Chapter 21).

References

Alexander, R., Greenswag, L., & Nowak, A. (1987). Ruminating and vomiting in Prader-Willi syndrome. *American Journal of Medical Genetics*, *28*, 889–895.

Afifi, A.K., & Zellweger, H. (1969). Pathology of muscular hypotonia in Prader-Willi syndrome: Light and electron microscope study. *Journal of the Neurological Sciences*, *9*, 49–61.

Bolanos, F., Lopez-Amor, E., Vasquez, G., Losker, R., & Morato, T. (1974). Hypothalmic-pituitary-gonadal function in two siblings with Prader-Willi syndrome. *Revista de Investigacion Clinica*, *26*, 53–62.

Bray, G., Dahms, W., Swerdloff, R., Fiser, R., Atkinson, R., & Carrell, R. (1983). The Prader-Willi syndrome: A study of 40 parents and a review of the literature. *Medicine*, *62*, 59–80.

Brissenden, J.E., & Levy, E.P. (1973). Prader-Willi syndrome in infant monozygotic twins. *American Journal of Diseases of Children*, *126*, 110–112.

Byrt, R. (1969a, September 25). A patient with suspected Prader-Willi syndrome at a mental subnormality hospital. 1. *Nursing Times*, *65*(39), 1234–1235.

Byrt, R. (1969b, October 2). A patient with suspected Prader-Willi syndrome at a mental subnormality hospital. 2. *Nursing Times*, *65*(40), 1260–1263.

Cassidy, S.B. (1984). Prader-Willi syndrome. *Curr Probl Pediatr*, *14*, 1–55.

Clarren, S.K., & Smith, D.W. (1977). Prader-Willi syndrome: Variable severity and recurrence risk. *American Journal of Diseases of Children*, *131*, 798–800.

Cohen, M.M., Hall, B.D., Smith, D.W., Graham, C.B., & Lampert, K.J. (1973). A new syndrome with hypotonia, obesity, mental deficiency, and facial, oral, ocular and limb abnormalities. *The Journal of Pediatrics*, *83*, 280–285.

DeFraites, E.B., Thurmon, T.F., & Farhadian, H. (1975). Familial Prader-Willi

syndrome. *Birth Defects: Original Article Series*, *11*(4), 123–126.
Dunn, H.G. (1968). The Prader-Labhart-Willi syndrome: Review of the literature and report of nine cases. *Acta Paediatrica Scandinavica Supplement*, *186*, 1–38.
Dunn, H.G., Tze, W.J., Alisharin, R.M., & Schulzer, M. (1981). Clinical experience with 23 cases of Prader-Willi syndrome. In V.A. Holm, S. Sulzbacher, & P.L. Pipes (Eds.), *The Prader-Willi syndrome* (pp. 69–88). Baltimore: University Park Press.
Endo, M., Tasaka, N., Matsuura, N., & Matsuda, I. (1976). Laurence-Moon-Biedl syndrome and Prader-Willi syndrome in a single family. *European Journal of Pediatrics*, *123*(4), 269–276.
Evans, P.R. (1969). The Prader-Labhart-Willi sydrome. *Developmental Medicine and Child Neurology*, *11*, 380–382.
Gabilan, J.C., Royer, P. (1968). Le syndrome de Prader, Labhart, et Willi (etude de onze observations). *Archives Francasises de Pediatrie*, *25*, 121–149.
Gorlin, R.J., Pindborg, J.J., & Cohen, M.M., Jr. (1976) Prader-Willi syndrome. In *Syndromes of the head and neck* (2nd ed., pp. 618–621). New York: McGraw-Hill Book Co.
Greenberg, F., & Ledbetter, D. (1988) Deletions of proximal 15 q without Prader-Willi syndrome (abstract). *Proceedings of the Greenwood Genetics Center*, *7*, 238–239.
Greenswag, L.R. (1984). The adult with Prader-Willi syndrome: A descriptive investigation. Doctoral thesis, The University of Iowa. (DA 056952, University Microfilms International, Ann Arbor, MI)
Greenswag, L.R. (1987) Adults with Prader-Willi syndrome: A survey of 232 cases. *Developmental Medicine and Child Neurology*, *29*, 145–152.
Hall, B.D., & Smith, D.W. (1972). Prader-Willi syndrome. A resume of 32 cases including an instance of affected first cousins, one of whom is of normal stature and intelligence. *The Journal of Pediatrics*, *81*, 286–293.
Hanson, J. (1981). A view of etiology and pathogenesis of Prader-Willi syndrome. In V.A. Holm, Sulzbacher, & P.L. Pipes (Eds.), *The Prader-Willi syndrome* (pp. 45–53). Baltimore: University Park Press.
Hoefnagel, D., Costello, P.J., & Hatoum, K. (1967). Prader-Willi syndrome. *Journal of Mental Deficiency Research*, *11*, 1–11.
Holm, V.A. (1981). The diagnosis of Prader-Willi syndrome. In V.A. Holm, S.J. Sulzbacher, & P.L. Pipes (Eds.), *The Prader-Willi syndrome* (pp. 27–44). Baltimore: University Park Press.
Holm, V.A., & Laurnen, E.L. (1981). Prader-Willi syndrome and scoliosis. *Developmental Medicine and Child Neurology*, *23*, 192–201.
Holm, V.A., Sulzbacher, S.J., & Pipes, P.L. (Eds). (1981). *The Prader-Willi syndrome*. Baltimore: University Park Press.
Ikeda, K., Asaka, A., Inouye, E., Kaihara, H., & Kinoshita, K. (1973). Monozygotic twins concordant for Prader-Willi syndrome. *Japanese Journal of Human Genetics*, *18*, 220–225.
Jancar, J. (1971). Prader-Willi syndrome (hypotonia, obesity, hypogonadism, growth and mental retardation). *Journal of Mental Deficiency Research*, *15*, 20–29.
Kollrack, H.W., & Wolff, D. (1966). Paranoid-halluzinatorische Psychose bei Prader-Labhart-Willi-Franconi-Syndrome. *Acta Paedopsychiatrica Scandinavica*, *33*, 309–314.
Kriz, J.S., & Clonninger, B.J. (1981). Management of a patient with Prader-Willi

syndrome by a dental-dietary team. *Special Care Dentist*, *1*(4), 179–182.
Laurance, B.M. (1961). Hypotonia, hypogonadism and mental retardation in childhood. *Archives of Disease in Childhood*, *36*, 690.
Ledbetter, D., Riccardi, V., Airhardt, S., Strobel, R., Kennan, B., & Crawford, J. (1981). Deletions of chromosome 15 as a cause of the Prader-Willi syndrome. *Medical Intelligence*, *304*(6), 325–329.
Lubinsky, M., Zellweger, H., Greenswag, L., Larson, G., Hansmann, I., & Ledbetter, D. (1987). Familial Prader-Willi syndrome with normal chromosomes. *American Journal of Medical Genetics*, *28*, 37–43.
Marshall, B.D., Jr., Wallace, C.J., Elder, J., Burke, K., Oliver, T., & Blackman, R. (1981). A behavioral approach to the treatment of Prader-Willi syndrome. In V.A. Holm, S.J. Sulzbacher, & P.L. Pipes (Eds.), *The Prader-Willi syndrome* (pp. 185–199). Baltimore: University Park Press.
Nugent, J.K., & Holm, V. Physical growth in Prader-Willi syndrome. In V.A. Holm, S.J. Sulzbacher, P.L. Pipes (Eds.), *The Prader-Willi syndrome* (pp. 269–280). Baltimore: University Park Press.
Prader, A., Labhart, A., & Willi, H. (1956). Ein Syndrom von Adipositas, Kleinwuchs, Kryptorchismus and Oligophrenie nach myotonieartigem Zustand in Neugeborenenalter. *Schweizerische Medizinische Wochenschrift*, *86*, 1260.
Prader, A., Labhart, A., Willi, H., & Fanconi, G. (1956). Ein Syndrom von Adipositas, Kleinwuchs, Kryptorchismus und Idiotie bei Kindern und Erwachsenen, die als Neugeborene ein myatonie-artiges Bild geboten haben. *Proceedings of the VIII International Congress on Pediatrics, Copenhagen.*
Prader, A., & Willi, H. (1961). Das Syndrom von Imbezillität, Adipostas, Muskelhypotonie, Hypogenitalismus, Hypogonadismus und Diabetes Mellitus mit "Myatonic"-Anamnese. In *Proceedings of the Second International Congress on Mental Retardation, Vienna, Austria, 1961*, Basel: S. Karger.
Prader, A., & Willi, H. (1963). Das Syndrom von Imbezillität, Adipositas, Muskelhypotonie, Hypogenitalismus, Hypogonadismus und Diabetes mellitus mit "Myatonie"—Anamnese. *Second International Congress on Mental Retardation, Vienna, 1961*. Basel and New York: S. Karger.
See C., (1976, January). For some children life is one endless meal. *Today's Health*, pp. 15–17, 50–51.
Schwarz, R., Brunzell, J., & Bierman, E. (1979). Elevated adipose tissue lipoprotein-lipase in the pathogenesis of obesity in Prader-Willi syndrome. *Clinical Research*, *27*(2), 137–143.
Tze, W.J., Dunn, H.G., & Rothstein, R.L. (1981). Endocrine profiles and metabolic aspects of Prader-Willi syndrome. In V.A. Holm, S.J. Sulzbacher, & P. L. Pipes (Eds.), *The Prader-Willi syndrome* (pp. 281–291). Baltimore: University Park Press.
Zellweger, H. (1969). The HHHO or Prader-Willi syndrome. *Birth Defects: Original Article Series*, *5*(2), 15–17.
Zellweger, H. (1981). Diagnosis and therapy in the first phase of Prader-Willi syndrome. In V.A. Holm, S.J. Sulzbacher, & P.L. Pipes (Eds.), *The Prader-Willi syndrome* (pp. 55–68). Baltimore: University Park Press.
Zellweger, H. (1984). The Prader-Willi syndrome. *Journal of the American Medical Association*, *25*(4), 18–35.
Zellweger, H., & Schneider, H.J. (1968). Syndrome of hypotonia-hypomentia-hypogonadism-obesity (HHHO) or Prader-Willi syndrome. *American Journal of Diseases of Children*, *115*, 558–598.

2 Differential Diagnosis in Prader-Willi Syndrome

HANS ZELLWEGER

Prader-Willi syndrome (PWS) is a complex clinical condition characterized by abnormalities of longitudinal and ponderal growth, central nervous system dysfunctions, endocrine disturbances, and dysmorphic features. In 50–70% of the cases the syndrome is associated with an abnormality of chromosome 15, most often a deletion of proximal parts of its long arm (del 15q11–q13). Signs and symptoms of PWS are listed in Table 2.1. PWS can be divided into two phases that present different diagnostic problems.

Diagnostic Considerations of PWS Phase I

Pregnancies resulting in the birth of a PWS child are often complicated by polyhydramnios. Fetal movements may be decreased. Dates of confinement vary more than usual and breech positions are often encountered. Newborns with PWS show signs of severe cerebral depression. They are unresponsive, motionless, and inactive for weeks or months. Their muscle tone is decreased, in many instances so much as to mimic paralytic hypotonia. Tendon reflexes are decreased or absent. Withdrawal and Moro's reflexes are absent. The facial expression is flat, and the mouth shows a triangular shape (fish-mouth). Sucking and swallowing difficulties may necessitate gavage feeding for an extended period of time. Other PWS infants have to be fed by spoon or by using a soft nipple with a widened hole.

The muscular hypotonia is comparable to that found in congenital diseases of the lower motor unit, in congenital lesions of the spinal cord, and in rare supranuclear hypotonias. The conspicuous hypogonadism of PWS males, consisting of micropenis, cryptorchidism, and in particular hypoplasia of the scrotum, is characteristic for PWS. Diagnosis of PWS females is more difficult, although hypoplastic labia majora and small or absent labia minora are noticeable in some instances. Acromicria (small hands, small feet, small fingers, and small toes) is also characteristic of, although not pathognomonic for PWS, since it appears in other conditions (e.g., Down syndrome) as well. Chromosome analysis may be helpful in at least some

TABLE 2.1. Signs and symptoms of the Prader-Willi syndrome.

Phase I
Severe cerebral depression
Muscular atonia
Areflexia or hyporeflexia
Sucking and swallowing difficulties
Hypothermia
Poor weight gain
Dry oral mucosa
Cryptorchidism
Scrotum hypoplasia
Hypoplasia of labia
Phase II
Delayed psychomotor development
Intelligence subnormal to borderline, rarely higher
Articulation defects
Behavior abnormalities
Emotional incontinence
Small stature
Hyperphagia
Obesity
Obesity-hypoventilation syndrome
Hypotonia
Periods of hyperthermia
Hypalgesia
Self-assaultiveness
Trichotillomania
Relative inability to vomit
Rumination
Hypogonadism
Infertility
Oligomenorrhea, anovulatory cycles
Decreased secondary sex characteristics
Increased glucose tolerance
Nonketotic diabetes
Convulsions (rare)
Dolichocephaly
Decreased bifrontal diameter
Strabismus, almond-shaped eyes
Microdontia, caries, enamel defects
Acromicria
Scoliosis, dislocated hips

cases of PWS, particularly if high-resolution chromosomes are studied. Molecular-genetic methods by using specific DNA probes may become helpful diagnostic tools in the near future.

Diseases of the lower motor unit, such as *infantile spinal muscular atrophy* (SMA, Werdnig-Hoffmann disease), congenital peroneal muscular atrophy, and various congenital myopathies, may show clinical features similar to those of PWS. Congenital diseases of the lower motor unit can be distinguished from PWS by electrophysiological studies of the muscle. The electromyogram, which is normal in PWS, is abnormal in all diseases of the lower motor unit. Furthermore, paralytic hypotonia in the early course of SMA is usually not as pronounced as in PWS. In fact, in most instances of SMA the muscular weakness becomes recognizable only after several weeks or months. Moreover, children with SMA are usually alert, take notice of their environment, and present feeding difficulties only in the terminal stages of their disease.

In contrast to SMA, severe paralytic hypotonia is present at birth in children affected with *congenital muscular dystrophy* and neuromuscular glycogenosis (Pompe's disease). Difficulties of sucking and swallowing are often early signs, although children afflicted with these conditions are usually alert and respond to external stimuli. The extreme cardiomegaly in Pompe's disease is of further help in the differential diagnosis. The 1-6-glucosidase deficiency that is the cause of Pompe's disease can be discovered by biochemical analysis of muscle tissue.

Severe paralytic hypotonia can also occur in the *benign congenital myopathies* such as fiber type disproportion, type 1 fiber hypotrophy with central nuclei, central core disease, nemaline myopathy, and centronuclear myopathy, although it is by no means a constant feature of these conditions. Most patients with benign congenital myopathy are only mildly hypotonic, yet serum creatine kinase, which is normal in PWS, may be elevated in some cases. Furthermore, the external ophthalmoplegia occasionally found in the nemaline and centronuclear myopathies is not a feature of PWS. The specific diagnosis of the benign congenital myopathies is ascertained by histochemical and electron microscopic studies of the muscle explant.

Newborns whose mothers have *myasthenia gravis* can develop severe and life-threatening hypotonia. Neonatal myasthenia develops in about 10–15% of the newborns of myasthenic mothers. Thus, every child of such a mother should be carefully watched during the newborn period. Neonatal myasthenia is a treatable condition and subsides within a few weeks of anticholinesterase treatment.

Peripheral neuropathy, especially its most frequent variant, peroneal muscular atrophy [Charcot-Marie-Tooth (CMT) disease], usually begins to show clinical signs in the second or third decade of life. In some exceptional cases of CMT, a severe infantile hypotonia may present that is comparable to the hypotonia in PWS. However, the infantile hypotonia associated with CMT resolves more rapidly. Hypesthesia cannot be tested at that tender age. Muscle biopsy and electrophysiological studies (motor nerve conduction velocity) may yield the correct diagnosis of CMT.

Muscular hypotonia is found in some cases of *birth-traumatic cord lesions*, which occur almost exclusively after breech deliveries. In severe cases, atonia and anesthesia are found below the lesion. Discrepancy between preserved motility in the segments above the lesion and paralytic hypotonia and anesthesia in the segments below the lesion as well as the presence of anal sphincter and bladder sphincter pareses distinguish birth-traumatic cord lesions from PWS. It should not be overlooked that tendon and withdrawal reflexes in the legs may be preserved if the spinal cord is injured above the level of the peripheral reflex arch. The incidence of birth-traumatic cord lesions has decreased since it has become customary to deliver breech positions by cesarean section.

A transient atonic phase is seen in some children with *prenatal or birth-traumatic brain lesions*, including intracranial hemorrhages and cerebral anoxia. Some of these patients are cerebrally depressed, at least in the beginning, yet in contrast to PWS patients they most often have hyperactive or exaggerated tendon reflexes after the initial Monakow diaschisis has subsided. Moreover, electroencephalography, computed tomography, and magnetic resonance imaging may disclose conspicuous brain pathology not seen in PWS.

Supranuclear or cerebral hypotonias are usually recognized by the presence of good strength during active movements, which contrasts with the decreased tone of the resting, non-α-innervated muscle. There are, however, some exceptions to this rule. Rare conditions of supranuclear hypotonia can mimic paralytic hypotonia similar to phase I of PWS. Such conditions are atonic diplegia, cerebrohepatorenal syndrome of Zellweger (ZS), congenital myotonic dystrophy (CmyD), and Down syndrome. Some newborns with Down syndrome are severely hypotonic, inactive, and motionless, with decreased or absent tendon, sucking, and swallowing reflexes. Yet this severe hypotonic condition lasts in most instances only a few days. It may last longer in those children with severe congenital heart malformation. Presence of mongoloid features and the result of the chromosomal analysis lead to the right diagnosis.

Atonia, areflexia, absence of sucking and swallowing reflexes, and severe cerebral depression are typical features of ZS and CmyD. Whereas these features disappear or alleviate in PWS and CmyD after a few weeks or months, they persist in ZS throughout life. In addition, ZS is characterized by several distinctive features such as high, receding or bulging forehead, wide-open fontanels and sutures, cataracts and/or glaucoma, hepatomegaly, and early-appearing convulsions. Laboratory findings in ZS include high serum iron, elevated levels of very long chain fatty acids, and absence of plasmalogen in plasma and cultured fibroblasts. Increased pipecolic acid in cerebrospinal fluid, blood, and urine is noticeable a few weeks after birth. Stippled calcifications of the patella can be seen in about 50% of the cases, and subcapsular renal cysts are a consistent finding in ZS. Electron microscopic studies show absence of peroxisomes in hepatocytes and renal tubular epithelial cells (Moser, 1987; Wilson et al., 1986; Zellweger, 1987).

The early phase of congenital myD cannot be clinically distinguished from the phase I PWS. Hypogonadism, notably scrotal hypoplasia, in PWS helps to differentiate the two conditions in males. The clinical differential diagnosis is more difficult or even impossible for PWS girls. Muscle biopsy may be of some help since it is normal in PWS, whereas some, but not all, infants with congenital myD show nonspecific histological features of a myopathy in this stage. The typical histological features for myotonic dystrophy, as well as clinical signs of myotonia, appear only later on in the course of the disease. Thus, the differential diagnosis between congenital myD and PWS is not always possible. The examination of the patient's mother may help in such cases. Signs of myotonic dystrophy (percussion myotonia, delayed relaxation of the fist, abnormal eye findings, including abnormal electroretinogram) in the mother suggest that the child has congenital myD. Early differentiation of congenital myD from PWS has merits since initiation of dietary treatment during the first phase of PWS holds some promise (Engel & Banker, 1986; Zellweger & Ionasescu, 1973). Table 2.2 describes differential diagnosis in phase I PWS.

Diagnostic Considerations of PWS Phase II

After some months, the symptoms of the first stage of PWS gradually subside; the children become more alert, take notice of their environment, begin to eat better, and soon cry for more food even immediately after a regular meal has been taken. They constantly appear to be hungry and eat whatever they can reach. This becomes particularly critical and disturbing after the child has learned to walk and to get around. Seeking and eating food becomes the major goal of life. PWS children will eat whatever is left on the table; they can consume anything in a freezer or pantry; and will pilfer in garbage, eat pet food, and even steal edibles from homes in the neighborhood. It is not surprising, therefore, that they become grossly overweight and their obesity often takes on grotesque, gargantuan dimensions. The characteristic small stature of PWS patients accentuates the obesity.

Delayed psychomotor development is another manifestation of PWS. Affected children rarely sit before the age of 1 year and rarely walk before the age of 2. Speech is also delayed and is frequently accompanied by articulation defects. Although intelligence is subnormal in the majority of cases, severe retardation is unusual; normal or borderline intelligence is found in about 10% of the cases. PWS patients display a peculiar emotional incontinence. On the one hand they are friendly, sociable, attached to their families, and show signs of extreme joy; on the other hand, they show bouts of anger, stubbornness, even uncontrollable rage. Essentially "good" children, they do try to please their parents, but when the parents try to control their food consumption they simply cannot comply. The urge to eat

TABLE 2.2. Differential diagnosis of phase I Prader-Willi syndrome versus other infantile hypotonias.

	Prader-Willi	Congenital myotonic dystrophy	Zellweger syndrome
Muscle tone	Atonia improving	Atonia improving, myotonia appears later on	Persistent atonia
Muscle strength	Slightly decreased	Decreased	Decreased
Muscle mass	Slightly decreased	Decreased	Decreased
Tendon reflexes	Initially absent, later on present	Initially absent, later on present	Absent or weak
Sucking/swallowing	Difficult for weeks or months	Difficult for months	Difficult throughout life in most cases
Mental status	Lethargic for weeks or months	Lethargic for months	Lethargic, nonresponsive throughout life
Electromyogram	Normal	Normal	Normal
Muscle biopsy	Normal	Normal or nonspecific myopathy	Normal; mitochondrial myopathy in exceptional cases
Other manifestations	Dysmorphic features, hypothermia, hypogonadism, microgenitale in boys, chromosome abnormality in over 50%	Clubfeet, abnormal diaphragm present	Clubfeet, hepatomegaly, abnormal ocular findings, convulsions, dysmorphic features
Infant mortality	Low	High	Very high, rarely survive to age of 2 years

is overwhelming. This discrepancy between what the PWS child wants to do and what he or she is able to do leads to frustrating conflicts that may result in depression and psychotic reactions. Obesity, always an emotional burden for anyone living in our society, is even greater for the emotionally labile PWS child. Another variant of PWS may be noted where the perception of satiety is lacking. In the author's opinion, these individuals will eat as long as food is in sight, but are not as distressed by a painful hunger feeling and have less violent outbursts of anger.

Hypogonadism is an important manifestation of PWS. In most cases hypogonadotropic hypogonadism, and in rarer instances hypergonadotropic hypogonadism, is found. Unfortunately, older individuals with PWS become unhappy and frustrated as they develop an awareness of how much they differ sexually from their normal peers; this sexual immaturity tends to compound problems of psychosocial adaptation in adolescence and adulthood. Precocious puberty has been observed in rare instances, yet no male or female PWS adult is known who has produced or borne a child.

Atonic diplegia	Werdnig-Hoffmann spinal muscular atrophy	Congenital myopathies	Benign congenital hypotonia
Atonia improving, spasticity appears later on in some cases	Progressively decreasing	Decreased but no progression	Decreased but improving
Very decreased	Progressively decreasing	Decreased	Good
Decreased	Progressive decrease to severe muscular atrophy	Decreased, often severe atrophy	Usually good, sometimes decreased
Hyperactive, Babinski positive	Weak, later absent	Absent or (rarely) weak	Normal but difficult to alicit
—	Good; difficulties may occur in advanced stages	Usually good, rarely difficult	Normal
Slow motor development	Alert	Alert	Alert
Normal	Abnormal	Abnormal	Abnormal
Normal	Abnormal	Abnormal	Abnormal
Convulsions present, slow development	Normal intelligence with severe muscle weakness	—	Normal development, easy fatigability
Low	High	Higher than usual	Not increased

PWS women may have menstrual cycles, yet some of these may be confounded with breakthrough bleeding, which is more likely to occur in obese women since body fat is said to enhance the conversion of androstenedione into estrone. Other manifestations of phase II PWS are listed in Table 2.1.

Obesity, hypogonadism, and the ensuing behavioral difficulties, with or without mental retardation, are important for the diagnostic and differential diagnostic considerations of phase II of PWS. Obesity and hypogonadism, not necessarily associated with mental retardation, occur in several conditions affecting the hypothalamic-pituitary system, such as tumors and less frequently inflammatory and traumatic lesions of that area. Such patients are hyperphagic as well, although their hyperphagia is less domineering than in PWS. Aggressiveness may occur in such conditions, but mood swings are not as prevalent as in PWS. Tumors in this region may induce symptoms that differ from PWS by several features, such as headache, disturbances of vision, enlargement of the sella turcica, and often diabetes insipidus. Genetic conditions with obesity and hypogonadism are the Bardet-Biedl and the Biemond syndromes. Both are autosomal recessive conditions and thus may affect more than one child in a sibship, whereas PWS in siblings is exceptional. In addition to the features that these aforementioned conditions have in common with PWS, they show a number of distinctive signs and symptoms. Patients with Bardet-Biedl syndrome have retinitis pigmentosa, decreased vision, night blindness, and polydactyly. They are somewhat small and mildly retarded. The Biemond syndrome is characterized by iris coloboma, mental retardation, and polydactyly. Conditions with obesity but normal intelligence and no hypogonadism are the Alström (retinitis pigmentosa and diabetes mellitus) and the Summit (craniosynostosis and syndactyly) syndromes. Both conditions are also autosomal recessive. Obesity, mental retardation, and hypogonadism are found in Carpenter's syndrome, which is also autosomal recessive (McKusick, 1986). Acrocephaly and polysyndactyly are distinctive features of Carpenter's syndrome.

Behaviors associated with PWS are unique and distinctive. None of the other conditions associated with obesity show the ongoing aberrant behaviors that torment PWS children and disrupt their families.

References

Dubowitz, V. (1980). *The floppy infant* (2nd ed.). London: Spastics International Medical Publications.

Engel, A.G., & Banker, B.Q. (1986). *Myology*. New York: McGraw-Hill.

Ionasescu, V., & Zellweger, H. (1983). *Genetics in neurology*. New York: Raven Press.

McKusick, V. (1986). *Mendelian inheritance in man* (7th ed.). Baltimore: Johns Hopkins University Press.

Moser, H.W. (1987). New approaches in peroxisomal disorders. *Developmental Neuroscience*, *9*, 1–18.

Smith, D.W. (1982). *Recognizable patterns of human malformations* (3rd ed.). Philadelphia: W.B. Saunders.

Volpe, J.J. (1981). *Neurology of the newborn*. Philadelphia: W.B. Saunders.

Wilson, G.N., Holmes, R.G., Custer, J., Lipkowitz, L., Stover, J., Datta N., & Hajra, A. (1986). Zellweger syndrome: Diagnostic assays, syndrome delineation and potential therapy. *American Journal of Medical Genetics*, *21*, 69–82.

Zellweger, H. (1983). The floppy infant: A practical approach. *Helvetica Paediatrica Acta*, *38*, 301–306.

Zellweger, H. (1987). Peroxisomal disorders. *Developmental Medicine and Child Neurology*, *29*, 821–829.

Zellweger, H., & Ionasescu, V. (1973). Early onset of myotonic dystrophy. *American Journal of Diseases of Children*, *125*, 601–605.

3
Hypogonadism and Osteoporosis

KAREN RUBIN and SUZANNE B. CASSIDY

Hypogonadism has been a recognized major feature of Prader-Willi syndrome (PWS) since it was first described (Prader, Labhart, & Willi, 1956). It has been shown to be hypogonadotropic in origin, and is manifested initially by small or poorly developed external genitalia and later by deficiencies of pubertal development, short stature, and infertility (Table 3.1). Osteoporosis is a recently described finding in PWS that is likely to be an additional consequence of hypogonadism, at least in part. There is presently no standard approach to the management of the hypogonadism, although recent reports suggest that treatment may have beneficial results.

Background

FEATURES OF HYPOGONADISM IN INFANCY

The hypogonadism in PWS is usually evident at birth. The initial findings are a small penis and undescended testicles in male infants and a small clitoris and rudimentary labia minora in female infants. The underdeveloped labia and/or clitoris often go overlooked in the female infant, unlike the small penis, which is almost uniformly noticed and may cause a great deal of concern on the part of the parents and/or physician. When careful measurements are performed (with a tongue depressor to push the suprapubic fat pad down to the pubic bone) most males are shown not to have true microphallus according to standards for stretched penile length (Winter & Faiman, 1972). In over 80% of males, one or both testes are undescended and the scrotum is underdeveloped (Bray et al., 1983; Hall & Smith, 1972).

HYPOGONADISM DURING ADOLESCENT AND ADULT YEARS

During adolescence, sexual maturation is usually delayed, incomplete, or disordered, although it may be normal or occur early (Holm, 1981; Ichiba

TABLE 3.1. Hypogonadism in PWS: clinical consequences.

From birth		
	Males	Small penis Small scrotum Cryptorchidism (80%)
	Females	Small clitoris Small labia minora
Puberty		
	Both sexes	Delayed, disordered, incomplete pubertal development (may be precocious or normal in onset) Pseudogynecomastia Scanty pubic and axillary hair Osteoporosis
	Males	Scanty beard and body hair No sexual interest or activity Infertility
	Females	Poor breast development Amenorrhea or oligomenorrhea Premature menopause ? Infertility

& Gardner, 1975). A pubertal growth spurt fails to occur, with resultant short stature. Pubertal development is more uniformly incomplete in males than in females. For example, it is rare that an untreated male becomes virilized to the degree that he needs to shave. Growth of the penis and testes are similarly subnormal in most PWS males. There have been no reports of a PWS male fathering a child.

In females, the degree of pubertal development is more difficult to assess since it may be difficult to distinguish true breast development from fatty tissue. Despite this, breast size and development of the areola and nipple are often subnormal. The labia minora and clitoris remain small and do not develop with exposure to higher endogenous or exogenous estrogen levels. The onset of menstrual periods is usually delayed and may not occur at all. A number of women with PWS initially have less than eight menstrual periods per year. Periods become progressively more infrequent with time until secondary amenorrhea develops. In addition, older adult female patients may experience episodes of irregular bleeding that are similar to the dysfunctional bleeding that occurs in menopausal women. It is unlikely that ovulation occurs on a regular basis in most women with PWS, although this has not been documented by appropriate testing. Finally, potential fertility has not been ruled out, although no definite cases have been reported in PWS women.

Causes of Hypogonadism in PWS

Over the past decade, refined endocrine laboratory measurements in diagnostic testing have made it possible to define the cause of hypogonadism in PWS individuals. Numerous studies have been done to identify the source of the hormone deficiency in the hypothalamic-pituitary-gonadal axis. Most studies have involved the administration to PWS individuals of human chorionic gonadotropin (hCG), luteinizing hormone–releasing factor (LRF), and/or clomiphene citrate (Bray et al., 1983; Jeffcoate, Laurance, Edwards, Besser, 1980; Linde, McNeil, & Rabin, 1982; Tolis, et al., 1974). The overall conclusion from these studies is that the most frequent cause of the hypogonadism in PWS is a hypothalamic deficiency or a deficiency in LRF.

The frequent observation of hypogonadism at birth suggests an intrauterine hypothalamic deficiency as well. In males, descent of the testes and growth of the penis occur in the last two trimesters. These late testosterone-mediated events in male development are dependent on pituitary gonadotropins and placental hCG. Although placental hCG levels are presumably normal, decreased gonadotropin release during these late events may result in a small penis and undescended testicles in PWS male infants. In the female a similar explanation may apply for the poorly developed clitoris and labia evident at birth.

Laboratory Findings

Serum estradiol levels are frequently low or low-normal for the follicular phase in adolescent and adult female PWS subjects, although they may be normal. In untreated PWS males, serum testosterone levels are uniformly low.

Basal luteinizing hormone (LH) and follicle-stimulating hormone (FSH) levels are usually low or normal, but on rare occasions may be elevated (Garty, Shuper, Mimouni, Varsano, & Kauli, 1982; Rudd et al., 1973). In most pubertal- and postpubertal-age subjects, injection of LRF produces only a small rise in either LH or FSH, suggesting a deficient gonadotropin reserve as a result of chronic LRF deficiency.

Subnormal response to provocative growth hormone (GH) tests are frequent in PWS individuals and are considered similar to the responses observed in obese subjects who do not have PWS (Tze, Dunn, & Rothstein, 1981). Somatomedin-C levels and 24-hour pulsatile secretory patterns of GH have not yet been reported in PWS subjects but are presently being studied.

Thyroid studies are usually normal, although tertiary hypothalamic hypothyroidism with a normal or low thyroid-stimulating hormone (TSH) level and a low thyroxine level is possible.

TABLE 3.2. Potential indications for hormonal intervention in PWS.

Microphallus
Cryptorchidism
Incomplete pubertal development
? Osteoporosis
? Short stature

Treatment of Hypogonadism

Hormonal intervention in PWS may be indicated for management of microphallus, cryptorchidism, and incomplete pubertal development. Intervention may also be considered in some cases of osteoporosis and short stature (Table 3.2).

TREATMENT OF MICROPHALLUS

Treatment of microphallus is sometimes recommended for psychological reasons alone and/or if the penis is small enough to prevent urination in the standing position, thereby interfering with social integration. Treatment with Depo-Testosterone 25 mg intramuscularly (IM) every 3 weeks for a total of five doses has produced a penis of normal size in several male children with PWS (Guthrie, Smith, & Graham, 1973).

MANAGEMENT OF CRYPTORCHIDISM

Opinions concerning management of descent of the testicles in PWS vary. In boys without PWS, the second year of life is believed to be the best age at which to initiate treatment for undescended testicles (Hadziselimovic, 1981). If a child does not respond to hormone treatment at that time, surgery is recommended early. Since fertility has not yet been reported in males with PWS, since the risk of testicular tumor does not decrease substantially after orchiopexy (Babata, Chu, Hilaris, Willet, & Golbey; 1982) and since there is no report of a testicular tumor in PWS, there is no compelling medical indication for surgery during childhood in PWS males. However, surgery may be considered early when there are psychological reasons. The most conservative approach is to wait until mid- to late adolescence for possible spontaneous descent, since late spontaneous descent during the adolescent years has been reported in PWS (Hamilton, Scully, & Kliman, 1972; Uehling, 1980). A trial of hCG therapy (3,300 IU/week for 4 weeks) or intranasal gonadotropin-releasing hormone (GnRH) (1.2 mg/day for 28 days alone or in combination with hCG) is recommended prior to contemplated surgery and may be initiated as early as the second year of life (Rajfer et al., 1986). Only a small percentage of testicles in high inguinal or higher positions respond to hormone therapy

(F. Hadziselimovic, personal communication). In cases in which hormone therapy does not work and the testicles have not descended spontaneously by midadolescence, surgery can be considered. However, every effort should be made not to remove the testicles at the time of surgery since the degree of hypogonadism is variable and the testicles might initiate some degree of spontaneous sexual development.

Sex Hormone Therapy

There are currently no well-established guidelines for if, when, or how to institute hormone therapy for people with PWS. Hormone intervention in PWS remains a highly controversial topic, with many physicians and/or parents regarding any kind of hormone therapy as unnecessary, potentially harmful, or inconvenient, whereas others believe that the benefits outweigh the problems. The associated risks and effects of hormone treatment and the variability of the PWS population are largely responsible for this dilemma. For example, the degree of hypogonadism varies from person to person, particularly among females with PWS. Differences in the level of intellectual and psychosocial functioning and degree of emotional lability are additional factors to be considered when making a decision regarding hormone therapy. The ability of a female to handle the hygienic aspects of menstruation is an important factor to be considered. A social setting that assures compliance should be prerequisite for treatment.

A strong indication for long-term hormone therapy is incomplete sexual development in an individual who desires further sexual development for social and psychological reasons. On occasion people with PWS will express a desire to more closely resemble their peers with respect to physical development. Table 3.3 summarizes a number of the advantages and disadvantages of hormone replacement therapy.

Male Sex Hormone Therapy

Information on the effects of long-term testosterone therapy in PWS males is lacking. Fear of intensifying the baseline behavioral lability in PWS males by increasing aggressive behavior and/or hostile feelings has led to a reluctance to initiate testosterone therapy. A careful prospective assessment of the effects of testosterone therapy in PWS on sexual activity, level of self-esteem, and various aspects of behavior is needed. Until this type of information becomes available, a more widespread acceptance of testosterone therapy is unlikely.

At the University of Connecticut Health Center PWS Clinic, the present philosophy is that, in most males, the potential benefits outweigh the risks. We have treated 10 males with Depo-Testosterone injections every 3–4 weeks and all have responded with voice changes; increased pubic, axillary, and facial hair requiring shaving; increased penis size; and an increased musculature. Testicular size may increase slightly in some patients.

TABLE 3.3. Sex hormone replacement therapy in PWS.

Female	Male
Advantages	
Improved self-esteem and/or other possible psychological benefits of increased secondary sex characteristics (e.g., improved family and peer interactions)	Improved self-esteem and/or other possible psychological benefits of increased secondary sex characteristics (e.g., improved family and peer interactions)
Predictable bleeding pattern in subjects with prior irregular menses	Increased muscle mass with positive effect on physical performance
? Increased bone density	Increased energy and activity levels
	? Increased bone density
Disadvantages	
Increased hygiene demand	? Intensification of aggressive behavior
? Increased libido	? Increased libido
Potential medical complications, especially in older subjects (e.g., diabetes, hypertension, clotting disorder)	Necessity for regular medical monitoring
Necessity for regular medical monitoring and regular pelvic exams	

Most patients have expressed an increased sense of well-being as a result of the increased virilization. A higher energy level that appears to be associated with increased participation in physical exercise has been observed in some patients.

In a manner similar to treatment for other testosterone-deficient states, testosterone therapy is optimally initiated during early to midadolescence (12–18 years of age) with low-dose Depo-Testosterone (approximately 50 mg) administered IM every 3–4 weeks. The dosage should be increased gradually to the average adult dose of 200 mg monthly by young adulthood, in an attempt to mimic normal pubertal development. Although peak serum levels of testosterone can be measured to titrate the dosage regimen, clinical assessment of the patient is usually all that is needed. Bone age should be monitored every 6 to 12 months prior to epiphyseal fusion to assure that accelerated bone maturation, and therefore decreased ultimate height, does not occur.

Female Sex Hormone Therapy

There are no reports of long-term estrogen therapy in PWS females despite the fact that the majority of adult females show evidence of chronic estrogen deficiency with incomplete sexual development. Estrogen therapy has more medical contraindications and potential risks (see Table 3.3) than testosterone therapy, and this has probably been the reason why there has been an even greater reluctance to treat PWS women with hormones than PWS men.

Prior to initiating estrogen therapy in a PWS female, control of obesity is extremely desirable. This would greatly reduce the potential for developing diabetes, hypertension, and clotting problems, all of which may be exacerbated by sex hormone therapy.

Estrogen therapy is administered to non-PWS, hypogonadic females in a cyclical fashion in combination with progesterone to mimic the normal menstrual cycle and to protect the endometrium. One commonly used regimen involves low to moderate doses of estrogen (0.625–1.25 mg Premarin) given alone from day 1 to day 12 of the cycle with progesterone (5–10 mg) added from day 12 to day 25 of the cycle. A withdrawal bleed occurs during the time when both hormones are stopped. This method minimizes the risk of developing uterine cancer. Nonetheless, all women on long-term estrogen therapy need to be followed with regular gynecological examinations.

Since PWS females are less uniformly hypogonadal than males, delaying hormone replacement therapy until late adolescence or young adulthood to ascertain if spontaneous sexual development occurs is suggested. Once a decision is made to initiate treatment, low-dose estrogen should be started and gradually increased to an adult dosage. After 6–9 months of unopposed estrogen, the patient should be started on cyclical therapy with progesterone.

A more physiological estradiol preparation, micronized 17β-estradiol, is now available to hypogonadal patients in doses to reproduce normal serum estradiol levels (Kastrup, 1985). Transdermal estrogen may represent the safest method of estrogen replacement therapy to date (DeLignieres, et al., 1986). There are no reports of the use of these newer preparations in PWS.

As with testosterone therapy, clinical assessment of secondary sexual characteristics and monitoring of bone age every 6–12 months prior to epiphyseal fusion is indicated. Individuals on estrogen therapy should have medical visits every 3–6 months to check for the development of potential complications such as diabetes or hypertension.

Discussion

A summary of the above-suggested possibilities for hormone therapies is presented in Table 3.4. Other regimens utilizing other hormone preparations can also be used for similar effects.

Pulsatile LRF agonist therapy is now being used to treat non-PWS males and females with hypogonadotropic hypogonadism (Leyendecker, Wildt, & Hansmann, 1980). Although this type of therapy can result in a smoother modulation of hormone levels and bypass the medical risks of

TABLE 3.4. Suggested sex hormone treatment regimens.

Abnormality	Hormone treatment approach
Microphallus	Depo-Testosterone: 25 mg IM every 3 weeks for 5 doses
Cryptorchidism	hCG: 3,300 IU IM/week for 4 weeks
	<and/or>
	Intranasal GnRH: 1.2 mg/day for 28 days
Sex hormone insufficiency	
Female	Premarin: 0.625–1.25 mg orally daily on days 1–25 of calendar month
	<with>
	Provera: 5–10 mg orally daily on days 12–25 of calendar month
Male	Depo-Testosterone: IM every 3–4 weeks
	early adolescence (12–14 years): 25–50 mg
	midadolescence (14–18 years): 50–150 mg
	adulthood (over 18 years): 150–200 mg

estrogen therapy, the potential for fertility in both sexes may make it a less desirable form of therapy in most PWS individuals.

In conclusion, although endocrine abnormalities in PWS are somewhat understood, experience with long-term hormone intervention to improve pubertal development is minimal, and the widespread reluctance to treat PWS individuals will likely remain until more information becomes available. It is hoped that collaborative studies on PWS individuals of both sexes receiving long-term hormone therapy will provide additional insight into the psychosocial, psychological, physical, and medical consequences of long-term hormone replacement therapy for individuals with PWS.

ROLE OF HORMONE TREATMENT FOR SHORT STATURE IN PWS

The mild short stature of PWS is believed to be largely due to the lack of a pubertal growth spurt. However, experience with growth-promoting agents such as oxandrolone (Anavar), low-dose estrogen, and/or GH is limited. Well-controlled clinical trials using such agents are needed to answer the questions of whether or not such treatment can enhance short-term growth and/or ultimate height in PWS.

Osteoporosis in PWS

People with PWS have a number of characteristic features that might predispose them to the early or later development of osteoporosis. The hypogonadism in PWS with its delayed and/or incomplete pubertal development may result in decreased bone mass. Prolonged marginal calcium intake may contribute another risk factor in PWS individuals. Those people with PWS on calorie-restricted diets with decreased intake of calcium-rich foods may experience prolonged periods of negative calcium balance. Another potential risk factor in PWS is inactivity related to obesity and hypotonia. Finally, fair coloring seems to be an additional risk factor for osteoporosis, and PWS individuals have been shown to have fair coloring for their families (Hittner, et al., 1982). In addition to the presence of some or all of these risk factors, a number of features of PWS may represent clinical manifestations of osteoporosis. These include an increased incidence of fractures with minimal trauma (Holm & Laurnen, 1981), an increased incidence of scoliosis, and, in our experience, frequent kyphosis in older PWS individuals.

Because of the presence of risk factors and suggestive clinical features, bone density measurements were obtained in 18 children and adults of both sexes ranging from 6 1/2 to 47 years of age who are followed regularly at the University of Connecticut Health Center PWS Clinic. We utilized the method of single-beam photon absorptiometry with iodine-^{125} as a source of photons. This method measures the amount of bone mineral in the distal radius, one third of the length from its distal end, a site comprised predominately of cortical bone.

The radial bone mineral (RMB) measurement in 17 of the 18 PWS subjects was at least 1 SD, and most were greater than 2 SD, below the mean. There was no correlation in either sex between the RBM measurement and the degree of clinical hypogonadism, presence of scoliosis or kyphosis, or presence or absence of the chromosome 15q deletion (Cassidy, Rubin, & Mukaida, 1985).

This preliminary study demonstrates for the first time that osteoporosis is a fairly consistent finding in PWS. Whether the low bone mass or osteoporosis in PWS is an intrinsic part of the disorder or it is the result of an interaction of a number of factors such as hypogonadism, inactivity, marginal calcium intake, subnormal levels of adrenal androgen, or an imbalance in the calcium-regulating hormones requires further investigation.

Treatment of Osteoporosis

Until a better understanding of the causes of osteoporosis in PWS is acquired, we recommend the encouragement of regular weight-bearing exercise with attention to posture control in order to prevent excessive stress on the spine. Adequate calcium intake of approximately 1000–1,200 mg of calcium/day with calcium supplementation if needed, is also recommended. Finally, if long-term estrogen and testosterone therapy can be shown to enhance bone mass in PWS, as it does in postmenopausal women or other hypogonadal men (Baran, Bergfeld, Teitelbaum, & Avioli, 1978; Lindsay, Hart, & Aitken, 1976), there would be a stronger indication for long-term hormone therapy in order to enhance bone deposition and thereby potentially prevent symptomatic osteoporosis with fractures.

References

Babata, A., Chu, F.C.H., Hilaris, B.S., Willet, F.W., & Golbey, R.B. (1982). Testicular cancer in cryptorchids. *Cancer, 49*, 1023–1030.

Baran, D.T., Bergfeld, M.A., Teitelbaum, S.L., & Avioli, L.V. (1978). Effect of testosterone therapy on bone formation in an osteoporotic hypogonadal male. *Calcified Tissue Research, 26*, 103–106.

Bray, G.A., Dahms, W.T., Swerdloff, R.S., Fiser, R., Atkinson, R., & Carrell, R. (1983). The Prader-Willi syndrome: A study of 40 patients and a review of the literature. *Medicine, 62*, 59–80.

Cassidy, S.B., Rubin, K.G., & Mukaida, C. (1985). Osteoporosis in Prader-Willi syndrome. *American Journal of Human Genetics, 37*, A49.

DeLignieres, B., Basdeoant, A., Thomas G., Thalabard, J., Mercier-Bodard, C., Conard, J., Guyene, T., Mairon, N., Corvol, P., Guy-Grand, B., Mauvais-Janis, P., & Sitruk-Ware, R. (1986). Biological effects of estradiol-17β in postmenopausal women: Oral versus percutaneous administration. *Journal of Clinical Endocrinology and Metabolism, 62*, 536–541.

Garty, B., Shuper, A., Mimouni, M., Varsano, I., & Kauli R. (1982). Primary gonadal failure and precocious adrenarche in a boy with Prader-Labhart-Willi syndrome. *European Journal Pediatrics, 139*, 201–203.

Guthrie, R.D., Smith, D.W., & Graham, C.B. (1973). Testosterone treatment for micropenis during early childhood. *Journal of Pediatrics, 83*, 247–252.

Hadziselimovic, F. (1981). Pathogenesis of cryptorchidism. In S.T. Kogan & E.S.E. Hafey (Eds.), *Pediatric andrology* (vol. 7, pp. 147–162). The Hague: Martinus Nijhoff.

Hall, B.D., & Smith, D.W. (1972). Prader-Willi syndrome: A resume of 32 cases including an instance of affected first cousins, one of whom is of normal stature and intelligence. *Journal of Pediatrics, 81*, 286–293.

Hamilton, C.R., Scully, R.E., & Kliman, B. (1972). Hypogonadotropinism in Prader-Willi syndrome. *American Journal of Medicine, 52*, 322–329.

Hittner, H.M., King, R.A., Riccardi, W.M., Ledbetter, D.H., Borda, R.P., Ferrell, R.E., & Kretzer, F.L. (1982). Oculocutaneous albinoidism as a manifestation of reduced neural crest derivatives in the Prader-Willi syndrome. *American Journal of Opthalmology, 94*, 328–337.

Holm, V.A. (1981). The diagnosis of Prader-Willi syndrome. In V.A. Holm, S.J. Sulzbacher, & P.L. Pipes (Eds.), *The Prader Willi syndrome* (chpt. 3). Baltimore: University Park Press.

Holm, V.A., & Laurnen, E.L. (1981). Prader-Willi syndrome and scoliosis. *Developmental Medicine and Child Neurology, 23*, 192–201.

Ichiba, Y., & Gardner, L.I. (1975). Metabolic and genetic syndromes of overgrowth. In L.I. Gardner (Ed.), *Endocrine and genetic diseases of childhood and adolescence* (2nd ed., pp. 1324–1328). Philadelphia: W.B. Saunders.

Jeffcoate, W.J., Laurance, B.M., Edwards, C.R.W., & Besser G.M. (1980). Endocrine function in the Prader-Willi syndrome. *Clinical Endocrinology, 12*, 81–89.

Kastrup, K.W. (1985). Effect of estradiol treatment monitored by serum concentration on growth and development in Turner syndrome. *Pediatric Research, 19*, 620.

Leyendecker, G., Wildt, L., & Hansmann, M. (1980). Pregnancies following chronic intermittent (pulsatile) administration of Gn–RH by means of a portable pump ("Zyklomat"). A new approach to the treatment of infertility in hypothalamic amenorrhea. *Journal of Clinical Endocrinology and Metabolism*, *51*, 1214–1216.

Linde, R., McNeil, L., & Rabin, D. (1982). Induction of menarche by clomiphene citrate in a 17-year-old girl with the Prader-Labhart-Willi syndrome. *Fertility and Sterility*, *37*, 118–120.

Lindsay, R., Hart, D.M., & Aitken, J.M., McDonald, E.B., Anderson, J.B., & Clark, A.C. (1976). Long-term prevention of post-menopausal osteoporosis by estrogen. *Lancet*, *1*, 1038.

Prader, A., Labhart, A., & Willi, H. (1956). Ein Syndrom von Adipositas, Kleinwuchs, Kryptorchismus und Oligophrenie nach Myotonicartigem Zustand in Neugeborenalter. *Schweizerische Medizinische Wochenschrift*, *86*, 1260–1261.

Rajfer, J., Handelsman, D.J., Swerdloff, R.S., Hurwitz, R., Kapan, H., Vandergast, T., & Ehrlich, R.M. (1986). Hormonal therapy of cryptorchidism. *New England Journal of Medicine*, *314*, 466–470.

Rudd, B.T., Rayner, P.H.W., Smith, M.R., Holder, G., Jivani, S.K.M., Theodoridis, C.G. (1973). Effect of human chorionic gonadotropin on plasma and urine testosterone in boys with delayed puberty. *Archives of Disease in Childhood*, *48*, 590–595.

Tolis, G., Lewis, W., Verdy, M., Friesen H.G., Solowon, S., Pagalis, G., Pavlatos F., Fessas, P.H., & Rochefort, J.G. (1974). Anterior pituitary function in the Prader-Labhart Willi syndrome. *Journal of Clinical Endocrinology and Metabolism*, *39*, 1061–1066.

Tze, W.J., Dunn, H.G., & Rothstein, R.L. (1981). Endocrine profiles and metabolic aspects of Prader-Willi syndrome. In V.A. Holm, S. Sulzbacher, & P.L. Pipes (Eds.), *The Prader-Willi syndrome* (chap. 22). Baltimore: University Park Press.

Uehling, D. (1980). Cryptorchidism in the Prader-Willi syndrome. *Journal of Urology*, *124*, 103–104.

Winter, J.S.D., & Faiman, C. (1972). Pituitary gonadal relations in male children and adolescents. *Pediatric Research*, *6*, 126.

4
Genetics Evaluation and Counseling for Prader-Willi Syndrome

ELIZABETH J. THOMSON

The provision of genetics evaluation and counseling services is one important aspect of comprehensive care for individuals with Prader-Willi syndrome (PWS) and their families. This distinctive counseling service should be offered to parents of children who are known or suspected to have PWS. It is best provided by a medical geneticist in conjunction with a genetics nurse specialist or a genetics counselor.

Unfortunately, the importance of genetics evaluation and counseling is frequently underestimated and, too often, the process itself is misunderstood. For example, some team professionals believe they can provide genetics counseling as well as a trained geneticist/counselor. Also, there are instances in which parents of affected children are not referred for genetics consultation because they do not plan to have more children; thus, the reproductive counseling aspect of services is not considered necessary. Understanding the genetic aspects of PWS and provision of reproductive information are just two parts of the total genetics evaluation and counseling process. It reaches beyond confirmation of diagnosis and informative counseling and includes both support and follow-up counseling as well.

Whereas it may appear that there is considerable overlap in the information provided by the genetics professionals and other members of the health care team, it is most likely that benefits accrue from purposefully repeated discussions of pertinent facts. Information about PWS restated in a variety of ways can enhance understanding. Certainly, qualified genetics professionals do provide a reliable resource and sensitive ongoing support for families over an extended period of time.

Genetics Evaluation and Counseling

Genetics counseling is defined as:

> . . . a communication process which deals with the human problems associated with the occurrence or the risk of occurrence of a genetic disorder in a family. This process involves an attempt by one or more appropriately trained persons (geneti-

cist, genetics nurse specialist or genetic counselor) to help the individual or family to:

1. comprehend the medical facts including the diagnosis, the probable course of the disorder, and the available management.
2. appreciate the way heredity contributes to the disorder and the risk of recurrence in specific relatives.
3. understand the options for dealing with the risk of recurrence.
4. choose a course of action which seems appropriate to them based on their perception of their risks, their family goals and values and to act accordingly.
5. make the best possible adjustment to the disorder in an affected member and/or to the risk of recurrence of that disorder. (Fraser, 1974, p. 637)

Some families will be referred for genetics evaluation in order to attempt to confirm or rule out the diagnosis of PWS. In other instances, the diagnosis will be well established and the family will be referred for genetics counseling so that they may receive further information and support regarding this diagnosis in their child.

Diagnosis

The first step in the genetics evaluation and counseling process is to establish or confirm a specific diagnosis. The clinical features and general diagnostic guidelines for making the diagnosis of PWS are described in Chapters 1 and 2. In addition, a chromosome analysis should be carried out when the diagnosis of PWS is suspected in a child. This is important because 50–60% of those children clinically diagnosed as having the syndrome will be found to have a chromosomal deletion in the long arm of chromosome 15 (Greenswag, 1987). It is not well understood why some children with PWS have a chromosomal deletion present while others do not, particularly since no clinical differences can be detected between the two groups. It has been hypothesized that perhaps all children with PWS have an alteration in their genetic material in the long arm of chromosome 15, but current laboratory capabilities do not allow for identification of the very small deletion or alteration that may actually be present (Latt et al., 1987). Although this chromosomal deletion does not seem to have substantial predictive value at this time regarding the prognosis of a child with PWS, nevertheless, chromosome analysis is an important test that is available for diagnostic purposes as well as for research regarding future characterization of PWS.

Although the genetic aspects of PWS are not as clearly defined as those seen in Huntington disease or cystic fibrosis, exciting progress is occurring in this area. The advent of newer molecular developments in genetics testing may, in the future, allow for the identification of genetic alterations or deletions at a molecular level rather than the chromosomal or cytogenetic level and may yield new information in the diagnosis and management of PWS.

Informative Counseling

Once the diagnosis of PWS is established, it is important to provide the family with information about the disorder, its pathogenesis, the specific risk of recurrence, and reproductive alternatives. Informative counseling is provided to the immediate family of the affected individual. They will be given information about PWS, its prognosis and management, and treatment programs available, if they are not already involved with such a program. Information will also be provided to the family regarding available resources, including alternative placement facilities and financial options available to them. When requested, this information is provided to extended family members, the local physician, members of the clergy, teachers, and other individuals who may be involved with the family in the future.

Specific recurrence risk information, currently estimated to be approximately 1.6% (Smith, 1982), is provided to the parents of a child with PWS. Despite this risk, which many couples interpret to be quite low, parents often appreciate having an opportunity to discuss available reproductive options. These include taking the risk and reproducing again or choosing not to reproduce any further and have other biologic children. If the latter alternative is chosen, couples may expand their family by adoption, although this option is becoming increasingly difficult in today's society.

Prenatal diagnosis is one other option that couples who have had a child with PWS may wish to consider. Prenatal diagnostic methods available include ultrasound evaluation, amniocentesis, and chorionic villi sampling. Although prenatal diagnosis cannot rule out the presence of PWS in an unborn child with a 100% degree of certainty, in some cases it may be reassuring to rule out the presence of a deletion in the long arm of chromosome 15, other chromosome abnormalities such as Down syndrome, and other structural defects such as spina bifida. Whereas the parents cannot be totally reassured that PWS has not recurred in their family, they may be relieved to know that their expected child has normal chromosomes and no significant neural tube defect present. Ruling out these birth defect problems brings the reproductive risks of parents of children with PWS very close to the general population risk (approximately 3%).

Supportive Counseling

The third component of the genetics evaluation and counseling process is the provision of supportive counseling. Support begins with a sensitive restatement to the family that their child's disorder is not due to anything they did or did not do. Support continues through helping families to process the normal grief response to having a child with PWS. Families of children with PWS may experience what Olshansky (1962) described as "chronic sorrow." They need help to understand that the grief process may be difficult and may last as long as their affected child is alive and even beyond that time. Referrals to parent support groups, the clergy, or a psychological/psychiatric counselor should be considered, and the parents are encouraged to identify their support people and to call on them when they feel in need of support.

Families involved in the reproductive decision-making process need support while weighing many factors. The couple's desire for children, their interpretation of their recurrence risk, their past experience with PWS, and their ethical, moral, and religious beliefs must be considered. Support by health professionals during this decision-making process should not be underestimated. It is vitally important that the couple feels comfortable to freely discuss these issues and choose a course of action that is best for them. They must be informed that the right decision for one couple may not be the right decision for another. In no case should genetics professionals or other health professionals attempt to influence a couple's reproductive decisions according to their own values or desires.

Follow-up Counseling

The final component of the genetics evaluation and counseling process is follow-up counseling. Follow-up allows counselors an opportunity to provide additional information to the family, to correct misunderstandings or misconceptions about the information the family has already received, and to continue to develop a relationship so that they can be an ongoing resource to the family. It allows for an opportunity to reinforce the information that they may have received and to answer new questions as they arise. The family may also request evaluation of other children or ask that other family members be allowed to attend subsequent genetics counseling visits so that they may have their questions and concerns addressed.

Assessment of the family's reaction to the presence of a child with PWS and the determination of the coping mechanisms of individual family members is also a vital aspect of follow-up. This assessment provides an opportunity for referral to other support services should they be needed or desired. Genetics counselors should point out that, despite the presence of PWS, affected individuals can, with appropriate supervision and guidance, lead productive lives.

Summary

When goals of the genetics evaluation and counseling process are met, families of children with PWS will have a better understanding of the disorder. The family will have received both verbal and written information about the disorder and about support services available to them. Referrals to other support services will be initiated as needed and/or desired. The family will also be better prepared to make informed reproductive decisions and, it is hoped, will be better able to cope with the presence of their child with PWS. Working together with the parents, genetics professionals can assist the family to make the best possible adjustment to the disorder.

References

Fraser, C. (1974). Current issues in medical genetics. *American Journal of Medical Genetics*, *26*, 636–659.

Greenswag, L. (1987). Adults with Prader Willi syndrome. *Developmental Medicine and Child Neurology*, *29*, 145–152.

Latt, S., Tantravaki, U., Neve, R., Nichols, R., Ringer, S., Stroh, H., Fuller, R., Donlan, T., Kaplan, L., & Worton, R. (1987, June). *New and better molecular probes for characterizing and ultimately understanding the consequences of number 15 deletions in Prader-Willi syndrome.* Paper presented at the Second Annual Prader Willi Syndrome Conference, Houston.

Olshansky, S. (1962). Chronic sorrow: A response to having a mentally defective child. *Social Casework*, *43*, 190–193.

Smith, D.W. (1982). *Recognizable patterns of human malformation.* Philadelphia: W.B. Saunders.

Part II A Case Presentation

5
A Case Study: A Chronology of Hope

Jack Sherman and Gerald Ente

As with most developmental disabilities, the presence of Prader-Willi syndrome (PWS) has a profound impact on the family system. It would be a disservice to both affected individuals and their families to ignore parental feelings. For this reason, the case presentation that follows integrates the medical, psychological, educational, and social history of a Caucasian female with personal, sensitive commentary from her parents. They assisted the case historians by sharing their recollections of their lifelong experiences and the endless frustrations as the parents of a disabled child whose diagnosis was delayed for over 26 years.

Case Study[1]

Miss M was born in 1957, just a year after the publication of the article by Prader, Labhart, and Willi (1956) that definitively described what has come to be known as PWS. Both the timing of her birth and the lack of physician awareness about this syndrome played a large part in the delay of accurate diagnosis. From the beginning, very early in her stormy neonatal period, M was evaluated by pediatricians, internists, endocrinologists, neurologists, and psychiatrists. All these specialists reported symptomatology now acknowledged to be some physical or emotional manifestation of PWS. Unfortunately, it was not the until M was 26 years of age and living in a home for the emotionally disturbed that a psychologist involved with

[1] For purposes of confidentiality, M's birthplace, current residence, and the identities of the medical centers where she was extensively evaluated are not disclosed. It is the opinion of the authors that, although lack of knowledge about PWS by the medical community contributed immeasurably to the 27-year delay in M's diagnosis, no purpose is served by lamenting past ignorance. It is hoped that through case descriptions such as this, the medical community will become increasingly familiar with PWS and consider it when confronted with the signs and symptoms of this disorder.

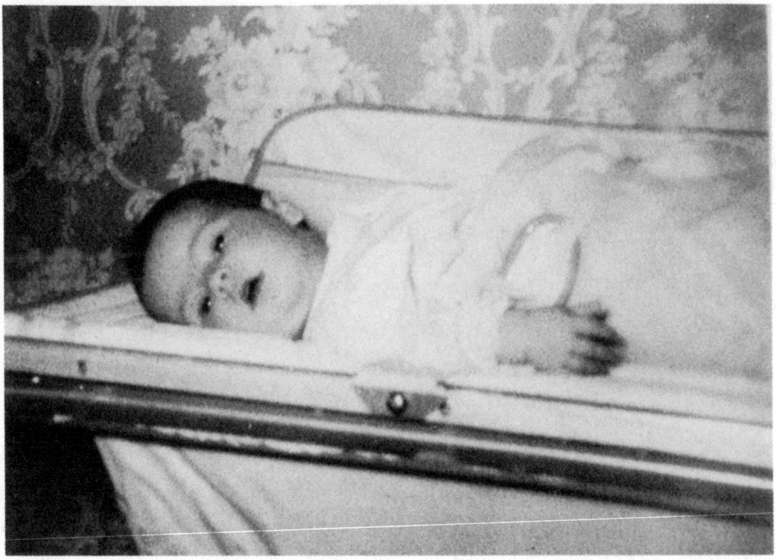

FIGURE 5.1. M at 2½ months.

her programming suspected that PWS might be the correct diagnosis. At his recommendation, M's parents sought a genetics center familiar with this disorder where a thorough assessment confirmed the diagnosis.

M was the fourth child born to a 38-year-old father and a 40-year-old mother who had three normal offspring, one miscarriage, and no stillbirths. There was no history of consanguinity nor exposure to teratogens prior to or during the pregnancy. History was also negative for birth defects or mental retardation. Her mother reported no discernible difference in M's fetal activity and that of her three previous pregnancies. The older siblings, ages 11, 9, and 6 at the time of the proband's birth, were all normal and healthy.

M was delivered vaginally 2 weeks postterm after an uneventful pregnancy and labor. She weighed 3.3 kg (7 lbs, 4 oz) and was 48.25 cm (19 in) in length. Apgar scores were not reported. Her neonatal course was marked by hypotonia and inability to take oral feedings because of poor suck. At 3 days of age she was transferred from the hospital where she was born to a university-based tertiary care center. She remained there 5 days and was discharged with a diagnosis of cerebral palsy of unknown origin.

Our story began when the doctor who delivered our daughter knew something was not normal and suggested immediate hospitalization for more tests at a children's hospital. After one week of tests, their findings were that our daughter had some form of cerebral palsy.

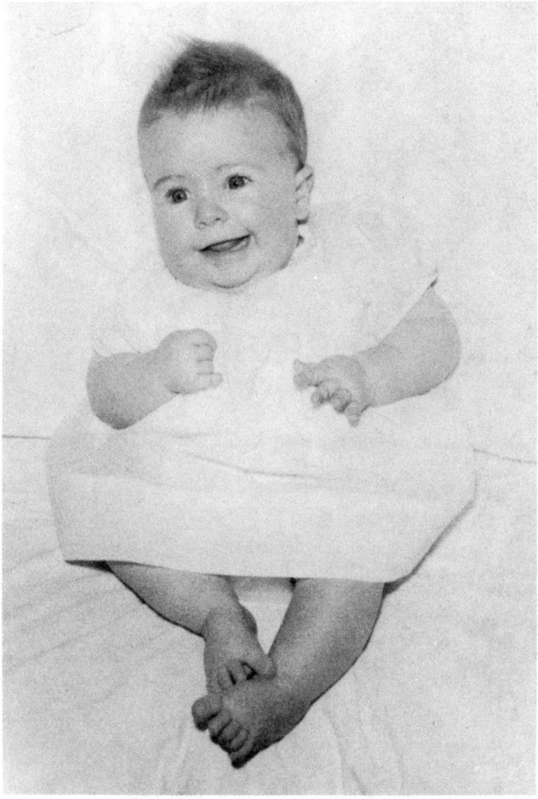

FIGURE 5.2. M at 6 months.

After her discharge to home care, M continued to require dropper feedings. Other than the prolonged feeding times, she was a quiet, placid infant who required little attention.

One of the most devastating medical contacts we had was when a consultant met with us at 4:30 on Christmas Eve, 1957. We appreciated his seeing us prior to the holidays. Then he said, "Your daughter would probably not survive six months because she could not overcome a simple cold." We were in tears. The timing and his lack of finesse were devastating. Of course, every day of those first six months was worrisome.

M's father, who traveled extensively for business, stayed in constant phone communication with his wife and said that the entire family prayed for a miracle. He spoke gratefully that they all survived the first 6 months and felt that the experience allowed him to be more willing to accept his daughter's problems because he had expected her to die in infancy.

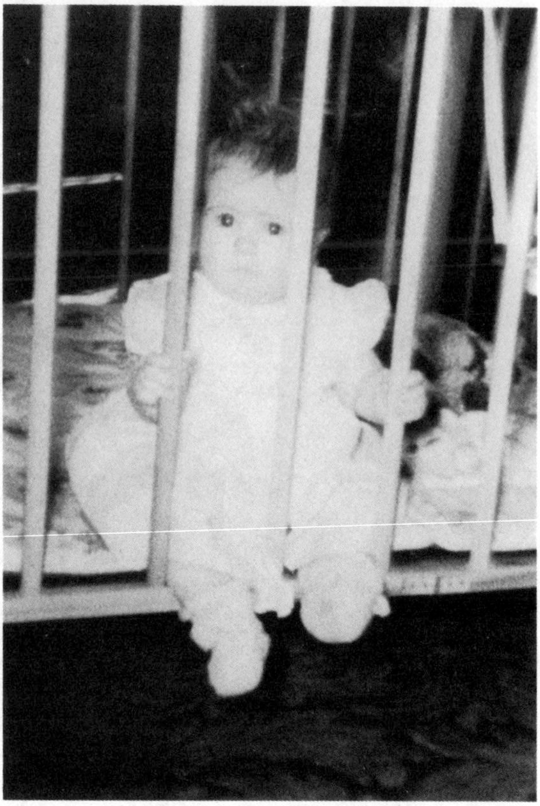

FIGURE 5.3. M at 9 months.

Yet every day that she survived was a boost to our morale. Somehow [after the 6 months had elapsed] whenever our daughter behaved abnormally, we would go back to that December day. . . . that always allowed me [her father] to be more understanding of her.

By 6 months of age her ability to take oral feedings and her appetite improved considerably, and from that time she demonstrated the voracious appetite consistent with PWS. No major illnesses were identified during her infancy and toddlerhood.

M's developmental milestones were delayed. She sat at 8 months, rolled over and stood with assistance at 10 months; she pulled herself up at 11 months but did not walk until 3 years of age. Speech began at age 2. Although she was reported to have been toilet trained at 3 years, nocturnal enuresis and occasional daytime "accidents" continued until age 8.

From a behavioral perspective, M's parents were disturbed at her weight gain in childhood despite their efforts to limit her food intake at meals.

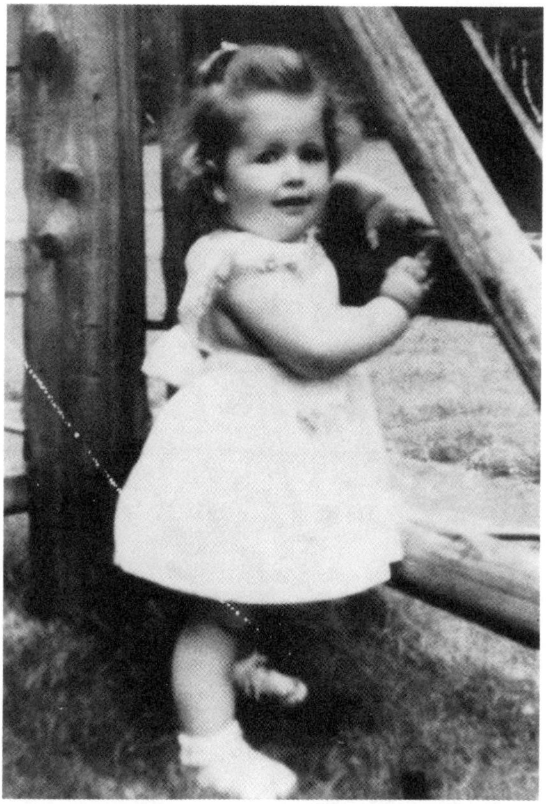

FIGURE 5.4. M at 22 months.

Initially, they thought the weight gain was due to her sedentary habits. They finally realized that she was stealing food. Her memory capacity was considered quite remarkable by her parents since she could remember people whom she had rarely seen and was able to identify the times and circumstances when she had seen them 2 or 3 years afterward.

Entering the educational system was difficult. M was teased, suffered from name-calling, and lacked friends. Her mother reported that she was pushed around frequently and sustained a fractured wrist when knocked down by another student. Her teachers repeatedly called on her parents to exercise more control over M because she continued to steal the lunches of other students and took leftover food from the garbage cans at school.

M's psychometric testing revealed that she had a verbal IQ of 102, a performance IQ of 95, and a full scale of 99. She was in the 47th percentile for reading and 42nd for spelling, but only the 18th for arithmetic. Her IQ scores were considerably higher than those of most individuals known to have PWS. However, her math skills were typical for affected individuals;

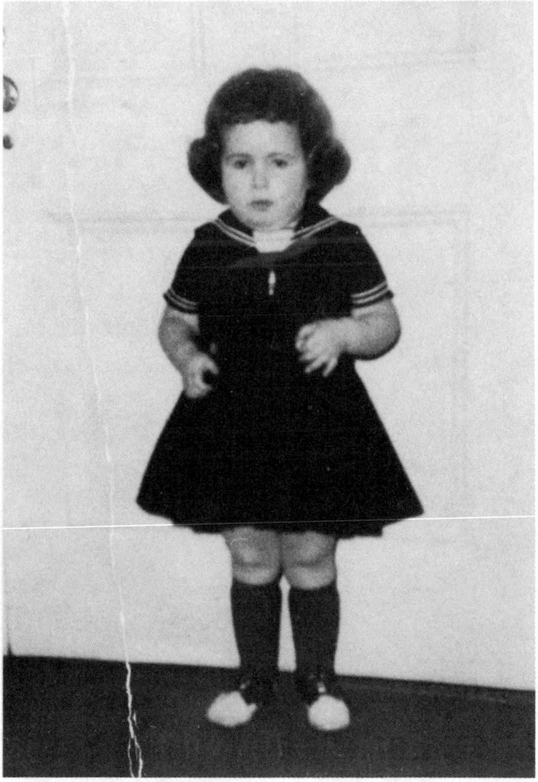

FIGURE 5.5. M at 5 years.

she maintained below-average scholastic performance throughout her childhood.

M's parents report that she was under extreme pressure to keep up with the other students when she entered high school. Furthermore, it was at this time of her life that she began to steal money, beginning with a few coins here and there but soon progressing to taking considerable sums from her parents and their house guests. She made no effort to hide the money she took.

At 17 years of age, while a sophomore in high school, M's emotional outbursts necessitated admittance to a psychiatric unit. After 10 days, the attending physician recommended that she be transferred to a psychiatric hospital for an extended stay. During the time M remained in this mental facility, her behavior deteriorated further. According to her parents," . . . she became very angry at us and learned at lot of bad habits."

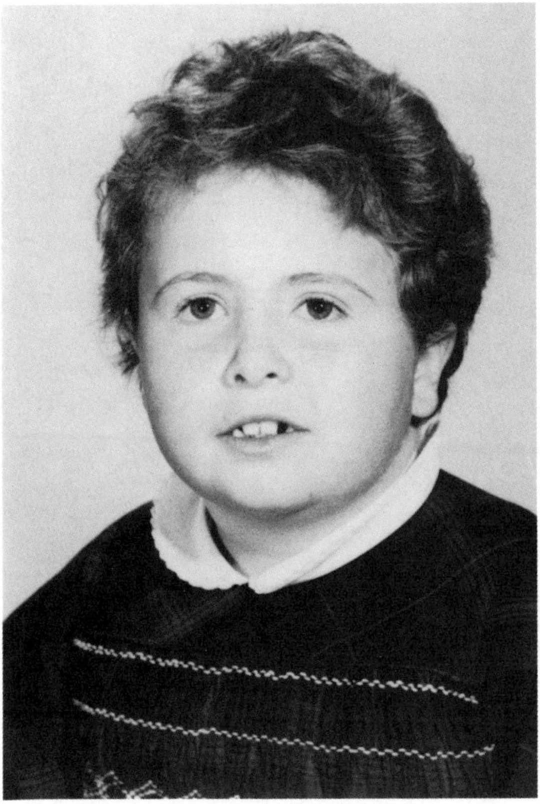

FIGURE 5.6. M at 8 years.

Four months later, M was transferred to a private school for troubled children. Interestingly enough, another student at the same private school had been diagnosed as having PWS. However, despite the marked similarities in their behavior and clinical appearance, M's parents were assured by the school's doctor and psychologist that she did not have PWS because her IQ was normal, she was a "good student," and she had no speech impairment.

During the time M lived in the private school, she was evaluated by an endocrinologist, who noted her hypogonadism, mild scoliosis, short stature, small hands and feet, obesity, amblyopia, and myopia. He initially entertained diagnoses of Froehlich syndrome, pseudohypoparathyroidism, pseudopseudohypoparathyroidism, and Turner syndrome, but PWS was not mentioned in the differential diagnosis.

After nearly 3½ years, M left the private school and went home to live with her parents.

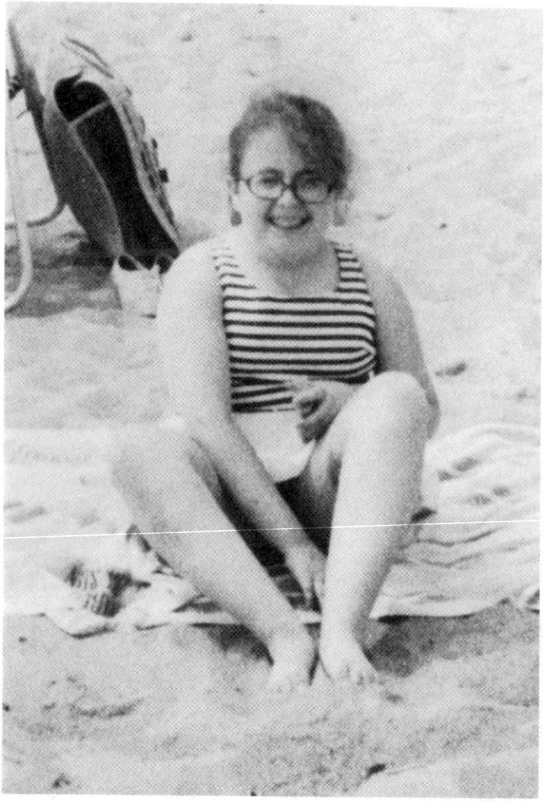

FIGURE 5.7. M at 12 years.

Our daughter received an equivalent to a high school diploma at this private school. She had far fewer tantrums and they were not as severe. Food was was still a problem, although at school she put on very little weight. She enjoyed the setting and the personnel and we felt she had progressed to the point where vocational training should be pursued.

Once home, M was placed under the care of a psychologist who diagnosed her obesity as "primarily psychiatric in nature." He further characterized her behavior as typical for a 7- or 8-year-old child (at this time, she was 22 years of age). He was impressed with her ability to crochet, hook rugs, and assemble jigsaw puzzles. He also commented on her "explosive emotional behavior" and her "habit of eating until she fell asleep." The psychologist suggested M start in a vocational program. She was referred to the state Division of Vocational Rehabilitation, which in turn referred her to Goodwill Industries for job training and placement.

Unfortunately, and unbelievably, M's vocational training started in a sheltered workshop as a cashier in the cafeteria. At the same time, she

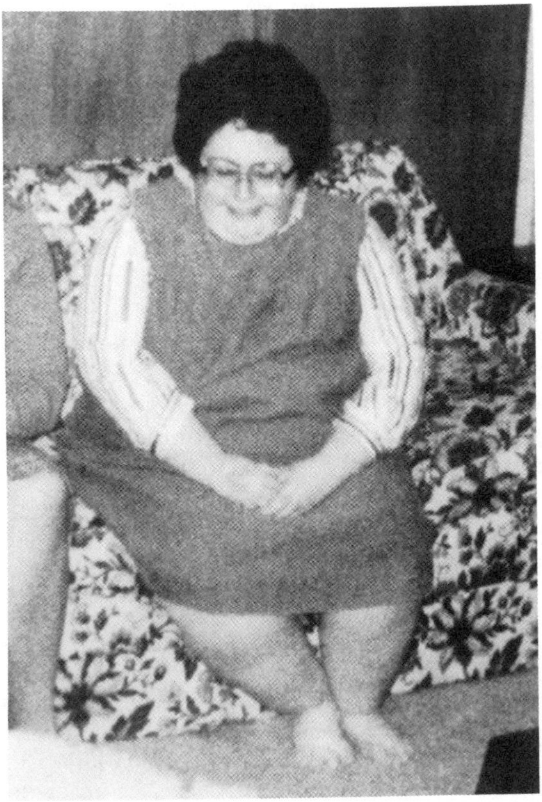

FIGURE 5.8. M at 24 years.

entered an independent living program at the sheltered workshop site. In this environment (unstructured and with food available), she gained weight rapidly. It reached an astronomical 131 kg (288 lbs); she could hardly walk and could not manage her personal hygiene. Very soon, she was denied employment "because of the severity of her psychophysiological problem."

M remained at home, but the conflicts that she had with her parents became intolerable. Her food-related tantrums continued to the point where her parents begged a psychiatric hospital to admit her. Her physical health was in jeopardy, her mental state fragile, and her parents exhausted. They knew she needed a well-structured facility where she could be cared for appropriately.

In March of 1980, M required admission to a small community hospital because of breathing difficulties. Her final diagnosis during this hospitalization was "Pickwickian syndrome."

In 1982, M was admitted to a home for the emotionally disturbed with a weight of 94.4 kg (207 lbs) and a height of 133 cm (52.5 in). During the third year of her stay in this facility, a psychologist noted her skin-picking behavior. He recalled that a patient known to have PWS whom he had seen at another hospital had the same habit. He recommended a genetic evaluation at a center experienced with PWS. M's diagnosis was confirmed on the basis of her history, previously mentioned physical findings, her highly arched palate, narrow forehead, almond-shaped eyes, and hands and feet that were below the third percentile in size. Cytogenetic analysis revealed a deletion on the 15th chromosome. Confirmation of the diagnosis of PWS was an emotionally charged event. The parents cried and were thankful that after nearly 26 years they "were not to blame."

Following the definitive diagnosis, M's parents quoted their daughter as saying "I am glad to know what I have. I will be glad to volunteer to go through any tests. I don't want another child to go through what I had to." Later in a newspaper story about the plight of individuals with PWS, she told a reporter that she wanted everyone to know about the condition.

In 1986, M achieved a long-awaited goal. She was transferred to a group home established exclusively for PWS adults through years of unrelenting effort and persistance by members of the state chapter of the national parent support group, the Prader-Willi Syndrome Association.

Four years later, 130 pounds less and over $600,000 in medical costs, our daughter entered a PWS group home. [Over the years] we were misguided and misinformed, which led to much confusion as to how to handle her, how to approach her eating habits, how to cope with her temper tantrums. We had many family problems, many debates, and heated discussions. The situation created more disorganized family conditions. Our other three children, who are older than M, would get upset due to our lack of control of her. Our being a very close and religious family had, no doubt, pulled us through some of these difficult periods. Our financial cost, due to her not being diagnosed, is close to $1 million. Fortunately, most of this was paid by personal medical insurance, but we as parents also paid a large amount. Our health suffered. We had high blood pressure, were depressed, nervous, upset, confused, disappointed, and just plain angry. All three of us struggled. . . but all three of us never gave up.

Summary

It is clear from this case history that delay in diagnosis caused many years of physical and emotional suffering for both M and her family. Moreover, it is evident that one of the issues that complicated the diagnosis in her case is her high level of cognition as indicated by her high IQ score and verbal skills. However, the medical community and allied health professionals can benefit by becoming familiar with the characteristics of PWS when confronted with the signs and symptoms suggestive of this disorder. Certainly, earlier identification is now a realistic expectation; it can lead to longer and more healthy lives for affected individuals and more stable family life for all concerned.

Reference

Prader, A., Labhart, A., & Willi, H. (1956). Ein Syndrom von Adipositas, Kleinwuchs, Kryptorchismus und Oligophrenie nach Mytonicartigem Zustand in Neugeborenalter. *Schweizerische Medizinische Wochenschrift*, *86*, 1260–1261.

6
A Team Approach to Case Management

LOUISE R. GREENSWAG and RANDELL C. ALEXANDER

Meeting the needs of children with Prader-Willi syndrome (PWS) and their families requires that the knowledge and skills of professionals who serve them be delivered through an efficient interdisciplinary system. The term "interdisciplinary" implies that health, educational, and social service specialists share information and work together. Ideally, this approach encourages collaborative development of appropriate assessment and management strategies.

Holm and McCartin (1978) pointed out that successful interdisciplinary teams believe in a comprehensive approach to serving the developmentally disabled and that team effectiveness depends on participation by competent professionals who have the ability to interrelate. Philosophically, this means that the members of such a team are capable of developing holistic interventions that optimize maximum growth based on a developmental model that targets normalization in the least restrictive setting. The developmental process model proposes that where services are appropriate, developmentally disabled individuals can continue to "learn and grow" throughout their lives. Normalization, in its broadest sense, refers to providing the handicapped with opportunities to live and work in environments as close as possible to typical community patterns (Wolfensberger, 1972). The concept of "least restrictive environment" supports the rights of the developmentally disabled to live as independently as possible, limited only by their individual capacity to make decisions.

The implementation of a team approach as a strategy for delivery of services to the developmentally disabled has been recognized by the public sector for over 25 years. Federal funding (Education for AU Handicapped Children Act of 1975 [PL 94–142]; Mental Health Facilities and Community Mental Health Centers Construction Act of 1963 [PL 88–164]) provided for interdisciplinary training, research, and delivery of services. As a result, programs currently exist that implement integrated services to the developmentally disabled far beyond the capacities of any one health/education discipline. In 1978, the federal government clearly defined "developmental disability" and established eligibility criteria (Developmental

Disabilities Act Amendments of 1978 [PL 95–602]). Clearly, by virtue of impaired cognition and the presence of limited functional capacity, individuals with PWS fall well within the guidelines established by law and are eligible for a broad range of services. The rights of this population to receive public funding and services are discussed in depth in Chapters 19 and 20.

Having discussed team intervention in general terms and acknowledged that there is formalized support of this service delivery model, the question arises, "Is a team approach appropriate in management of PWS?" Our answer to this query is a firm "Yes."

A team approach is sensible simply because PWS presents a constellation of symptoms that require the expertise of many disciplines for management. Diagnostic, medical, nursing, and nutritional issues predominate early in life, and all but the diagnosis remain constant concerns throughout life. Language, education, activity therapies, and social services become greater issues as the child grows older. Behavioral and social problems become a major source of family stress; vocational guidance and appropriate living arrangements become the cornerstone of adaptation to adulthood.

In more specific terms, concepts identified previously (e.g., developmental processes, normalization, and least restrictive environment) offer the prospect for team members to think "futuristically." Assessment and case management based on developmental stages are critical since, as with other mental retardation conditions, the discrepancy between chronological and mental age in individuals with PWS becomes more pronounced over time. Certainly, the acquisition of social skills becomes increasingly difficult where the cognitive capacity to make decisions is diminished and the maturity to set goals is rarely achieved.

When applying the definition of normalization to this population it becomes apparent to anyone familiar with PWS that to "normalize" life for many individuals means encouraging a move away from a dependent and relatively restricted life in the family unit into a community living facility where opportunities exist for peer interaction and development of social and work skills.

For affected individuals, the concept of "least restrictive environment" has a purposefully narrow framework. Realistically, for the individual with PWS, the term "least restrictive" means constant supervision to prevent death from overeating.

Each of the succeeding chapters in Part III contains sharply defined specialist procedures that, at the same time, represent the integral components of a comprehensive, interdisciplinary team approach to case management.

References

Developmental Disabilities Act Amendments of 1978, 42 U.S.C. §6000–6081 (1982).

Education for All Handicapped Children Act of 1975, 20 U.S.C. §1400–1420 (1982).

Holm, V., & McCartin, R. (1978). Interdisciplinary child development team: Team issues and training in interdisciplinariness. In K.E. Allen, V. Holm, & R. Schiefelbusch, (Eds.), *Early interventions—A team approach* (pp. 99–102). Baltimore: University Park Press.

Mental Retardation Facilities and Community Mental Health Centers Construction Act of 1963, 42 U.S.C. §6000–6081 (1982).

Wolfensberger, W. (1972). *Normalization: the principle of normalization in human services.* Toronto: National Institute on Mental Retardation.

7
Medical and Nursing Interventions

RANDELL C. ALEXANDER and LOUISE R. GREENSWAG

Historically, physicians have been perceived as diagnosing, treating, and if possible, curing disease states. Nurses have been viewed as providing holistic case assessment, care, and patient education. However, in recent years there has been a blurring of traditional physician/nurse roles in response to the need for ongoing interventions for individuals with chronic disabling conditions. Nowhere is the importance of such a physician/nurse primary health team effort more apparent than in the delivery of care to individuals with Prader-Willi syndrome (PWS).

This chapter indicates the respective responsibilities of the physician and nurse, and focuses on the potential for collaborative efforts in case management that ensure optimal growth and development for this population.

Medical Intervention

The initial problem for the physician in the primary health care team is the establishment of a correct diagnosis of PWS. Zellweger (Chapter 2) clearly points out indications for differential diagnosis. Frequently a referral will be made to a genetics (or sometimes endocrinology) clinic before a firm diagnosis is made. Typically, a single symptom (e.g., hypotonia, hypogenitalism, developmental delay, or gross obesity) is the initial rationale for seeking care from a primary physician or pediatric nurse-practitioner. All too frequently the syndrome itself goes unrecognized for some time. However, once the proper diagnosis has been made it is critical that the presenting symptoms be understood both within the framework of PWS and as individual problems requiring appropriate management.

The age at which the individual is diagnosed varies considerably. Awareness of the syndrome's characteristics and its traditional delineations as a two-phase clinical course is important (Table 7.1). Although this two-phase conceptualization is a convenient clinical guide, it should be kept in mind that not all characteristics of PWS show a two-phase progression. For example, changes do not occur in the level of cognitive impairments or structural features.

TABLE 7.1. The two clinical phases of Prader-Willi syndrome.[a]

Phase I	Moderate to severe neonatal hypotonia
	Poor suck
	Difficult feeding
	Hypogonadism
	Marked delay in motor milestones
Phase II	Much less hypotonia
	Short stature
	Hyperphagia
	Increasing obesity
	Labile emotions, stubbornness
	Cognitive limitations

[a] See Chapter 2 for additional details.

Medical management of PWS requires a clear understanding of the characteristic signs and symptoms. The developmental course of specific signs and symptoms should be considered in order to better assess their impact on the child and family. This also aids the physician in determining an appropriate course of treatment and in evaluating the prognosis for specific symptoms. Many of the characteristics of PWS, their individual developmental courses, and current management concepts are indicated in Table 7.2.

Developmental Stages of PWS

Although there may be substantial variations, most individuals follow a characteristic developmental course. This perception could change if large numbers of atypical cases are identified in the future. These developmental stages can be divided into: fetal, neonatal/infancy, early childhood, late childhood, adolescence, and adulthood periods. Child development within this conceptual framework represents a "cross-section" of the changing and interwoven strands of development in much the same way that knowledge of a cross-section of the spinal cord complements the knowledge gained about individual longitudinal neural pathways. In practice, the physician uses both strategies to provide anticipatory guidance and plan for future management.

Fetal

Mothers have frequently reported a decrease in fetal activity when compared to other pregnancies. This may reflect the onset of both hypotonia and decreased activity levels. The index of suspicion for PWS is quite low at this time and it is only through incidental amniotic or chorionic chromosomal analysis that the 15th chromosome deletion (noted in 60% of the

TABLE 7.2. Characteristics, developmental sequence, and intervention for Prader-Willi syndrome.

Characteristic	Developmental sequence	Intervention
A Structural		
1. Facial: almond-shaped eyes, triangular-shaped mouth ("fish-mouth"), narrow bifrontal diameter.	Present at birth but more noticeable by several years of age. Nonprogressive and persistent.	Cosmetic surgery not necessary since appearance is not distinctively "abnormal"; contraindicated because of diminished intellectual understanding.
2. Small hands and feet.	Most noticeable by 3–4 years of age. Persists, but nonprogressive.	No problems finding shoes or gloves. No orthopedic shoes.
3. Central fat distribution. Obesity most prominent around stomach, hips, and thighs.	Begins at 18–36 months with noticeable hyperphagia. Prominence depends partly on weight control.	Diet (see Chapter 9). To a mild extent, will have this abnormal fat distribution even when weight is "normalized."
4. Hypogonadism. Males: cryptorchidism; small testes; short, underdeveloped penis and scrotum. Females: flattened, hypoplastic labia.	Present at birth. Nonprogressive but a more marked contrast with normal individuals during teenage years and beyond.	(See Chapter 3.)
5. Short stature. Average adult height: males, 5′0″; females, 4′8″.	May be slightly smaller at birth but more noticeable during elementary school age. Very noticeable during teen years and beyond (no potential "growth spurt").	(See Chapter 3 and Appendix A.)
6. Eye problems. More likely to have myopia, strabismus	May present at any age. Course similar to that of normal peer group.	Index of suspicion. Should have preschool vision screening and periodic school screening. Surveillance.
B. Regulatory/Functional		
1. Hypotonia.	Decreased fetal movements. May be severe at birth. Often low Apgars. Poor suck. May need gavage feeding in first 1–2 months. Failure to thrive concern diminishes with age; feeding improves by 12–18 months. Hypotonia persists to mild degree even as adult.	Relationship to possible articulation problems, scoliosis, and respiratory problems likely. Child abuse may be alleged in early failure to thrive stage. May lead to misdiagnosis in infancy (e.g., muscular dystrophy), but obesity and lessening of the hypotonia with age rules out neuromuscular diagnoses. Symptomatic treatment.

TABLE 7.2. *Continued.*

Characteristic	Developmental sequence	Intervention
2. Decreased motor skills. Probably combination of hypotonia, decreased cognitive abilities, and deficits in motor planning.	Delayed motor milestones even for mental age. May not walk until 2–3 years. Gross motor skills tend to be more affected than fine motor skills. Tend to "catch up" somewhat during elementary school years, but always remain behind the norm.	Special physical education adaptations useful. Anticipatory guidance for safety issues where motor skills are a factor, such as bicycle riding (see Chapter 13).
3. Thermoregulation. Poor temperature control, usually hypothermia. May have cool hands or feet at times. Poor ability to compensate for heat stress reported anecdotally.	Most troublesome in neonatal period. Can prove fatal. Less problematic after several months of age; can have high fevers when ill.	Symptomatic treatment. Isolette to maintain temperature is common for newborns.
4. Hyperphagia. The feeding drive often appears insatiable; affected individuals describe it as "hunger."	Not clinically evident for first 18–24 months (possibly masked by the increased hypotonia at earlier ages?). Develops during 18–36 months of age in most cases. Persistent, but nonprogressive beyond midchildhood.	Diet and external behavioral controls (see Chapters 9 and 10). Weigh weekly (school nurse may help with this). Medications to control appetite have not proven useful to date. Gastric bypass has been successful in some severe cases. Watch for ingestions (poisoning). Locks on refrigerator and cupboards may be necessary. Keep child from eating garbage, dog food, and other atypical "foods." Stealing food may occur and sometimes leads to legal problems (see Chapter 10).
5. Higher vomiting threshold (less likely to vomit). May not vomit when ill or overeating at the point when others will. However, at least 36% vomit at some point in their life.	May be somewhat more likely to spit up as an infant than later. About two thirds of those who vomit first do so under 6 years of age.	Ipecac works about 50% of the time—use with caution and watch for toxicity. Consider gastric lavage as an alternative.
6. Rumination (at least 10–17%)	No age relationship known.	Behavior modification. Overly strict weight control may induce or aggravate rumination.

TABLE 7.2. *Continued.*

Characteristic	Developmental sequence	Intervention
7. Hypoactivity. Physical activities are slow and without wasted efforts.	Begins with decreased fetal activity. Decreased activity at all ages.	Calories not consumed as quickly. Diet must contain fewer calories (see Chapter 9). Exercise programs less effective for weight regulation and cardiovascular fitness (see Chapter 13).
8. Decreased sex hormones. No pubertal growth spurt. Sterility. Little or no menstrual flow in female teens and adults. (About Tanner Stage 2.)	Decreased at all ages, although most noticeable difference when teenage and older (essentially no pubertal development).	Affects psychosexuality. Exogenous hormones may affect activity level and/or behavior in unpredictable ways (see Chapters 3 and 17).
9. Sleep/respiratory disturbances. May fall asleep in classrooms (especially in afternoons). Sleep apnea, Pickwickian-like syndrome, and respiratory failure have been observed where weight is not controlled. Snoring may have multiple etiologies (sleep apnea, hypotonia).	Daytime sleepiness more apparent in school-age patient. May increase with age and/or weight.	Weight control may help. Small changes may lead to large effects on day and night disturbances (more so than expected on a "Pickwickian" basis alone.) Awareness of sleepiness as a feature of the syndrome is very helpful. Watch for scoliosis leading to respiratory compromise. Sleep apnea testing and tracheostomy may be warranted in extreme cases.
10. Decreased pain responsiveness. Not known if this is a decreased sensitivity to pain, a decreased affect toward pain, or some combination of both.	Apparently constant throughout life.	Expect more minor accidental injuries (bruises, burns), especially given the poorer gross motor skills. In light of decreased cognitive skills, safety issues must be discussed with the care providers.
11. Skin picking. Very frequent; arms, hands, and feet most commonly affected. Stimulus unknown, but decreased pain responsiveness may be an associated factor.	Rare before 5 years of age. Tends to persist at same frequency in a given individual.	Self-injurious behavior modification programs can help. Cut fingernails short and often. Watch for secondary infections.
C. Cognitive		
1. Decreased intelligence. Most often mildly retarded. Parental intelligence may have at least some effect on the levels.	Nonprogressive, but may be difficult to assess at early ages when confounded with poor motor skills and hypotonia.	Appropriate educational programming (see Chapters 10 and 11). Early referral helpful.

TABLE 7.2. *Continued.*

Characteristic	Developmental sequence	Intervention
2. Speech/language deficits. Controversial: language problems may be a symptom of decreased intelligence. Speech may be affected by structural and/or hypotonic abnormalities.	Speech delays typical because of decreased intelligence. Speech/language problems are apparent at early ages. Variable causes.	Appropriate speech/language programming (see Chapter 12). Early referral helpful.
3. Behavior problems. Stubbornness, emotional lability, food-seeking–related behaviors. Often major family stressor.	Unusual before 3 years of age. Tend to intensify over time and then plateau as an adult. Considerable individual variations.	Coupled with the constant food seeking, problem behaviors frequently are the reasons teenagers and young adults go to a supervisored group home. Anticipatory guidance regarding residental care. However, behaviors seldom cease entirely and goals must be modest. Psychology referral (see Chapter 10).
D. Probable secondary effects		
1. Poor dentition. Cause frequently controversial; many believe there are enamel deficits, xerostomia, differences or decreases in saliva. Decreased IQ, poor eating habits, possible rumination, and poor brushing secondary to poor motor skills may contribute.	Multiple caries during early early childhood. Progressive.	Floride supplementation as indicated. Watch for rumination. Early referral to dentist (see Chapter 8).
2. Scoliosis. Occasional. Probably a result of hypotonia.	Cases seen in late childhood but most as teenagers. Follows typical pattern and course of idiopathic scoliosis in normals.	Yearly exam from 10 years of age until skeletal growth stops (often early 20s). X-rays if significantly obese or any question. Orthopedic referral if detected.
3. Undescended testes universal in males. Likely due to lack of neonatal/postnatal sex hormones.	Present at birth. Do not spontaneously descend.	Surgery at 4–5 years of age may be considered. No known cases of cancer with untreated cases (see Chapter 3).
4. Diabetes (Type II). Rare; undoubtably due to obesity.	With significant obesity. More likely at older ages, as with normal persons.	Urine screening for all patients beyond 5 years old on a yearly basis. Weight management. Standard diabetic treatment.

TABLE 7.2. *Continued.*

Characteristic	Developmental sequence	Intervention
5. Heart disease/ respiratory compromise. Occasional. Usually because of morbid obesity, although severe scoliosis may contribute.	In the past, teenagers and young adults died of this. Still more frequent in these ages and beyond.	Weight management. Orthopedic management if appropriate. Symptomatic treatment.
6. Increased bruisability. Often pale skin, poor gross motor skills, decreased IQ, poor muscular fitness, and decreased pain reponsiveness may all contribute. Coagulation studies are normal. Bruisability most likely at extreme end of "normal range," not pathological.	Seen with the ambulatory child. May increase when placed in unstructured environments.	Heals normally. Anticipatory guidance regarding safety issues. May complicate any child abuse concerns.

cases) might be detected. Should a fetus have this chromosomal deletion, there is no known treatment, but genetics counseling is advised (see Chapter 4). It has been estimated that 10–40% of PWS births are breech, which may indicate decreased motor and cognitive abilities. Polyhydramnios is often present. Although the length of gestation is normal, birth weight may be slightly less than average. The birth process itself is relatively unremarkable, with no known reports of increased fetal distress or delivery complications.

Neonatal/Infancy

Thermoregulation may be a significant problem in the newborn with PWS, and use of an isolette is frequently necessary. The neonate usually manifests moderate to severe hypotonia at birth, and Apgar scores may be low. Initially, poor suck, "floppiness," and consequent failure to thrive may suggest a variety of diagnostic possibilities. Gavage feeding may be necessary for the first several weeks of life. Gradually the infant develops sufficient muscle tone to suck efficiently, although increased feeding time and limited consumption may necessitate smaller and more frequent feeds. Occasionally, child abuse (failure to thrive) has been inappropriately considered. However, recognition of the hypotonia, which affects the infant's feeding and may continue into the second 6 months of life, usually alters concerns about abuse. Unfortunately given the feeding difficulties, it is possible that a care provider might neglect to feed a child adequately. Confounding organic complications like gastroesophageal reflux and iron-deficiency anemia should always be considered and appropriate therapeutic interventions made. Proper nutrition and specific feeding methods should be reviewed with the care providers at each visit. Regular immunization should begin, but no special indication exists for influenza or pneumococcal vaccines during infancy or childhood.

Early Childhood

By 18 months to 3 years of age feeding difficulties have been replaced by hyperphagia. Initially this increased appetite is welcomed by parents, physicians, and nurses, who vividly recall earlier feeding problems. This sense of relief may delay the recognition of the emerging problem of obesity. The combination of short stature, hyperphagia, and obesity frequently results in a referral to medical specialists, who then make the diagnosis of PWS. As the hypotonia diminishes to milder levels, children with PWS increase their motor skills and learn to walk between 2 and 3 years of age. During this time consideration may be given to surgery for undescended testes in preschool males. Dental problems often begin to appear as well; they may be related to poor brushing skills (due to decreased cognition and fine motor skills), intrinsic defects, type and amount of consumed food, and, in some instances, rumination.

Early educational planning is important in order to address cognitive delays, motor delays, and possible speech/language difficulties. Most children begin to display stubbornness and other behavior problems by 3–5 years of age. Anticipatory guidance should include education of the care provider about potential obesity and behavioral issues, and appropriate referrals for behavior management and nutritional counseling are often made. Marked dietary restrictions necessitate supplemental vitamins and iron; cases of iron-deficiency anemia have been seen in balanced diets that are very limited in quantity.

Late Childhood

Without careful management, there will be excessive weight gain. Some children get up at night to forage for food, and with their increased motor skills they may be able to climb or defeat simple attempts at restricting access to food. Close observation sometimes works, but during this age many families resort to chains or locks on refrigerator and cupboards.

Behaviors such as stubbornness and temper outbursts usually intensify. School becomes a prime focus of activity in late childhood, and appropriate classroom placement (usually special education) may be confounded by problems such as verbal or physical aggressiveness. Often children with PWS are given food by their peers or find some other way to obtain it. Such behavior can alter social settings such as the school lunchroom. Short stature, poor gross motor skills, obesity, and mental retardation can result in teasing by other children, causing further isolation and stigmatization of the PWS child. Skin picking and falling asleep in the classroom may be noted.

Anticipatory guidance should include appropriate counseling of parents and school personnel. The school psychologist frequently will need to coordinate behavior management at school and home.

Obese children should have periodic urinalyses to check for proteinuria or glucosuria, and blood pressure should be monitored. Weekly weight checks are appropriate, and any significant deviations should be reported. Weight-for-height curves are particularly useful, and successful weight management results in a child within at least the upper-normal percentiles.

The effects of the child with PWS on general family functioning, particularly in regard to other siblings, may be detrimental, and family counseling or support groups can avert more serious difficulties.

Adolescence

Unlike their peers, teenagers with PWS do not have a "growth spurt" or surge of sex hormones. Without exogenous hormones, males and females will usually not progress beyond pubic hair development consistent with a Tanner Stage of 2. Females may have occasional spotting but true menstrual periods do not occur. The increasingly obvious physical differences between PWS and normal teenagers frequently causes emotional distress. For boys, testosterone supplementation may reduce the appearance of immature genitalia, although problems with short stature remain. The lack of reproductive capacity for both sexes is discussed in Chapter 3. Although this simplifies concerns about birth control for this mentally handicapped population, sexual education is still important. Management should be developmentally appropriate, with the focus on interpersonal skills and relationships (see Chapter 16) and incorporation of parental values (see Chapter 17). School problems (academic and sometimes behavioral) also continue (Chapters 10 and 11). Vocational training is important (Chapter 14). As teenagers become physically larger, they may intimidate other family members or prove more difficult to control, and many parents begin to recognize the need for out-of-home placement. Anticipatory guidance should emphasize the need for care providers to make legal preparations (wills and assignment of guardianship prior to the age of majority). Attention to secondary effects of obesity should continue. Scoliosis may be observed, and usually follows the same course of "idiopathic" scoliosis seen in normal teenagers. However, there may be a somewhat longer period of risk because skeletal maturation may not be complete until the early to mid-20s.

Adulthood

Although an increasing proportion of the PWS population is reaching adulthood, information about this age range is only beginning to accumulate. In the past, complications of morbid obesity (e.g., diabetes, cardiac or respiratory complications) doomed nearly all victims to die young. Increased awareness of the syndrome and more aggressive attention to its management have significantly reduced the likelihood of early death. It is no longer inevitable that adults with PWS will be obese. However, skin picking, behavior problems, and food seeking persist. Sometimes in the search for food, the adult with PWS may steal money or, more likely, food. To avoid jail, it is necessary to explain to proper authorities the "addictive" nature of the condition, the individual's cognitive limitations, and the undesirability of prison as an effort to remediate these behaviors. Greenswag (1984, 1987), in a survey of 232 individuals with PWS ages 16 years and beyond, found that those few who attempted to live independently were significantly more obese than those living in a more restrictive setting. In most instances the persistence of food-seeking behaviors, the need for peer stimulation and work, and the stress to the family result in a residential or out-of-home placement. Just as with any other developmentally disabled adult, psychosexual adaptation, interpersonal relationships, and vocational training are important. Meaningful opportunities to contribute to society should be encouraged.

The elderly adult with PWS is not well understood. The impact of the lifelong fight with obesity, the hypotonia, the difficulty in attaining cardiovascular fitness, and the natural history of the syndrome itself will become more apparent in the decades to come. Although one woman with PWS lived to be 65, life expectancy probably is shorter than normal, as is true for other cognitively limited populations. It is possible that specific medical problems may emerge in the elderly PWS population.

Nursing Interventions

As professionals who "care for" and "teach," nurses incorporate concepts of physical and emotional growth and development, family, environment, and society into intervention strategies. Whether in a tertiary, regional, community, or school setting, pediatric nurse-practitioners (PNPs), school nurses, or public health nurses, with their wholistic perspective on health care, are in an optimum position to aid in coordination of case management to ensure that children with PWS are appropriately served. They may also function as a resource for information and support.

Once the initial diagnosis of PWS is made, attention should be directed not only to current symptomatology and medical treatment, but also to the development and maintenance of the optimum health of the affected child and enhancement of family stability. The nursing interventions that best meet these goals are based on:

1. Documentation of the child's physical and behavioral condition.
2. Recognition that the developmental processes of affected children differ significantly from the majority of children.
3. Ongoing assessment of health needs throughout the life span.

4. A clear understanding of how the physical and mental dimensions of PWS impact on the family system.
5. Evaluation of family dynamics and potential problem areas.
6. An awareness that in addition to alterations in life-style, problems with social interactions, spousal difficulties, and indifferent public attitudes, the presence of PWS imposes considerable financial burdens.
7. An awareness that many disciplines are involved in providing care, that confusion about delivery of services can occur, and that the nurse can help "make sense of it all."

Strategies for nursing interventions begin with a compilation of a nursing history. This process, initiated during the first visit, includes a review of the diagnosis of PWS and a baseline health assessment that takes into account growth parameters, a physical examination, and a review of laboratory studies. Observation should incorporate photographing the child; this provides a permanent record that is useful in future consultation and retrospective review. Next, data collection should focus on feeding problems and interventions, since weight/height information is critical to nutritional planning. Personal hygiene, grooming, skin care, and any indications of self-mutilation (skin picking or hair pulling) should be noted along with assessment of the child's capacity for self-health care. Careful evaluation of adaptive function is necessary since emotional lability, inappropriate behaviors, alterations in thought processes, and poor social skills are requently observed and provide important background for psychological management.

Assessment of parent/care provider knowledge and perceptions about PWS is critical and requires that the nurse evaluate parenting skills. Safety factors in the living environment and the child's cognitive capacity for judgment in hazardous situations require ongoing review. Certainly, availability of food is a major issue that affects the child's health status and the family's ability to cope. Nursing diagnosis, interventions, and indications of positive outcomes to presenting problems are described in Table 7.3.

Counseling and anticipatory guidance for health-related matters are essential nursing interventions. This includes teaching about routine health issues such as feeding, toilet training, accident prevention (particularly since there is evidence that many children with PWS have decreased response to pain), personal hygiene, skin care, and emotional lability. Teaching guidelines are listed in Table 7.4.

Family stability and parental coping mechanisms require sensitive management. Both the PNP, as a member of a tertiary clinic team, and the community nurse should look for opportunities to organize and facilitate parent discussion groups. Follow-up visits allow the nurse to collect interval health history information, monitor growth and development, assess current status, and detect any new health problems. Any family problems and/or new concerns should result in appropriate referral to medical and other allied disciplines.

TABLE 7.3. Nursing diagnosis, interventions, and indications of positive outcomes with individuals with Prader-Willi syndrome.[a]

Nursing diagnosis	Nursing interventions	Indications of positive outcomes
Alterations in nutrition: caloric intake greater than body requirements	Lock, refrigerators, freezers, and any cabinets where food is stored. Search for hidden food. Weigh daily until food goals are reached, then weekly. Supervise and observe frequently. Collaborate with dietary specialists.	Maintains reasonable weight.
Impairment of skin integrity, both actual and potential	Provide skin care. Encourage personal hygiene. Discourage self-mutilating behaviors.	Wounds heal completely. Good hygiene is maintained. Patient demonstrates decreased self-mutilation.
Self-concept disturbances in body image and self-esteem	Encourage self-care and responsibility. Offer positive reinforcement for successful behaviors.	Verbalizes improved feelings of self-worth. Demonstrates pride in self-care. Demonstrates ability to cope with limitations at highest level of functional ability. Family participates in socialization experiences. Patient participates in IQ- and age-related activities with others.
Alterations in thought processes.	Reduce confusing stimuli. Set limits. Provide a safe environment. Structure daily living activities.	Behaviors are appropriate for identified level of cognitive function. Remains free of harm to others, property, and self. Demonstrates social behavior and positive coping mechanisms related to intellectual and emotional age.

[a]From "Endocrine and Metabolic Systems" by Linda D. Anderson et al., 1986, in June M. Thompson et al., *Clinical Nursing* (pp. 908–909), St. Louis: C.V. Mosby. Adapted by permission.

The Physician/Nurse Primary Health Care Team

Delivery of primary health care to individuals with PWS is the responsibility of the physician and nurse team, and the multidimensional aspects of the syndrome call for a wholistic approach based on the collaborative efforts of both disciplines. Such a team, which integrates the expertise and skills of both professions, is concerned with achieving workable case management strategies. Examples of teamwork include comparing physical assessment data, exchanging historical information, discussing laboratory

TABLE 7.4. Teaching guidelines for nurses who care for individuals with Prader-Willi syndrome.[a]

1. Instruct care providers for newborns in methods of administering nasogastric feedings or use of other feeding aids.
2. Assist in teaching prescribed diet to care providers.
3. Stress importance of maintaining diet and reporting of signs and symptoms of exacerbation of weight.
4. Instruct care providers in maintaining skin integrity and daily hygiene.
5. Teach integration of exercise into overall care program.
6. Stress importance of the following and assist in planning for:
   a. continual supervision and observation.
   b. educational and environmental stimuli.
   c. setting of behavioral expectations and limits.
7. Inform care providers about and encourage use of support and counseling groups.
8. Ensure that care providers know about community resources available to assist with compliance.

[a]From "Endocrine and Metabolic Systems" by Linda D. Anderson et al., 1986, in June M. Thompson et al., *Clinical Nursing* (p. 922), St. Louis: C.V. Mosby. Adapted by permission.

results, and identifying the need for other interdisciplinary services. Whether focusing on a specific symptom over time or a set of symptoms at a given age, the physician and nurse can aid the patient and family by supplying information, guarding against fads or "cures" (e.g., eliminating sugar in the diet to control behavior), supporting other family members, and intervening at the early stages of specific symptoms. It should also be pointed out that the primary health care team process need not be limited to tertiary clinic settings. The physicians and nurses at the community level should plan to network their services.

In summary, the importance of a physician/nurse primary health team cannot be understated. Clearly the professional tasks of each discipline complement one another and collaboration provides the basis for optimal case management.

REFERENCES

Anderson, L., Bosmaas, C., Boykin, P., Choate, T., DiGiorgi, D., Drass, J., Hench, K., Long, J., McAtee, A., Robbins, P., Solomon, R., & Wells, M. (1986). Endocrine and metabolic systems. In J. Thompson, G. McFarland, J. Hirsch, S. Tucker, & A. Bowers, *Clinical Nursing* (pp. 823–942). St. Louis: The C.V. Mosby Co.

Greenswag, L.R. (1984). The adult with Prader-Willi syndrome: A descriptive investigation. Doctoral thesis, University of Iowa. (DA 056952, University Microfilms International, Ann Arbor, MI)

Greenswag, L. (1987). Adults with Prader-Willi syndrome: A survey of 232 cases. *Developmental Medicine and Child Neurology*, *29*, 145–152.

Part III The Interdisciplinary Process

No one who has ever worked with D had ever even seen a PW person before (school, activity center, workshop, doctors, no one). We have found that people, even professionals who work with retarded people, do not understand his drive for food. They think it is a matter of training or discipline or an emotional problem. He has never fit into any program, even for the retarded, because of this drive to get food. He is ingenious at getting it. And it causes all kinds of problems. It is all he really cares about. We wonder if all PW adults are like he is—or if many of his behavior problems have been caused because we didn't know what was the matter with him until he was 21. And even since then, professional people who have worked with him haven't really been able to accept and believe the extent of his handicap.

When J is feeling well, she is pleasant to get along with. But there is much of the time she is so listless. She doesn't want to do anything but eat and sleep. This makes life miserable not only for her but everyone around her.

If permitted, L would watch TV continually. She is difficult to motivate. Her disposition is usually good till someone tries to get her to change what she is doing or disagrees. Then she flares up.

At age 10 we were able to secure speech therapy. Until that time we were rebuffed due to his retardation. Today S can carry on a conversation quite well using many words.

Our main concern for P is that he will be able to function is a sheltered workshop. There is no one in the voc[ational] training program that understands that he can't be around food and that he will steal it.

8
Dental Manifestations and Management

ARTHUR J. NOWAK

Dentists and their staffs should be active members of all interdisciplinary health teams serving Prader-Willi syndrome (PWS). Interaction with the patient and family should begin no later than the time of the eruption of the first tooth. Only then can the benefits of a comprehensive dental health program be fully enjoyed and the effects of oral disease reduced or even eliminated. The major role of the dental team is to provide early preventive counseling, indicated treatment, and periodic follow-up. Too frequently the dental team is called upon to interact with the patient only after complaints of oral discomfort or just prior to entering the educational system, when an oral examination is requested.

As an active member of the health team, the dentist provides comprehensive evaluation of the oral-facial system. Because this system is associated with many important physiological processes it is important that it be maintained in an excellent state of health and, if already ravaged by disease, restored to health. The patient must be evaluated during the initial team interaction, not as a secondary examination. The results of the dental examination then become part of the initial assessment of the patient and can be included in the individualized plan and prioritized.

Compromising conditions and limitations imposed by the presence of PWS increase the risk of dental disease. The syndrome requires modification of diet and may have direct oral manifestations. Medical therapy may alter expected growth and development, and required dental care may be delayed or withheld because of social and financial considerations.

Dental interaction continues throughout the patient's involvement with the team. Because dental disease is a continuing risk that varies with age and medical status, PWS patients require evaluation and continuing supervision that is best monitored by the dentist during periodic visits.

Dental-Oral Characteristics of PWS

The literature is void of any comprehensive studies of the dental characteristics of the PWS patient. The few references available are primarily case studies. The most frequently reported findings are delayed eruption, hypoplastic enamel, and rampant caries. Secondary findings include micrognathia (small jaw), high arched palate, microdontia (small teeth), and xerostomia (dry mouth). Fourteen patients with the diagnosis of PWS are currently being followed at the dental clinic of the University of Iowa. They consist of seven males and seven females, ranging in age from 3 to 24 years. Ten of the 14 patients reside in communities with optimally fluoridated water. The most common oral finding is generalized marginal gingivitis secondary to poor oral hygiene. Dental caries is a minor problem, with most patients having decay rates similar to non-PWS patients. However, one male had all of his teeth removed and dentures inserted at 19 years of age, as a result of caries and fractured teeth. Other common findings in this group have been crowding, malocclusions, enamel attrition, and grinding.

Rumination and vomiting have recently been reported as a finding in patients with PWS (Alexander, Greenswag, & Nowak, 1987). In these cases enamel decalcification and erosion may have placed the teeth at greater risks for caries. Additionally, with loss of enamel tooth sensitivity has been reported, especially to acidic foods and cold liquids. Non-oral/dental characteristics of PWS may affect the oral health and management of the patient, both in and out of the office. The characteristic constant eating by PWS patients greatly increases the availability of fermentable carbohydrates necessary to the development of dental caries. Increased dietary intake coupled with crowded dental arches results in food retention and increased plaque formation, leading to gingival irritation and inflammation.

Developmental delay and/or mental retardation in PWS compromises management. The patient may not be able to comprehend how to practice daily oral hygiene, manual dexterity necessary to manipulate the toothbrush and dental floss may be minimal, and modification of dietary practices may be impossible—all of which increase the risk for oral disease.

Assessment

Assessing the dental health status of the PWS patient requires an oral examination, since no laboratory or diagnostic tests are available. Only through evaluation of the hard and soft tissues will it be possible to determine the presence or absence of disease.

It has been suggested that certain populations are at higher risk for dental disease. Although PWS patients have many high-risk characteristics, the literature remains inconclusive as to their actual oral problems. The one major PWS characteristic, overeating, undoubtedly is the major risk factor.

A thorough history is important. Information on the eruption dates and sequencing of the erupting teeth is helpful. History of trauma to the face and mouth should be obtained. Dietary habits, especially eating frequencies and types of foods consumed, are important. Fluoride intake, either from the community water or through supplements, should be reviewed, as should oral hygiene practices, including the number of times each day brushing takes place, the kind of brush, the type of dentifrice, and whether it is supervised or performed by a parent. Question whether the patient has any sucking, chewing, or swallowing problems. Are some foods more difficult than others? Does the patient appear to have or complain of a dry mouth? Does the patient demonstrate habits such as nonnutritive sucking or tooth grinding (day, night, or both)? Does the patient complain of facial muscle pain or discomfort in the area anterior to the ear? Is there a history of repeated vomiting and holding food in the mouth? A family dental history, including siblings and parents, is important.

If the first oral examination happens to occur at or around the time of eruption of the first primary tooth, the examination is relatively short and will be a pleasant experience for the infant. If the diagnosis is not made until after all the teeth erupt, and if the patient has had some unpleasant experiences in the health delivery setting, the oral examination may be more difficult.

The developmental and mental status of the patient will thus influence the examination process. Some patients may be combative or resistant. The length of appointments may have to be decreased because of short attention spans and overactivity. Obesity may make it be difficult for patients to be comfortable in the dental chair, and because of the reported micrognathia, small oral opening, and the increase in adipose tissue around the face, oral examination may be compromised. Nevertheless, PWS patients should be able to be managed with minimal difficulty by a knowledgeable team, regardless of age. The older patients (school age) are more inquisitive and require additional explanations, a little more time, and considerable positive reinforcement. For patients with extensive needs, management may consist of treatment in the dental office with local anesthesia and/or conscious sedation management. Finding the necessary landmarks for the administration of local anesthesia may be difficult because of the limited oral openings and the excessive oral tissues. Treatment with general anesthesia in the hospital or ambulatory surgical center may be necessary.

As with all patients, a dental team familiar with PWS will make the visit pleasant, efficient, and productive. Parents/guardians should inform the clinic or office coordinator of the child's diagnosis, the developmental level, whether the patient has ever had an oral examination (and if so, where and when), if the patient is presently in any oral pain, and if there are any additional medical problems present. This information allows the dental staff to prepare for the visit, and, if the patient was examined previously, contact the previous office for past history and radiographs.

When examining infants, the knee-to-knee position (between the dentist and parent), with the patient straddled in the cradle developed by the upper legs, is ideal. The parent will have an excellent view of the examination as well as be able to participate in the exam. With increasing age, positioning the patient in a dental chair is appropriate. It may be difficult for obese patients with PWS to lie in a supine position because of the weight and pressure on the upper body; reclining the chair slowly, allowing the patient to adjust, may help. It may be necessary to keep the chair at a 45° angle to the floor rather than the traditional 180°. With time, most patients gain confidence and adjust very nicely to the traditional position.

If the oral opening is limited, and if the excessive tissues intrude into the mouth, additional time will be necessary to complete an examination. If radiographs are indicated, the age-appropriate size of film may not be able to be used. Use the next smallest film size instead.

Treatment and Follow-up

After completion of the examination, an individualized treatment plan is developed. A comprehensive preventative program is initiated, including use of optimal systemic and topical fluorides and daily oral hygiene by the patient and/or parent/guardian. Because dietary intake and frequency are major findings that affect not only the patient's general medical status but oral health as well, discussion with the rest of the members of the team is indicated. Dietary guidelines must be developed that will respond to both the medical and dental concerns.

If dental treatment is indicated, the patient's behavior needs to be anticipated. The use of local anesthesia, mouthprops, and a rubber dam will assist the team to isolate the areas to be treated and help the patient keep his or her mouth open. If administration of the local anesthetic, especially the inferior alveolar and the posterior alveolar nerve blocks, is difficult, consideration should be given to alternatives, including the periodontal ligament injection. As indicated earlier, for extensive treatment and/or the apprehensive or uncontrollable patient, consideration should be given to a general anesthetic.

Follow-up should be scheduled as per the individual needs of the patient, but at least semiannually. Because poor oral hygiene is widespread, parents/guardians must be involved with the patient daily in preventing it. They should participate *actively* in cleaning the teeth, not just in passively observing that the patient is brushing. In addition to the use of the toothbrush, dental floss, and a dentrifice, consideration should be given to other plaque-reducing methods. Oral rinses with bactericidal properties are now available that may be indicated as a supplement to daily oral hygiene. If the patient has a history of vomiting and rumination, extra attention should be paid at home to additional cleaning and frequent rinsing to rid the mouth of stomach acids and partially digested foods. If decalcification is noted, topically applied fluoride should be considered on a daily schedule. If the decalcified areas progress to cavitation, full coverage with stainless steel crowns (in the primary dentition) may be indicated. Periodic follow-ups should be scheduled no less than every 6 months, and more frequently if other risk factors are identified, such as hypoplastic enamel, rumination, vomiting, or poor oral hygiene.

If the health care of the patient is managed by a team, communication between members is facilitated by the usual reporting process. If treatment is performed independently, changes in history or any treatments should be reported to the primary health care provider, who must keep the dental team informed of the patient's systemic conditions as well as of major changes taking place in medications and diet.

Conclusions

It has been reported that dental caries is generally decreasing in school-age children in the United States, due largely to fluoridation and increased awareness of the importance of oral health. PWS patients can enjoy the same benefits if modifications in oral management can be recommended and carried out. It is important for the dentist, as a member of the health team, to be able to make appropriate recommendations. Early intervention, initiation of a comprehensive preventative program, and scheduled follow-up may ensure that PWS patients can enjoy optimal oral health.

References

Alexander, R.C., Greenswag, L., & Nowak, A. (1987). Rumination and vomiting in Prader-Willi syndrome. *American Journal of Medical Genetics*, *28*, 889–895.

Foster, S. (1971). Prader-Willi syndrome; report of cases. *Journal of the American Dental Association*, *83*, 634–638.

Krautmann, P.J., Barenie, J.T., & Myers, D.R. (1981). Clinical manifestations of Prader-Willi syndrome. *Journal of Pedodontics*, *5*, 256–261.

Kriz, S., & Cloninger, B.J. (1981). Management of a patient with Prader-Willi syndrome by a dental-dietary team. *Special Care in Dentistry*, *1*, 179–182.

9
Nutritional Management

DIANE D. STADLER

Two extremes of inappropriate growth impact on the nutritional management of individuals with Prader-Willi syndrome (PWS): failure to thrive and morbid obesity. Infants with PWS present to parents and medical personnel as hypotonic, with insufficient suck and swallow reflexes, and failure to thrive. Sometime after 1 year of age, children display the features of short stature, hyperphagia, and obesity, and demonstrate insatiable, nonselective appetites. Left untreated, adolescents or adults may develop respiratory distress, cyanosis, or sleep apnea secondary to massive obesity.

Individuals with PWS, at any age, benefit from nutritional intervention to optimize growth and development. The nutritionist interfaces with the interdisciplinary health care team to assess the nutritional status of individuals with PWS, to develop dietary recommendations that promote appropriate linear growth and weight gain, to educate the care providers so they may successfully implement dietary recommendations, and to provide follow-up support.

Typical Findings

The feeding of neonates and young infants not affected with PWS revolves around regular periods of sleep and wakefulness. Normally, neonates demonstrate pronounced rooting and coordinated suck and swallow reflexes, and show signs of hunger and satiety. Infants initially require small, frequent feedings of breast milk or infant formula. As stamina develops and the stomach grows to accommodate increased food volume, the time interval between feeds increases.

In contrast, infants with PWS usually experience feeding difficulties throughout the first year of life. They often fail to awaken for feeds, and when finally aroused are listless and demonstrate poor rooting reflex, weak suck at breast or bottle, and poor head and neck control. (Note: No instances of breast feeding were reported in a survey of 700 cases conducted by the Prader-Willi syndrome Association.) Unfacilitated nutriture often results in insufficient caloric, macro-, and micronutrient intakes and insufficient weight gain. The feeding of infants with PWS is best facilitated by early transition from breast to bottle feeding, enlarging the openings of nipples, using nipples designed for premature infants, scheduling short and frequent feeds, increasing the caloric density of formula, and initiating short-term nasogastric or orogastric tube feedings.

Between 1 and 2 years of age children with PWS gradually develop the musculature, the coordination, and the stamina to complete feeds and to consume sufficient calories for growth. Once weight gain commences, care providers (usually parents) become very pleased with the ease and the success of feeding and mealtimes become positive experiences for the family. Unfortunately, however, if the strategies just described to promote initial weight gain continue into the hypertrophic period, massive obesity results within months. Obesity usually results because of the care providers' emotional need to continue a regimented feeding schedule, and the child's lack of satiety and his ability to gain weight on significantly low-caloric intakes.

Obesity persists among older individuals with PWS because they have extreme difficulty controlling food intake and seldom use discretion when making food consumption choices. The consumption of excessive amounts of food and nonfood items (pica) is not uncommon. In addition, any one or a combination of the following inappropriate behaviors may be exhibited and contribute to excessive caloric intake: creative food seeking, stealing, foraging, hoarding, and gorging. Environments or work conditions that predispose to aberrant behavior around food or its inappropriate consumption must be avoided.

Nutritional Intervention

Nutritional management of infants, children, and adults with PWS should include 1) complete nutritional assessment (Figure 9.1), 2) design of an appropriate diet, 3) nutrition education of care providers, and 4) follow-up nutritional support.

Weight, height, skinfold thickness and body circumference measurements, and nutrient analysis of food intake records are important parameters for assessing and monitoring nutritional status of individuals with PWS. This information allows the nutritionist to monitor linear growth and weight gain, to assess body fat distribution and utilization, to evaluate the adequacy of diets and the appropriateness of food intake schedules, and to assess the capability and willingness of care providers to comply with nutritional recommendations.

The growth parameters of individuals with the syndrome are used to determine the dietary recommendations for weight management. Therefore, the need for accuracy in making these measurements cannot be overstated. Infants should be weighed on a calibrated pan-type infant beam scale with nondetachable weights, without clothes or diaper and when the child is calm and still. Length should be measured on a recumbent stadio-

NAME: ______________________ Present Address: ______________________
DATE OF BIRTH: ______________ ______________________
DATE OF EVALUATION: ______ Telephone No: ______________________
CHRON. AGE: ______________
HEIGHT AGE: ______________

DIAGNOSIS: ____

Weight: ___ kg, ___ %ile; increase/decrease of ___ kg in ___ days.
Length (Height): ___ cm, ___ %ile; increase of ___ cm in ___ days.
WT/LT (Height): _____ %ile.
% IBW/LT _____.
Rt. Arm Circumference _______ cm _______%ile.
Rt. Triceps Skinfold __________ mm _______%ile.
Rt. Subscapular Skinfold ______ mm _______%ile.
Arm Muscle Area ____________ mm^2 _______%ile.
Arm Fat Area ______________ mm^2 _______%ile.

ESTIMATED CALORIC REQUIREMENT: _____ kcl/cm.

ESTIMATED PROTEIN REQUIREMENT (RDA): _____ g.

FOOD INTAKE HISTORY (24-hour food recall):

ESTIMATED CALORIC INTAKE: _____ Kcal _____ Kcal/cm.

ESTIMATED PROTEIN INTAKE: _____ g.

MULTIVITAMIN/MINERAL SUPPLEMENT: ____________________

HOME ENVIRONMENT:
Which meals are eaten at home? ______________________
Are meals eaten as a family? ______________________
Are serving bowls placed on the table? ______________________
What size serving is offered? Meat _____, Starch _____,
Vegetable _____, Fruit _____,
Dairy _____, Other _____
How many servings are offered? _____
How long does it take child to compete meal? _____

Does child participate in a school lunch program? hot _____, cold _____
Is the lunch room supervised? Y/N _____
Are snacks available at school? _____

Is food available at other times of the day? _____
Are cabinets/refrigerator locked? _____
Do you nave a garbage disposal? _____
Do you own a pet? _____
How is pet food stored? ______________________

Do you own a home scale? (Y/N) ___ If yes, do you weight child? (Y/N) ___
How often? _____

PROBLEM BEHAVIORS:
- Food preferences ___
- Food foraging ___
- Food stealing ___
- Rapid consumption ___
- Pica ___
- Nondiscriminatory ___
- School concerns ___
- Other ___

PHYSICAL CONCERNS:
- Constipation/diarrhea ___
- Vomiting, gagging, choking ___
- Sleep apnea ___
- Drowsiness ___

ACTIVITY (note time spent on activity per day and number of days per week);
Walking ___ Swimming ___
Bicycling ___
Jogging ___ Other ___

INVOLVEMENT OF LOCAL SERVICES (list names of therapists):
___ WIC
___ Visiting Nurses Association
___ Area Education Agency
___ Other

FIGURE 9.1. Nutritional assessment sheets.

meter (length board). Two people are usually required to meaure length accurately. Position the infant on the length board with his or her head against the nonmoveable right-angle headboard, trunk and pelvis aligned perpendicularly to the head board, and legs straightened with feet positioned with toes pointed up. Place the moveable footboard at the infant's feet and read the rule to the nearest 0.05 cm.

Children and young adults should be weighed on a calibrated single-beam scale while wearing undergarments and paper gowns. Height should be measured using a wall-mounted vertical stadiometer. The individual should stand as straight as possible, in bare feet with heels together, weight evenly distributed, and looking straight ahead. The measuring bar should be brought to the top of the individual's head and the rule read to the nearest 0.05 cm. The same scale, stadiometer, and measuring techniques should be used at each visit.

Weight and height measurements as well as weight-for-height ratio should be recorded and plotted with respect to age on standardized growth charts (Hamill et al., 1979). Although adolescents and adults with PWS are not expected to follow the linear growth patterns of nonaffected individuals, these charts may be used to monitor individual growth patterns. PWS-specific growth charts have been designed to describe linear growth during childhood, adolescence, and early adulthood in affected individuals (Holm & Nugant, 1982). These charts take into account the lack of, or diminished, adolescent growth spurt and provide a means for detecting inappropriate linear growth of individuals in this population. It is suggested that the reader take note of these charts (see Appendix A).

Skinfold thickness and body circumference measurements performed over time provide information about the regional deposition and utilization of somatic protein stores and subcutaneous fat stores during periods of weight gain and weight loss. Like weight and height measurements, skinfold and circumference measurements may be compared to normal values established for non-PWS children (Frisancho, 1981). Ideally, skinfold measurements should be taken at multiple sites, including the triceps, biceps, subscapular, suprailiac, midaxillary, abdominal, thigh, knee, and calf sites.

Getchell (1983) indicated that an examiner may best measure skinfold thicknesses by grasping with his or her left thumb and forefinger a fold of nonmuscular tissue at each designated site. A calibrated Lange skinfold caliper (Cambridge Scientific Instruments, Cambridge, MD) or a Harpenden skinfold caliper with a standard pressure of 10 g/mm should be used. Plastic calipers are available but do not provide reproducible measurements and therefore should not be used. The caliper should be positioned approximately 1 cm below the grasped point at a depth equal to the thickness of the fold. Each skinfold should be measured on the right side of the body, in the vertical plane, while the subject stands at ease, except for subscapular and suprailiac skinfolds, which are taken following the natural fold of the skin. Measurements should be performed in triplicate after which the average of the three values is recorded to the nearest 0.5 mm.

Circumference is best measured with a metal or nonstretch flexible fiberglass tape measure. Measurements should be taken on the right side of the body while the patient stands tall and relaxed with weight evenly distributed between the feet. Keep the tape measure in contact with the skin, but without constriction, and read each measurement to the nearest 0.1 cm. Common sites for circumference measurement include: chest, waist, hips, midthigh, midcalf, ankle, upper arm, wrist, and head.

Dietary Guidelines

In general, the dietary management of infants and young children with PWS should follow the recommendations developed by the Committee on Nutrition of the American Academy of Pediatrics. Breast milk or infant formula should remain the primary source of nutrition during the first 6 months of life. Beikost (any food product other than milk or formula) should be introduced no sooner than 5–6 months of age. Introduction of strained foods should progress from iron-fortified cereals to fruits, vegetables, and meats. Desserts and high-calorie solids should not be provided because their nutrient-to-calorie ratio is low.

During the first 2 years of life, or prior to the onset of obesity, caloric intake should be adjusted to promote growth within the 50th to 75th percentile weight for height (Hamill et al., 1979). Once weight gain becomes a problem, the ultimate goal of dietary intervention is to restrict weight to the 75th percentile weight for height, or, more realistically, to achieve weight maintenance and allow linear growth into the stabilized weight. However, because many children with PWS are massively obese, weight loss programs may need to be initiated immediately to achieve a desirable body weight as soon as possible. The severe caloric restriction required to induce weight loss in children with PWS should only be done under the supervison of a qualified nutritionist or medical personnel.

Attempts to manage the weight of individuals with PWS include caloric restriction with behavior management (Kriz & Cloninger, 1981); hypocaloric diets (Evans, 1964; Jancar, 1971; Juul & Du Pont, 1967; Holm & Pipes, 1976); hypocaloric-protein sparing diet (Bistrian, Blackburn, & Stanbury, 1977); 1,000 calorie-ketogenic diet (Nardella, Sulzbacher, & Worthington-Roberts, 1983); and a balanced macronutrient diet devoid of simple sugar (MacReynolds, 1972, cited in Coplin, Hine, & Gormican, 1976). Each dietary regimen required frequent intervention over a long period of time and unfortunately resulted in only limited ability to maintain weight goals.

Explanations for the difficulty in achieving weight loss are provided by Holm and Pipes (1976) and Coplin, et al. (1976), who reported that caloric requirements of PWS individuals to maintain weight are 50–75% and 37–77%, respectively, of nonPWS individuals. In addition, a second characteristic of PWS is the desire to consume massive amounts of food. Bray et al. (1983) reported that, when unsupervised, the ad lib caloric intake of these individuals reached 5,167 ± 503 kcal/day. Thus, the ease with which PWS individuals gain weight and their drive to seek out and consume large amounts of food often make weight management a frustrating battle requiring continuous external supervision.

Determination of Caloric Requirement

It is the responsibility of the nutritionist to determine the dietary prescription; to calculate average intakes of calories, protein, fluid, and micronutrients from diet records; and to keep accurate records that document anthropometric measurements and nutritional status. Figure 9.2 provides a

NAME: ____________________ DIET PRESCRIPTION:
DATE OF BIRTH: ______________ Kcal ______________
DX: ______________________ Kcal/cm ______________
Protein (g) ______________

DATE							
AGE							
WT (kg)							
HT (cm)							
IBW/HT (kg)							
% IBW							
Calories							
kcal							
kcal/cm							
kcal/kgIBW							
Protein (g)							
g/kgIBW							
% kcal							
Carbohydrate (g)							
% kcal							
Fat (g)							
% kcal							

Comments:

FIGURE 9.2. Nutritional management record sheet.

recording sheet that may help to organize growth and nutritional information in an easily retrieved fashion.

The caloric requirement of nonaffected, healthy individuals is associated with a rate of linear growth and weight gain expected within a specific age range. Because individuals with PWS demonstrate patterns of growth different from nonaffected individuals, their caloric requirement cannot be estimated by traditional methods: Recommended Dietary Allowance (RDA), (NAS-NRC, 1980), or basal metabolic rate. Height and chronological age, however, do provide indices for determining the caloric needs of an individual with PWS.

Holm and Pipes (1976) first described the caloric requirement of individuals with PWS in terms of kilocalories per centimeter of height (kcal/cm). A compilation of the results of weight management attempts of individuals with PWS is presented with respect to age, kcal/cm, percentage weight loss, and length of dietary intervention in Table 9.1. Although all data points are not available, the information presented supports, objectively, the principle that individuals with PWS require few calories to maintain weight. It appears that individuals with PWS at any age can lose weight when maintained on a calorie-restricted diet of 7 kcal/cm. Significant weight loss, up to 43% of total body weight, over a 13-month period has been documented (Marshall et al., 1979). Weight maintenance has been reported with diets that provide 8–11 kcal/cm.

Depending upon the individual's height and dietary goal, daily caloric intake may range from 600 to 800 kcal among young children and from 800 to 1,100 kcal among older children and adults. If an individual gains weight on an appropriately restricted caloric intake unaccounted food may be available from additional sources: school cafeterias, snack machines, fast food restaurants, neighbors, and food stealing. Management strategies that restrict food accessibility include: 1) locking the refrigerator, freezer, and other food sources such as cabinets and pantries; 2) disposing of leftover foods immediately into trash compacters, garbage disposals, or inaccessible garbage cans; 3) locking away pet foods; 4) locking kitchen doors; and 5) following a regular meal pattern. Additional suggestions are presented in Table 9.2.

The composition of the diet should approximate 25% protein, 50% carbohydrate, and 25% fat. Protein intake should meet the RDA and be of high biological value (contain all of the essential amino acids), carbohydrate should be complex carbohydrate, and fat should be limited to that found naturally in foods (Figure 9.3). Because prolonged caloric restriction predisposes any individual to insufficient intakes of micronutrients, a multiple vitamin and mineral supplement becomes an inevitable component of the diet. Table 9.3 provides information on available multiple vitamin and mineral preparations and their nutrient compositions.

Nutrition Education

As soon as the diagnosis of PWS is made, care providers must be taught to complete accurate records of food intake that include the meal/feeding time and the types, amounts, and caloric contents of the foods consumed (Figure 9.4). Solid food intake is best described using common household measurements (e.g., cups, teaspoons, fluid ounces), or standard or metric weights. To familiarize care providers with standard portion sizes, and to increase awareness of the caloric density of various foods, the first 2 months of nutritional intervention should begin with encouraging the primary care provider to monitor and to weigh or measure all foods provided.

When solid food becomes the child's primary nutritional source, the care providers should be given instructions and appropriate resources to provide adequate nutrition. This includes teaching the design of meals that meet the child's nutritional needs while complying with the necessary caloric restriction. The choice of instructional model is dependent upon the primary care provider's understanding of the individualized dietary guidelines and his or her ability to follow the recommendations.

TABLE 9.1. Individual caloric requirements.

Age (years)	Sex	Weight (kg)	Height (cm)	Caloric intake: Diet order (kcal)	Actual intake (kcal)	Kcal/kg	Kcal/cm	Weight change (percentage)	Time interval (weeks)
1 8/12[a]	M	—	86.1	775	800	—	9	(−0.6 kg)	3
2[a]	M	—	—	—	815	—	9	(−1.4 kg)	12
2[b]	M	—	—	—	800	—	8	0	—
3[b]	M	—	—	—	950	—	10	0	—
3 4/12[c]	F	13.6	—	—	715	53	—	0	24
4 3/12[c]	M	31.4	—	—	863	28	—	+1	24
4[b]	M	—	—	—	990	—	10	0	—
4 9/12[c]	F	23.1	—	—	560	24	—	+1	24
4[a]	F	—	—	—	880	—	9	(−1.6 kg)	12
4[d]	M	29.7	101	protein sparing fast	—	—	—	—	deceased
4[b]	M	—	—	—	880	—	10	0	—
5 1/12[c]	F	27.7	—	—	890	32	—	+1	24
6[a]	M	—	—	—	980	—	9	(−3.6 kg)	12
6[a]	M	—	—	—	690	—	6	(−4.8 kg)	approximately 1
6 5/12[c]	M	24.5	—	—	1060	43	—	−10	24
6 5/12[c]	M	29.1	—	—	755	26	—	−11	12
6[d]	M	56.6	122	1000	—	18	18	(−5.6 kg)	—
7[b]	—	—	—	—	1020	—	9	0	—
7[b]	—	—	—	—	1280	—	11	0	—
7[d]	M	47.5	116	1.5 protein/kg	—	—	—	(−6.8 kg)	0.1 yr
7[d]	M	99.0	81	protein sparing fast restricted fluid	1200	—	—	(−22 kg)	—
8[d]	—	59.4	124	protein sparing fast	1200	20	10	—	—
9[b]	M	—	—	—	1180	—	10	0	—
9 3/12[c]	M	41.4	—	—	938	23	—	−11	24
10 8/12[c]	F	107.7	—	—	600	6	—	−26	24
11[b]	M	—	—	—	1990	—	15	0	—
11[e]	M	57.2	142.2	1000	—	17	7	−4	2

12[e]	F	28.1	125.1	1000	—	36	8	0	1
12[e]	M	36.3	146.7	1000	—	28	7	−2	2
12[e]	M	46.3	142.2	1000	—	22	22	−2	1
12[f]	M	95.3	147	1.4 g protein/kg protein sparing fast	—	—	—	—	—
12[d]	—	107	147	1.5 g protein/kg	—	—	—	—	—
13[e]	M	45.8	140.3	1000	—	22	7	−1	1
13[e]	M	60.8	146.1	1000	—	16	7	−4	2
14[e]	F	61.7	140.3	1000	—	16	7	−3	2
15[e]	M	51.7	143.4	1000	—	19	7	−3	1
17[e]	M	68.0	151.8	1000	—	15	7	−3	2
17[f]	M	118.7	150	1.5 g protein/kg protein sparing fast	900	8	6	−53	40
18[e]	M	54.9	133.9	1000	—	18	7	−2	2
18[e]	M	66.2	150.5	1000	—	15	7	−5	2
19[f]	F	124.2	155	1.9 g protein/kg protein sparing fast	1100+	9	7	−36	112
20[g]	F	90.1	132	1000		11	7	−37	72
21[g]	F	77.3	142	1000		13	7	−40	52
21[g]	M	81.8	142	1000		12	7	−43	52
22[e]	M	122.9	148.0	1000 kcal		8	7	−3	2
24[f]	F	97.7	137	1000 kcal 2.1 g protein/kg protein sparing fast		10	7	−32	44
26[g]	M	107.7	147	1700	—	16	12	−58	52
20[h]	F	—	142.2	900	—	—	—	(−7.7 kg)	32
								(−12.7 kg)	72

[a] Pipes and Holm (1973).
[b] Holm and Pipes (1976).
[c] Coplin et al. (1976).
[d] Bye et al. (1983).
[e] Nardella et al. (1983).
[f] Bistrain et al. (1977).
[g] Marshall (1978).
[h] Kriz and Cloninger (1981).

TABLE 9.2. Weight reduction and dieting tips.

1. Establish a consistent meal pattern immediately. Do not deviate from the meal pattern. The calorically restricted diet should become a way of life rather than a burden or punishment for the individual.
2. Provide three meals daily. If food is inappropriately consumed between meals, subtract an equal amount of calories from the next meal.
3. Include the individual with PWS in family social and holiday activities. However, be prepared to provide appropriate supervision.
4. Small portion sizes of the family meal may often be provided to the individual with PWS. Discretion must be used and alternatives provided when necessary.
5. Limit the use of food as a reward. Instead use a book, record, TV time, or activity as positive reinforcement for appropriate behavior (see Appendix C).
6. Set restrictions on the types of foods purchased (do not purchase ice cream, peanut butter, cookies, or candy if these foods are inappropriately consumed).
7. Measure average portion sizes of food to be served; divide in half and serve the second half as a second portion. If a second portion is not requested, do not offer the remaining food.
8. Serve food on a smaller plate (8 inch vs. 10 inch). Offer fluids in a 6-ounce glass.
9. Serve food in the kitchen, away from the table, and leave remaining food in kitchen. Do not set serving dishes on the eating area.
10. Cut meat in small pieces.
11. Snack suggestions: Provide a variety of fresh fruits and vegetables or use canned fruits and vegetables *packed in their own juice.* Prepare large quantities of tossed salads to have available for immediate consumption after school, or as an evening or night-time snack. Always provide a salad with the evening meal and at lunch if possible. Lettuce takes up space but has few calories.
12. Dilute fruit juices. An increased volume may be offered if this is done. Use only *unsweetened* juices.
13. Consider purchasing Dole Fruit-N-Juice Bars or Jello Gelatine Pops as a substitute for ice cream or as a birthday/holiday treat.
14. Send a sack lunch to school, day care, or workshop to avoid excessive or unintended caloric consumption. *Make sure that appropriate supervision is provided during each meal.*

One commonly used model for diet planning is the exchange system, which divides foods into six groups: milk, meat, fruit, vegetable, bread, and fat. The distribution of calories from the total daily recommendation into specific food groups, or exchanges, is designed to assure adequate micro- and macronutrient intakes. Portion sizes are assigned to foods in each group to provide equal amounts of protein, carbohydrate, fat, and calories (Table 9.4). Using this model, foods within a group may be substituted or "exchanged" freely. Exchanges are allocated into a specific meal plan to meet the needs of the child while attempting to conform to the family's life-style (see Appendix B for an example of a 1-week meal pattern based on the food exchange system and a sample menu). Verbal and written instructions on using the exchange system for meal planning must be provided and the design of daily menus must be practiced with the nutritionist as a resource. Following dietary instruction, nutrition monitoring should take place at intervals that assure that the recommendations are appropriate.

1. Estimated caloric requirement based on age and height (table 9.1): ______ kcal/cm. ______ kcal/day.

2. Protein requirment (RDA): ______ g.
   Kcal from protein: ______ kcal.
   Percent of total kcal: ______ %.

3. Kcal from carbohydrate (approximately 50% total kcal): ______ kcal.
   Grams of carbohydrate: ______.

4. Calories from fat (total kcal – [kcal from protein and carbohydrate]): ______ kcal.
   Grams of fat: ______.

5. Multivitamin/mineral supplement: ______________ (brand/dose).

6. Allocation of calories into food groups (refer to Table 9.4 for macronutrient values):

FOOD GROUP	No. of Exchanges	Kcal	PRO (g)	CHO (g)	FAT (g)
Bread	____	____	____	____	____
Fruit	____	____	____	____	____
Vegetable	____	____	____	____	____
Meat	____	____	____	____	____
Dairy	____	____	____	____	____
Total	____	____	____	____	____
% Kcal			____	____	____

7. Distribution of food exchanges into meal pattern:
   Breakfast ______________
   ____
   ____
   ____
   Lunch ______________
   ____
   ____
   ____
   Dinner ______________
   ____
   ____
   ____
   Snacks ______________
   ____

FIGURE 9.3. Diet prescription worksheet.

TABLE 9.3. List of multivitamin and mineral supplements and their contents.

Product (distributor, dose)	Vitamins													
	A (IU)	D (IU)	E (mg)	B_1 (mg)	B_2 (mg)	B_3 (mg)	B_5 (mg)	B_6 (μg)	B_{12} (mg)	C (mg)	Fe (mg)	FA[a] (mg)	Biotin (μg)	Other (mg)
RDA for infants and children 1–3 years of age	*400*	*400*	*5*	*0.7*	*0.8*	*9*		*0.9*	*2.0*	*45*	*15*	*0.1*	*65*	
Poly-Vi-Sol (Mead Johnson, 1 ml)	1,500	400	5	0.5	0.6	8		0.4	2	35				
Poly-Vi-Sol With Iron Drops (Mead Johnson, 1 ml)	1,500	400	5	0.5	0.6	8		0.4	35	10				
Theragran Liquid (Squibb, 5 ml)	10,000	400		10.0	10.0	100	21.5	4.1	5.0	200				
Tri-Vi-Sol With Iron (Mead Johnson, 1 ml)	1,500	400.								35	10			
Vi-Daylin Drops (Ross, 1 ml)	1,500	400	5	0.5	0.6	8		0.4	1.5	35				
Vi-Daylin Liquid (Ross, 5 ml)	2,500	400	15	1.0	1.2	13.5		1.0	4.5	60				
Vi-Daylin Plus Iron ADC Drops (Ross, 1 ml)	1,500	400								35	10			
Vi-Daylin Plus Iron Drops (Ross, 1 ml)	1,500	400	5	0.5	0.6	8		0.4		35	10			
RDA for children 4–6 years of age	*2,500*	*400*	*9*	*0.9*	*1*	*12*	*3–4*	*1.3*	*2.5*	*45*	*10*	*0.2*		
Bugs Bunny Plus Iron (Miles Labs)	2,500	400	15	1	1.2	13.5		1	4.5	60	15	0.3		

Bugs Bunny With Extra C (Miles Labs)	2,500	400	15	1	1.2	13.5		1	4.5	250		0.3		
Centrum (Lederle)	5,000	400	30	2.25	2.6	20	10	3	9	90	27	0.4	45	Ca (162), P (125), Mg (100), Zn (22.5), I (150), Cu (3), Mn (7.5), K[b] (7.5)
Centrum, Jr. (Lederle)	5,000	400	15	1.5	1.7	20	10	2	6	60	18	0.4	45	Cu (2), Mn (1), K (1.6), Ca (108), I (0.1), Mg (25), Zn (10)
ET Chewable With Iron (Squibb)	5,000	400	30	1.5	1.7	20		2	6	60	18	0.4		
ET Children's Chewable (Squibb)	5,000	400	30	1.5	1.7	20		2	6	60		0.4		
Flinstones Chewable (Miles Labs)	2,500	400	15	1	1.2	13.5		1	4.5	60		0.3		
Flinstones Complete (Miles Labs)	5,000	400	30	1.5	1.7	20	10	2	6	60	18	0.4	40	Ca (100), P (100), Mn (2.5), Zn (15), Mg (20), I (150)
Flinstones Plus Iron (Miles Labs)	2,500	400	15	1	1.2	13.5		1	4.5	60	15	0.3		
Flinstones With Extra C (Miles Labs)	2,500	400	15	1	1.2	13.5		1	4.5	250		0.3		
One-A-Day (Miles Labs)	5,000	400	30	1.5	1.7	20	10	2	6	60		0.4	30	K: 0.05μg^{b}
One-A-Day Plus Extra C (Miles Labs)	5,000	400	30	1.5	1.7	20	10	2	6	500		0.4	30	K: 50μg^{b}
One-A-Day Plus Iron (Miles Labs)	5,000	400	30	1.5	1.7	20	10	2	6	60	18	0.4	30	K[b], tartrazine
One-A-Day Plus Minerals Maximum Formula (Miles Labs)	5,000	400	30	1.5	1.7	20	10	2	6	60	18	0.4		Ca, Cl, Cr, Cu, Zn, L, K, Mg, Mn, Mo P, Se, biotin, Vit. K
One-A-Day Stressgard (Miles Labs)	5,000	400	30	15	10	100	20	5	12	600	18	0.4	30	Cu, Zn, K[b]

TABLE 9.3. *Continued.*

Product (distributor, dose)	Vitamins													
	A (IU)	D (IU)	E (mg)	B_1 (mg)	B_2 (mg)	B_3 (mg)	B_5 (mg)	B_6 (μg)	B_{12} (mg)	C (mg)	Fe (mg)	FA[a] (mg)	Biotin (μg)	Other (mg)
Pac-Man Chewable Iron (Rexall)	5,000	400	30	1.5	1.7	20		2	6	60	18	0.4		
Pac-Man Pre-schooler's With Iron (Rexall)	2,500	400	10	0.7	0.8	9		0.7	3	40	10	0.2		
Poly-Vi-Sol Chewable (Mead Johnson)	2,500	400	15	1	1.2	13.5		1	4.5	60		0.3		
Poly-Vi-Sol With Iron Chewable (Mead Johnson)	2,500	400	15	1	1.2	13.5		1	4.5	60	12	0.3		
Popeye Chewable Multivitamin (Beecham)	2,500	400	15	1.05	1.2	13.5	2.5	1.05	4.5	60	15	0.3	37.5	Mg (40), I (0.1), Zn (12), Cu (1.5)
Smurf Chewable (Mead Johnson)	2,500	400	15	1	1.2	13.5		1	4.5	60		0.3		
Smurf With Iron & Zinc (Mead Johnson)	2,500	400	15	1.05	1.2	13.5		1.05	4.5	60	12	0.3		
Spider-Man Chewable (Hudson)	2,500	400	15	1	1.2	13.5		1	4.5	60		0.3		
Spider-Man Plus Iron (Hudson)	2,500	400	15	1	1.2	13.5		1	4.5	60	15	0.3		
Stress Formula Vitamins (various)		30	15	15	100	20	5	12	600	0.4			45	
Theragran-M Tablets (Squibb)	10,000	400	15	10	10	100	20	5	5	200	12			Cu, I, Mg, Mn, Zn

Theragran Tablets (Squibb)	10,000	400	15	10.3	10	100	18.4	4.1	5	200				
Unicap (Upjohn)	5,000	400	15	1.5	1.7	20		2	6	60		0.4		
Unicap M (Upjohn)	5,000	400	15	1.5	1.7	20	10	2	6	60	18	0.4		K[b] (5), Zn (15), Cu (2), I (150 μg), Mn (1)
Unicap Plus Iron (Upjohn)	5,000	400	15	1.5	1.7	20	10	2	6	60	18	0.4		
Unicap T (Upjohn)	5,000	400	15	10	10	100	10	6	18	300	18	0.4		Cu, I, K, Mn, Zn
Vita-Lea Chewable for Children (Shaklee)	2,000	400	10	1.1	1.2	14	4	1.5	3	60	10	0.3	10	Ca (130), P (100), Mg (60), Zn (1.5), Cu (0.2), I (15 μg)
Vi-Penta Multivitamin Drops (Roche, 0.6 ml)	5,000	400	2	1.0	1.0	10	10	1		50			30	
Vi-Penta Infant Drops (Roche, 0.6 ml)	5,000	400	2							50				
Vi-Daylin Chewable (Ross)	2,500	400	15	1.05	1.2	13.5		1	4.5	60		0.3		
Tri-Vi-Flor With Iron Drops (Mead Johnson 1 ml)	1,500	400								35	10			Fl (0.25 μg)

Note: Adapted from Arizona Department of Health Services, Office of Nutrition Services, Multivitamin Reference Chart (81/86) by Maria Navdella, M.A, R.D., Phoenix, AZ.
[a] Folic acid.
[b] Potassium.

NAME: ______________________
DATE: ______________________
WEIGHT: ________lb __________kg

TIME OF DAY	FOOD OFFERED	AMOUNT CONSUMED	CALORIE (kcal)	(Parents leave blank) PRO (g)	CHO (g)	FAT (g)

Was this a typical day? ____ If no, please comment ______________________

Did you observe any of the following events? (If so, please indicate and comment):

____ Food foraging
____ Consumption of nonfood items
____ Consumption of unauthorized food

FIGURE 9.4. Twenty-four hour food intake record.

TABLE 9.4. Macronutrient content for standard portion sizes of foods in each food group.

Food group	Calories (kcal)	Protein (g)	Carbohydrate (g)	Fat (g)
Dairy (nonfat)	80	8	12	—
Fruit	40	—	10	—
Vegetable	25	2	5	—
Starchy vegetable	70	2	15	—
Bread/cereal	70	2	15	—
Meat (lean)	55	7	—	3

a sample menu). Verbal and written instructions on using the exchange system for meal planning must be provided and the design of daily menus must be practiced with the nutritionist as a resource. Following dietary instruction, nutrition monitoring should take place at intervals that assure that the recommendations are appropriate.

Follow-up

The plan for nutrition follow-up of children with PWS should be discussed and presented in writing to the primary care providers. Follow-up plans should be individualized to meet the needs of the child and his or her family. Food intake should initially be recorded daily and sent, together with the child's weight, to the nutritionist on a weekly basis. If the care providers comply with the recommendations and the weight goal is met, 3-day food records and weekly weight measurements should continue for 2 more weeks. If after 4 weeks goals are met, a 72-hour food record and weekly weight measurements should be submitted to the nutritionist monthly. When all the above goals are met, formal nutritional follow-up should take place every 4–6 months.

Where compliance with dietary recommendations is good, but the weight goal is not met, the nutritionist will be required to reevaluate the diet. If the weight goal is not met because of lack of compliance, additional nutritional counseling will be necessary. This may include a home visit to evaluate whether the environment is conducive to the diet protocol, or, in other instances, a referral to a primary health care agency.

Case Study

The following information is presented as a case study to illustrate the successful dietary management of a young child with PWS. It is essential to keep in mind that each person with PWS is unique and will require indi-

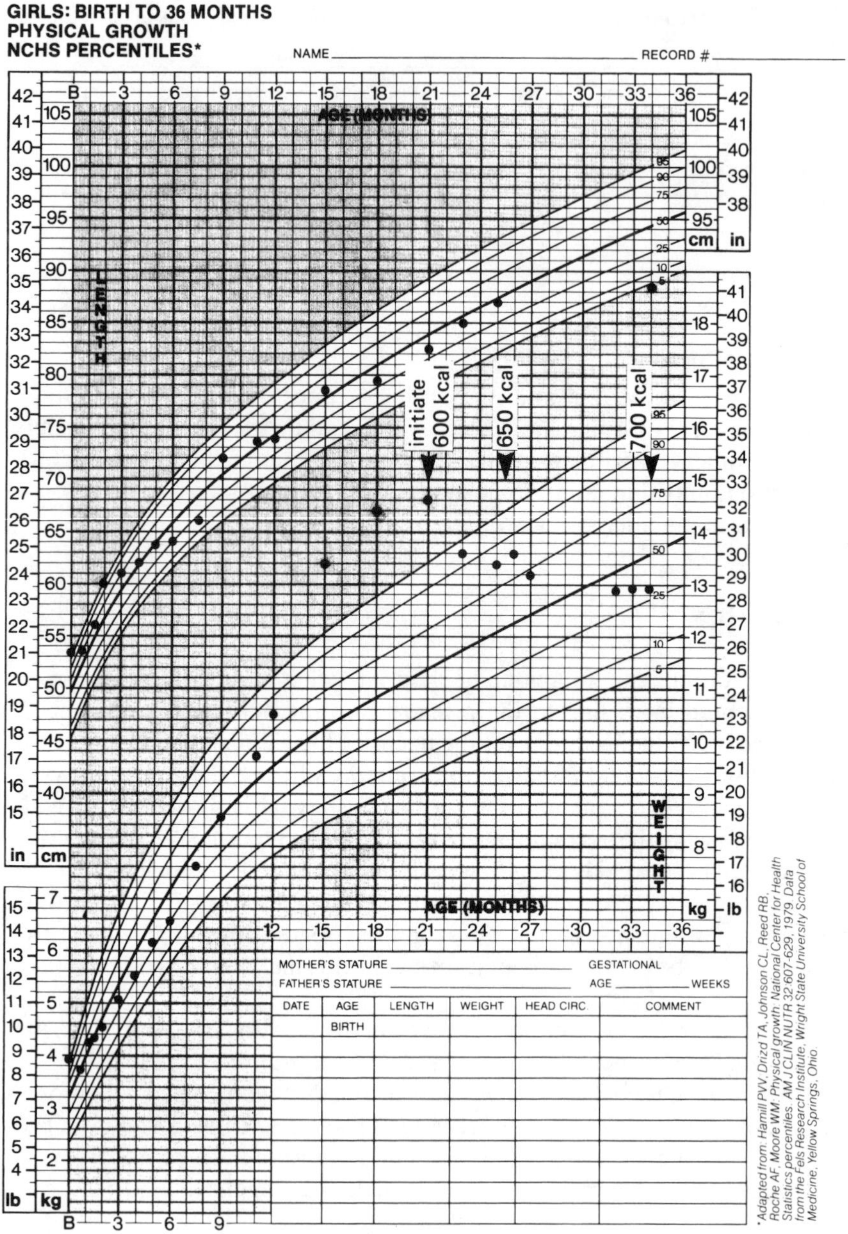

FIGURE 9.5. Linear growth (*top curve* and weight gain (*bottom curve*) plotted over time for TR. Dietary caloric levels indicated on weight gain curve by arrowheads. Chart reprinted by permission of Ross Biomedical Publications.

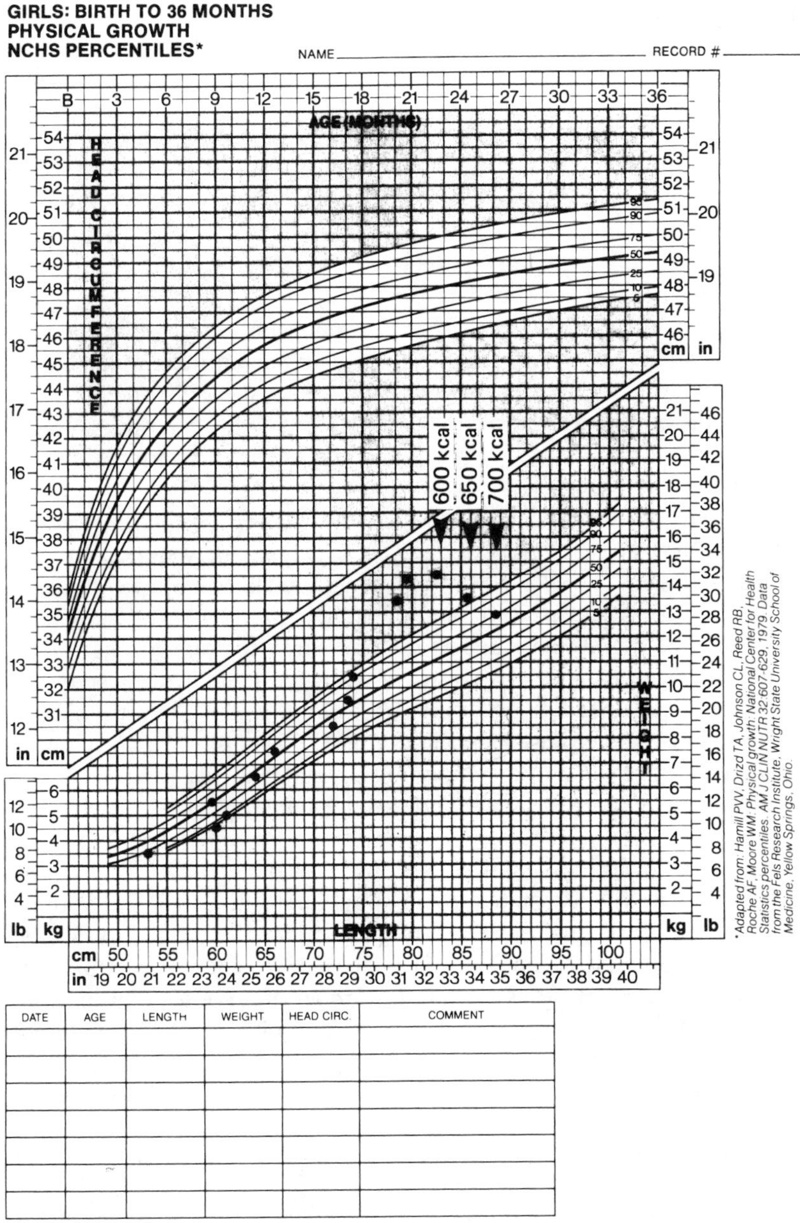

FIGURE 9.6. Weight for age measurements plotted over time for TR. Dietary caloric levels indicated by arowheads. Chart reprinted by permission of Ross Biomedical Publications.

vidualized management. Similarly, each family environment is unique, and the content of counseling sessions and the type and amount of reinforcement will be different. Frequent contact by the nutritionist and effective communication skills are essential to provide the family with the knowledge and support necessary to meet the dietary needs of their child.

TR carries the medical diagnosis of PWS. She weighed 3.96 kg (95th percentile) and was 53.3 cm in length (95th percentile) at birth (50th percentile weight for length; refer to Figures 9.5 and 9.6). TR tracked along the 50th percentile weight for age between 1 and 3 months of age, and along the 25th percentile weight for age between 3 and 6 months of age. She demonstrated accelerated weight gain between 6 and 21 months of age, during which time she crossed from the 25th percentile to much above the 95th percentile. Her linear growth progressed along the 90th percentile until 3 months of age, was below the 25th percentile at 7.5 months of age, and tracked within the 25th to 75th percentile between 8 months and 21 months of age.

TR was referred to the Division of Developmental Disabilities by her local pediatrician at 21 months of age. At that time she weighed 14.6 kg (>95th percentile) and was 82.4 cm in length (25th to 50th percentile). TR's food intake included soft mashed table food, diluted juices, and whole milk. She consumed three meals and three to four snacks a day. Computer nutrient analysis of a typical 24-hour food intake suggested that TR consumed approximately 785 kcal (9.5 kcal/cm) and 34.4 of protein per day. The following micronutrients did not meet 66% of the RDA: vitamin D, vitamin E, vitamin C, zinc, iodine, niacin, and iron. By report, TR did not demonstrate hunger or satiety and she consumed all foods provided to her.

Dietary intervention was initiated at 21 months of age and was designed to restrict caloric intake while providing adequate nutrition for optimal linear growth. Caloric intake was restricted to 575–600 kcal/day (7–8 kcal/cm) to initiate gradual weight loss. Specific dietary recommendations included: limiting food portion size and the number of servings, diluting fruit juices with water in a 1:4 ratio, providing skim milk and cheeses made of skim or low-fat milk, substituting bite-sized pieces of fresh fruit for dried fruit, providing a multivitamin and mineral supplement daily, and providing food in three meals and two snacks daily. Written information on the caloric contents of foods was provided to enable accurate calculation of total caloric intake.

Arrangements were made to have TR weighed at her local pediatrician's office, and a 72-hour food intake record was to be completed and returned for analysis as soon as possible. Telephone contact was made with her mother following the receipt of the diet record to provide additional recommendations. Diet records and weight measurements were requested on a monthly basis and frequent telephone contact was made to discuss changes in dietary recommendations.

At 26 months of age, 5 months after dietary intervention, TR weighed

13.6 kg (75th to 90th percentile) and was 85.8 cm in length (25th percentile). Her desirable body weight estimated at the 75th percentile weight for height was 12.5 kg. Her mother reported that TR consumed 100% of the foods offered and that she did not demonstrate hunger or satiety, nor inappropriate food-seeking or food consumption behaviors. Her caloric intake was adjusted to 650 kcal (7.6 kcal/cm) per day. Food intake records and monthly weight measurements were continued.

At 34 months of age, 13 months after her initial evaluation, TR weighed 12.9 kg (25th to 50th percentile) and was 88.5 cm in length (<5th percentile). Her weight-for-length ratio was at the 75th percentile, her desired body weight. Upper arm skinfold thickness (50th to 75th percentile) and circumference (90th percentile) and subscapular skinfold thickness (90th to 95th percentile) were measured. Arm muscle area (90th to 95th percentile) and arm fat area (50th to 75th percentile) were calculated. TR had been maintained on a diet of 650 kcal (7.3 kcal/cm) and had lost an average of 0.08 kg/month. TR's protein intake exceeded the RDA and a multivitamin and mineral supplement was provided to meet micronutrient needs. TR's caloric intake was increased to 700 kcal/day (7.9 kcal/cm); meat and dairy products were to comprise the additional calories. Weight and length will be measured monthly, and caloric intake will be adjusted as necessary to promote appropriate growth. Formal evaluation, including anthropometric assessment, will take place every 6 months.

Conclusion

Nutritional intervention for individuals with PWS is indicated at any age and continues throughout life. Infants with PWS may fail to thrive and children, adolescents, and adults may be massively obese. Older children and adults with PWS require significantly fewer calories to maintain weight than non-PWS individuals. This, in combination with a need to satisfy an uncontrollable hunger, results in massive obesity. Weight management of this population is difficult and requires continuous external supervision. The nutritionist works with the interdisciplinary team and the primary care providers to assess and monitor the nutritional status of individuals with PWS, to develop appropriate dietary recommendations, to teach providers how best to implement recommendations effectively, and to provide follow-up services.

References

Altman, K., Bondy, A., & Hirsch, G. (1978). Behavioral treatment of obesity in patients with Prader-Willi syndrome. *Journal of Behavioral Medicine*, *1*, 403–412.

Bistrian, B.R., Blackburn, G.L., & Stanbury, J.B. (1977). Metabolic aspects of protein-sparing modified fast in the dietary management of Prader Willi obesity.

New England Journal of Medicine, *296*, 774–779.

Bray, G.A., Dahms, W.T., Swerdloff, R.S., Fisher, R.H., Atkinson, R.L., & Carrel, R.E. (1983). The Prader-Willi syndrome: A study of 40 patients and a review of the literature. *Medicine*, *62*, 59–79.

Bye, A.M., Vines, R., Fronzek, K. (1983). The obesity hypoventilation syndromea and the Prader Willi syndrome. *Australian Paediatric Journal*, *19*, 251–255.

Caldwell, M.L., & Taylor, R.L. (1983). A clinical note on food preference of individuals with Prader-Willi syndrome: The need for empirical research. *Journal of Mental Deficiency Research*, *27*, 45–49.

Coplin, S.S., Hine, J., & Gormican, A. (1976). Out-patient dietary management in the Prader-Willi syndrome. *Journal of the American Dietetic Association*, *68*, 330–334.

Crnic, K.A., Sulzbacher, S., Snow, J., & Holm, V.A. (1980). Preventing mental retardation associated with gross obesity in the Prader-Willi syndrome. *Pediatrics* *66*, 787–789.

Evans, P.R. (1964). Hypogenital dystrophy with diabetic tendency. *Guy's Hospital Reports*, *113*, 207–222.

Frianscho, A.R. (1981). New norms of upper limb fat and muscle areas for assessment of nutritional status. *American Journal of Clinical Nutrition*, *34*, 2540–2545.

Getchell, B. (1983). *Physical fitness, a way of life* (3rd ed.). New York: John Wiley & Sons.

Hamill, P., Drizd, T., Johnson, C., Reed, R., Roche, A., & Moore, W. (1979). Physical growth: NCHS percentiles. *American Journal of Clinical Nutrition*, *32*, 607–629.

Holm, V.A., & Nugent J.K. (1982). Growth in the Prader-Willi syndrome. *Birth Defects: Original Articles Series*, *18*, 93–100.

Holm, V.A., & Pipes, P.L. (1976). Food and children with Prader-Willi syndrome. *American Journal of Diseases of Children*, *130*, 1063–1067.

Holm, V.A., Sulzbacher, S.J., & Pipes, P.L. (Eds.). (1981). *The Prader-Willi Syndrome.* Baltimore: University Park Press.

Jancar, J. (1971). Prader-Willi syndrome. *Journal of Mental Deficiency Research*, *15*, 20–29.

Juul, J., DuPont, A. (1967). Prader-Willi syndrome. *Journal of Mental Deficiency Research*, *11*, 12–20.

Kriz, S.J., & Cloninger, B.J. (1981). Management of a patient with Prader-Willi syndrome by a dental-dietary team. *Special Care in Dentistry*, *1*, 179–182.

Laurance, B., Brito, A., & Wilkinson, J. (1981). Prader-Willi syndrome after age 15 years. *Archives of Disease in Childhood*, *56*, 181–186.

Marshall, B.D., Elder, J., O'Bosky, D. Wallace, C. & Liberman, R. (1979). Behavioral treatment of Prader-Willi syndrome. *Behavior Therapy*, *2*, 22.

Nardella, M.T., Sulzbacher, S.I., & Worthington-Roberts, B.S. (1983). Activity levels of persons with Prader-Willi syndrome. *American Journal of Mental Deficiency*, *87*, 498–505.

Food and Nutrition Board, National Academy of Sciences–National research Council (1980). *Recommended dietary allowances* (9th ed.).

Pipes, P.L., & Holm, V.A. (1973). Weight control of children with Prader-Willi syndrome. *Journal of the American Dietetic Association*, *62*, 520–524.

10 Psychological and Behavioral Management

STEPHEN SULZBACHER

Important issues face psychologists evaluating individuals with Prader-Willi syndrome (PWS). They include school placement, management of food-related behaviors, and problems such as stubbornness and temper tantrums. PWS families need guidance as they look beyond current crises and address their feelings and plans about where their children will live and work when they reach adulthood. The need for psychological advice seems to occur at predictable intervals as PWS individual grow up. Establishing a general intelligence level is important in the preschool years, and appropriate educational placement requires psychological evaluation and recommendations. In most cases, once the transition into elementary school is completed, the need for psychological services diminishes until the child is about 10 years old, the time at which stubbornness and temper tantrums generally intensify and require intervention. The transition to junior high school, where students are often less directly supervised by a single teacher, is another point at which educators frequently seek psychological advice.

Since the syndrome was first described in 1956, there have been important and predictable changes in concerns about the PWS population. In the late 1970s, services focused on earlier identification of the syndrome, refinement of the diagnostic criteria, and implementation of a variety of psychological diagnostic procedures and behavioral interventions, primarily with younger children. The emphasis was on dissemination of information to practicing pediatricians and school district personnel unfamiliar with the disorder. This entailed extensive travel and in-sevice training. In almost every case the psychologist was obliged to spend several hours explaining the nature of the disorder to allied health disciplines and school personnel, who were understandably skeptical about what parents told them.

Now, nearly 10 years later, the level of understanding about PWS in the community is relatively more sophisticated. New referrals to the Prader-Willi clinics indicate that, in many states, community physicians are increasingly able to make the diagnosis themselves and schools and state agencies now require less extensive documentation to support the diagnosis.

The focus of presenting problems at PWS clinics has also shifted recently. In the past, psychological services emphasized early diagnosis, cognitive assessment, behavioral management, education of professionals, and support of families who had finally discovered what was wrong with their child. Now, new clinic referrals tend to be cases correctly diagnosed and who face problems rarely addressed in professional literature or even mentioned in previous references to the syndrome (e.g., Holm, Sulzbacher, & Pipes, 1981). As the treatment advances of the past decade have improved the health and longevity of this population, psychological issues associated with adolescents and young adults have emerged. Appropriate programming and out-of-home residential care are now major concerns.

The first question generally asked of a psychologist on an interdisciplinary team is, "What is the patient's IQ?" This is a relatively important question for individuals with PWS who are younger than 9 years of age or are being evaluated for the first time. IQ scores in the population reflect a wide range of abilities, but nearly all cases are below average intellectually. In a sample of 232 cases, 63% were borderline or mildly retarded, 31% were moderately retarded, and 3% were severely retarded (Greenswag, 1987). In evaluating individuals with disorders other than PWS, it is often very important to establish the exact nature of subtle, cognitive malfunctions, which are usually revealed through an analysis of subscale scores on the Weschler Intelligence Scales and may require the administration of a complete neuropsychological battery (Reitan & Boll, 1973). However, current experience and understanding of the nature of PWS have not suggested any indications for neuropsychological testing or sophisticated brain scanning techniques (Gabel et al., 1986). Although neuropsychological testing is not usually necessary, there are unique features of the syndrome that become more apparent in adolescence and young adulthood (Bransen, 1981; Sulzbacher, Crnic, & Snow, 1981; Turner & Ruvalcaba, 1981).

The second question often directed to the psychologist is, "How can inappropriate behavior be changed?" A request for a clinical reevaluation or referral to a psychologist is generally precipated by a behavioral crisis, either at home or at school. Several emotional and behavioral characteristics distinguish individuals with PWS from others with comparable developmental delay:

1. Individuals with PWS generally have higher interest and skill in reading.
2. PWS individuals tend to be more talkative, although they have a lower level of abstraction and a relatively higher level of argumentativeness.
3. Although quite clever and often devious in developing schemes to obtain food, these individuals typically show very poor judgment relative to their IQs.
4. Impulse control is low and frequently leads to unpredictable behavior outbursts.

5. Tantrums, verbal and physical aggression, and irritability tend to be more frequent, whereas inappropriate sexual behavior is relatively rare in this population (see Chapter 17 for further discussion of psychosexual development).
6. Most of the time (when not tantruming) these people are socially engaging, conversational, well groomed, and friendly.
7. In a work setting where access to food is controlled and supervision is constant, persons with PWS can be diligent and reliable model workers who take pride in their work.

A Developmental Perspective

Preschool Children

As previously reported (Sulzbacher et al., 1981), weight management has serious cognitive implictions in PWS. In that retrospective study, children who were diagnosed in infancy and who were never allowed to become obese had significantly higher average IQ scores than those who became obese and then lost weight or those who remained obese. Dunn, Tze, Alisharan, & Schulzer (1981) also reported a downward trend of IQ scores before the age of 10, further evidence that age and weight may affect cognitive function. Of course, the families who are successful in weight management are also usually more consistent in general behavior management. Careful weight and behavior management may lead to a more favorable intellectual prognosis.

The use of consistent positive and negative consequences and strict parental control over access to food is very effective with preschool children. However, the degree of "control" that will be necessary throughout the life of a person with PWS (particularly around food) is so much greater than what is needed for the average child that it is important to look for opportunities, even in the preschool years, to allow the child to "call some shots." Parent-child play sessions allow the psychologist to observe the parents' style of interaction (Slater, 1986) and point out how parents can reduce their own "directiveness" and encourage the child to direct the play (Eyberg & Robinson, 1982). Finding times for the child to be "in charge" often reduces noncompliance in other situations in which the parent must be in control.

Elementary School-Age Children

A difficult decision for many parents and school administrators is determining the best classroom placement. Most, if not all, children with PWS appear to benefit from contact with unaffected age peers in "mainstream" class placement. For some, regular kindergarten followed by a 50% resource room placement in first grade has been beneficial. Obviously, the regular class teacher needs to make adjustments to assure that other childrens' lunches are inaccessible to the PWS child. Classmates should be told about the syndrome and discouraged from sharing food, even if asked. A sensitive discussion of health problems that other classmates may have is a good pedagogical technique within which PWS can be explained.

Most children with PWS begin school in special education, however, and may have as little as 20% mainstream experience. Thus, it is particularly important for their social development that they be exposed to organized social groups outside of school, such as parks department programs, church groups, and swimming club/team activities.

At home, behavior problems centering on food begin to escalate during this age period. The child has increased freedom to move about, but lacks judgment or self-control regarding food. One way to foster the feeling of self-control is to rearrange the environment to reduce the potential for confrontations between parent and child. Initially, the major recommendation is to lock the kitchen or refrigerator. Contemporary technology can be used in the form of burglar alarm "motion sensors" that sound an alarm whenever anyone enters the kitchen, signalling the child to get out on his or her own and also notifying the parents.

When confrontations over food can be minimized, many parents report this age to be a period when they particularly enjoy their interactions with their children.

Preadolescents

Psychologists can help families of preadolescents by explaining the exact nature and implications of PWS to the affected individual, extended family, friends, and babysitters. In some cases, once this information has been shared, it can be relayed by the parents to other family members. In other instances, psychotherapeutic group sessions are indicated. The psychologist should ask both parents to describe how they explain their child's disorder to friends. When parents disagree about this, other underlying spousal relationship issues may require more in-depth counseling. Similarly, it is important to learn how individuals with PWS describe their condition to peers. They need to learn to be able to provide accurate, dignified responses to questions. It is common for siblings to be embarrassed and/or angry about their handicapped brother or sister. The psychologist can assist them in understanding the genetic implications of the disorder for sibs (essentially none) and to help them overcome embarrassment and express their anger in constructive ways. A very useful technique is to arrange small group sessions for siblings from several families where they can learn that they are not alone in their feelings and can discuss mutual concerns. Siblings typically have many unanswered questions, and support groups formed at several clinics have met with great success in ensuring a more complete understanding of PWS and their own role in helping the family to cope (LeConte, 1981). Genetic counseling issues as they relate to future children of siblings are typically discussed, and in the case of Prader-Willi syndrome, these discussions can lead to relief of unvoiced anxieties (see Chapter 4).

Adolescents

In adolescence, behavioral crises are frequently precipitated by tantrums or stealing of food or money and usually involve strangers, neighbors, or shopkeepers. Stringent behavior modification programs can be effective at this point, but typically do not have longlasting effects on behavior unless the programs are strictly maintained. Even with careful supervision, a significant proportion of older adolescents have had contact with police as a result of theft (usually food), running away from home, or complaints to children's protective agencies by strangers who observe parents engaged in management procedures that, although not appropriate for most children, are necessary for those with PWS. In addition, the unpredictable outbursts of rage observed in many cases (which are probably directly attributable to the syndrome itself) have resulted in police involvement on charges of assault. Parents should be advised to have preventative contacts with police and neighborhood shopkeepers to explain the syndrome and provide a photo of their child while still very young (in elementary school). Law enforcement agencies tend to be grateful for such advance input so that they can be aware of potential problems and can react accordingly. This policy can prevent situations such as the one that occurred when a PWS individual was kept overnight in jail and "kindly" jailers provided far too much for him to eat.

Ten years ago, the lack of knowledge about PWS caused serious problems in the public schools. Today, the judicial system is faced with the same challenge to learn about this condition. Psychologists who treat affected individuals should be prepared to appear at court hearings to explain the syndrome and, when necessary, testify to the inappropriateness of incarceration. However, probation officers usually are very helpful in monitoring young adults with PWS who have committed crimes.

Family Issues

Individuals with PWS and their families need to agree upon consistent descriptions of problems associated with the syndrome. Families differ widely in their respective value systems, which must be taken into account when helping a family decide how to describe the syndrome to others. Some families feel that it is necessary to minimize the handicap, whereas others feel it is important to educate the public about the syndrome. For others, religious values are closely intertwined and must be considered. The answer to the question, "Who am I?" cannot be taken lightly. It may be a recurring theme over several years or may be the subject of a short-term intensive psychotherapeutic intervention.

Explanations to grandparents and other members of the extended family usually involve issues of disbelief, distrust of the parents, and/or fault-finding. It is not a joking matter when grandparents find it difficult to refrain from "spoiling their grandchildren" with extra treats.

The psychologist is often the first to approach sensitive family issues of guardianship, wills, and trusts. Even though specific arrangements and drafting of such documents is clearly a matter for a lawyer experienced in developmental disabilities, this topic often provides the opening for discussion and better understanding of family dynamics. Siblings, in particular, should be consulted about the question of who will manage the affairs of the PWS individual when the parents are gone.

Components of Successful Behavioral Programs

Although certain elements of behavior management programs are presented as nonnegotiable by the psychologist, PWS clients are encouraged to understand that they can adjust key elements of the programs, such as the nature of rewards and punishments, the setting of weight goals, and the right to manage certain aspects of their parents' behavior. Rewards and punishments of the behavior modification approach are central to any program, but it is also essential that the family "empower" the patient with a feeling of some degree of control over important events in the patient's life and in the operation of the family unit. The use of the "family council" approach (Dreikurs, Gould, & Corsini, 1974; Dreikurs & Soltz, 1964) is recommended. It emphasizes the importance of the patient's feelings of self-worth and personal power as important long-range deterrents to socially unacceptable means of manipulating the behavior of others.

Behavior modification procedures have been shown to be successful with a wide variety of problem behaviors of children without PWS (Daniels, 1974; Lovitt, 1984), and these same principles have been applied to those with PWS (Thompson, 1985). A practical, inexpensive handbook for parents that incorporates behavior modification with some family systems concepts is *Without Spanking or Spoiling* by Crary (1979). Although PWS presents some unique problems, the methods for management differ very litte from those used with other children and adolescents. For example, food can be used as a reinforcment for those with PWS, provided low-calorie foods are used in small portions and are included in calculating total daily caloric intake. A program to reduce tantrums might employ a glass of diet pop as a bedtime treat (or at the end of the school day for a classroom program). The treat is prepared at the beginning of the day and, whenever a tantrum is imminent, the child is warned that unless the behavior stops, some pop will be poured down the drain. If the behavior persists, a small amount of pop is poured out. The child loses small increments of pop for each subsequent infraction, but there is still some pop left as an incentive for self-control later in the day. Obviously, such behavior management techniques must be individually tailored to the needs and interests of each child. A list of suggested positive reinforcements/rewards may be found in Appendix C. Once the PWS population reaches adolescence and adulthood, residential services become a consideration, and behavioral modification techniques using a token economy have proved effective (see Appendix I).

A daily personal exercise program should start when children are as young as 7 or 8 years of age. Exercise should be viewed in the same way as toothbrushing, something to be done regularly once or twice each day. A 5–10 minute session with a parent or other care provider as co-participant, conducted each day before breakfast, is an ideal arrangement for young children. Televised or videotaped low-impact aerobics lessons tend to be enjoyable, as is a brisk walk around the block with a parent or other companion. The obvious reinforcing contingency to this activity is that it is followed by breakfast. For the initial year or two of such a program, building an enjoyable exercise habit is the main goal, rather than building muscle or burning calories. Over time, emphasis can shift to more strenuous activity and serious conditioning. A major additional benefit of such a structured program is that the young adolescent may be able to build a repertoire of conversational topics around sport and exercise that may encourage socially appropriate peer interactions. For example, considerable satisfaction could result from managing a high-school athletic team where interest in sport and exercise is reinforced by the friendships with nonhandicapped athletes.

Programming self-restraint is a difficult but important component of an overall strategy of building a feeling of personal worth and self-control. For example, giving the child several days' "ration" of snacks to manage as he or she sees fit seems to be of some value. Food should be left in a separate bowl to which the child has free access with the understanding that the bowl will be refilled only every third day. It is the child's responsibility to manage the snacks so they last 3 days. If the child is successful at managing this ration of snacks the amount may be expanded to a week's supply. Avoid negative comments if the entire supply is eaten in 1 day. Express sympathy over the choice, which results in no more snacks until the bowl is scheduled to be refilled.

Power sharing, as a preventative approach, should begin at 6 years of age or even younger. This approach teaches by example that it is better to negotiate than to use force, even if it is obvious that the negotiator could win by force alone. At the simplest level, it involves encouraging children to voluntarily give up food, rather than taking it away from them. It involves giving individuals choices wherever possible, even if these choices are limited. During normal development between the ages of 6 and 12, children experience and experiment with increasing degrees of autonomy in a process called "individuation" (Adler, 1963). For many developmentally disabled individuals this process is disturbed. Many experiences through which a sense of personal power may be gained are denied, because care providers must continue to rule arbitrarily, as in the case of food intake. If subsequent stubbornness and tantrums are to be diminished or avoided, it is imperative that individuals be given as many opportunities as possible to develop feelings of autonomy and personal power in other domains so that they can develop a sense of control and still be able to "go along with" dietary restrictions.

A convenient mechanism for beginning this power-sharing process with a very young child is to suggest that "we need to do something about [food stealing]." Even though a parent has a fairly clear agenda, it is usually possible to discuss and lead the child into being a partner is setting up contingency arrangements. As the child gets a little older, it is useful to ask which behaviors of his or her parents he or she would like to see changed so that a contingency on the behaviors of the parents can be managed by the child. The process can be a fairly pleasant, game-like situation. If a chart is being kept, allow the child to put the stars marks on the chart himself or herself. Because of the power of the reinforcers and the efficiency of most behavior modification procedures, the process of including the child in setting up the program is frequently forgotten. Because the behavior modification procedures themselves usually work very well in the short term, the effects of neglecting to include the child in planning them are generally not noticed until months or years later. Benefits of early negotiation practices become apparent when the parent is faced with a 15-year-old who doesn't really "have to" go along with the program but has developed the habit of making adjustments through negotiations rather than outright refusal.

Some limited success in using relaxation techniques has been reported with children with PWS, such as methods of self-management to control anger and hunger impulses (Nielsen & Sulzbacher, 1981). Similar techniques have been successful for impulse control with other handicapped youngsters (McMahon & Sulzbacher, 1980). Teaching individuals with PWS how to do self-relaxation should be viewed as an adjunct to other, more effective methods of behavior control, but the relaxation training reemphasizes the personal responsibility of individuals for their own behavior. Relaxation techniques are more effective for management of anger than for reduction of hunger impulses and are more appropriate for cases with mild to borderline intellectual functioning than for those with greater degrees of retardation.

In a survey of 200 families with a PWS child, two thirds had tried medication to control behavior and/or appetite (Holm, 1987). Seventy-two percent of the males and 57% of the females had been given psychotropic medication. In only 15% of the cases was such medication tried in individuals under 12 years of age. Trials with a great variety of medications were reported, including psychostimulants (Ritalin, dextroamphetamine, and Cylert), major tranquilizers (e.g., Thorazine, Stelazine, Navane, Haldol, Mellaril), antidepressants (e.g., imipramine, amitriptyline), and others (e.g., lithium, Atarax). Holm interpreted the results of this survey as indicating no consistent benefit from any of these medications for the behavioral symptoms associated with PWS. However, individual cases of hallucinations and paranoia were successfully treated with medication. Such psychiatric problems may be seen in individuals with PWS, but are probably best viewed as an unrelated disorder.

Only in rare instances have parents reported any beneficial effects of medication on appetite control or sleep disorders. A number of other studies reported the use of naloxone to reduce hunger intensity (Krotkiewski, Fagerberg, Bjorntrop, & Terenius, 1983; Kyriakides, Silverstone, Jeffcoate, & Laurence, 1980), but none have been successful in altering hunger or weight in persons with PWS.

The overall lack of major beneficial effects of medication in PWS noted in Holm's survey is consistent with the results of a study of the effects of Ritalin and dextroamphetamine in children with PWS conducted by Sulzbacher and Holm (1977). Five boys ranging in age from 4 to 11 years were enrolled in a classroom where daily measurements were taken of behavior and of academic progress. During the 2-month study, parents recorded occurrences of specific behavior problems at home. Data recording was double-blind and each child had two dosage levels of medication and a placebo condition. Behavior management in the class consisted of a point system for staying on task and in seat. Points were exchanged for free-time activities at the end of each day. Time-out for tantrums was used with only one child, and inappropriate behavior such as talking out was systematically ignored for the class. Talking-out, out-of-seat, and tantrum behavior were independently recorded by two observers. The data indicated no consistent drug effect on any of these behaviors, and medication was discontinued in all five cases at the conclusion of the trial. In each case, progress was noted in reading and math skills, but there was no significant differential effect of medication levels on either performance rates or accuracy. Data collected at home also reflected no meaningful drug effect on the behaviors of concern to the parents. In summary, a simple but consistent classroom behavior management system was effective in these cases, and psychostimulant medication provided no additional benefit.

Case Studies

Case Study #1

BJ has been one of the most successful cases followed at our clinic. Since he first came to our attention at about the age of 8 years, his history and subsequent course of development have been what one would expect from an individual diagnosed with PWS, except that he has consistently scored above 90 on standardized intelligence tests. As a result of diligent monitoring by BJ's parents and teachers, his weight has always been kept within acceptable limits. He was mainstreamed throughout his high school career, with 50% or less of his classes in the resource room. The psychologist was called on at fairly regular intervals to arrange cooperative weight and behavior management programs for his parents and junior high school teachers. BJ persisted in foraging for food during any unsupervised time at school, including begging from classmates. This required psychological intervention with BJ, his parents, peers, and teachers. Although he was unsupervised for a period of more than an hour from the time he arrived at home until his mother came home from work, the behavior management system prevented food stealing during this period.

BJ's primary weight management program involved weekly weigh-ins on Saturday mornings followed by a discussion between BJ and his mother about his "menu" for the following week. If BJ had maintained progress along the weight projections plotted by his nutritionist, caloric intake for the remaining week remained the same. If BJ had exceeded his projected weight for that Saturday, his mother made a downward adjustment in total calories and discussed the matter with him. If BJ's weight dropped below projection, a more flexible discussion took place, where BJ and his mother decided whether to provide some extra treat or to continue on the maintenance diet and engage in some nonfood activity as a reward. An important rule for these Saturday morning discussions was that arguments or excuses about weight gain were not acceptable topics of conversation. If BJ's weight had increased, it meant that an adjustment had to be made the following week. If BJ protested that there had been no food stealing violations, his mother pointed to the scale and said that she was making no accusations nor was she interested in excuses; an adjustment simply had to be made because of the weight gain. BJ was not being punished but it was made clear to him that when his weight went up or down the rules would call for caloric intake adjustments.

It should be noted that BJ and his mother joined in a daily exercise program of brisk walking, an important feature in their personal fitness program. In BJ's case, adjustments for weight gain by increasing energy output were not part of his program since his mother felt that changes in their exercise program would be too complicated. (In other cases, the program has included an option of increased exercise the following week when a weight adjustment was indicated.)

An important feature of BJ's behavior management program, which should be incorporated into all such programs, is the emphasis on shared control between the patient and his or her parents. If a parent also has some weight loss goals, for example, it would seem cooperative and fair to let the individual with PWS monitor contingencies on the parent's weight loss program.

Problems arose in junior high school when BJ literally fell upside down into a waste can in the school lunchroom while trying to steal garbage. He needed assistance to be extricated from the can. Some of his nonhandicapped peers also discovered that they could get BJ to make a fool of himself by dancing or saying silly things in exchange for a tidbit of food. Since there was no way to reasonably modify the normal junior high school situation nor was there a convenient way to supervise BJ during his entire day, a series of psychotherapeutic sessions was used to help him overcome the judgmental deficits associated with PWS (even seen in those whose IQs approach normal). Over a period of months, it was possible to instill some degree of self-control over the specific situations causing difficulty. With increased vigilance by the high school staff, these problems diminished. The gist of the psychotherapeutic intervention was to point out more efficient ways of stealing food without accompaning social indignity. BJ's cravings for food were acknowledged, and by helping him to figure out better ways to filch food, his social functioning improved *without* reducing the food stealing. Of course, a goal of the therapeutic intervention was to begin the process of shifting responsibility for self-management onto BJ's shoulders. Unfortunately, there are no reports of anyone with PWS ever being able to effectively self-manage their hunger. In fact, BJ may have been our most successful attempt in that he lived in a tenant support apartment situation for 2 years. Temper management problems, rather than unacceptable weight gain, ended that experiment and BJ is now living in a group home. At this time, BJ travels independently on a bus to a sheltered workshop situation, where he is an exemplary worker and is only slowly gaining weight. Crises of one sort or another arise over his living situation at the rate of one or two a year, and are expected to continue.

Other Case Examples of Young Adults with PWS

Despite obvious individual differences in personality, interests, and skill levels, there seem to be some common developmental milestones and problem areas unique to PWS that occur during adolescence and the young adult years. Without exception, in every case behavioral problems associated with food and diet have necessitated a more restricted environment at school, work, and home than the individuals would otherwise be capable of enjoying.

Many states provide developmentally disabled persons with apartment living arrangements called Tenant Support Programs. Case workers make regular visits to these semi-independent settings. Attempts at tenant support living by young adults with PWS in our clinic have resulted in unacceptable weight gain, and parents should be counseled to accept the fact that independent living is not a realistic option for any individual with PSW. However, careful dietary management and strict behavioral controls can be instituted in a group home living situation for young adults, which allows them to participate in a considerable variety of work situations and leisure time activities. Appropriate residential programming is discussed in depth in Chapter 20.

Case Study #2

C2 lived at home until he was 21, when he moved into a Prader-Willi group home. Although there were many difficulties with C2 at home, his parents only reluctantly agreed that it was time for him to leave. In the 2 years he has lived at the group home he has lost 60 pounds. He enjoys an occasional light beer and rides public transit on his own to his evening work shift as a janitor in a downtown office. He often spends weekends with his parents (who now realize that the move was absolutely the best thing for them and him), but knows that he can lose this privilege for violations of his behavior contract at the group home.

Case Study #3

C3 experienced a more circuitous route to his eventual placement in the same group home. In high school, C3 became the manager for one of the school's regular athletic teams, which enabled him to count many of the highest status boys at the school as his friends. This was a very positive feature of his high school years. However, he still had problems with stealing food and running away from home. Gradually he began traveling further from his own neighborhood, where he was known to the police, and was eventually arrested and jailed for theft in another community. He was placed in a state institution for the mentally retarded, where a trial of psychotropic medication at the institution proved ineffective. After several years of behavioral interventions his behavior improved, and he has been successfully placed at the group home and continues to maintain good weight control.

Clearly, institutional placement is not ideal for individuals with PWS, but it does remain the only option for several cases, to prevent stealing and running away. These individuals are in the institutional setting at this time primarily because not enough group homes are available.

Summary

A meaningful and productive adult life, with mutually satisfying social relationships, is clearly possible for many individuals with PWS. Regardless of their tested IQ level, people affected with this syndrome have significant disabilities in learning and judgment that can be treated with psychoeducational practices. Individuals with PWS will typically require psychological assistance throughout their lives in order to come to terms with their disability and to improve their self-esteem. Even the most effective and caring of families need assistance at those critical transition times between elementary and junior high school, when formal schooling is completed (around the age of 21), and when the individual leaves the home. With very few exceptions, it is in the best interest of both young adults with PWS and their families that the affected person live in a group residence. Clearly the psychologist's role is to guide the parents' thinking in this direction well in advance of the time when the move should occur. Planning for this transition should begin when the child enters adolescence. Although parents may find this separation process very difficult, the transition should be viewed as an opportunity for individuals with PWS to grow and develop expanded social and psychological horizons.

References

Adler, A. (1963). *The problem child.* New York: Capricorn Books.

Bransen, C. (1981). Speech and language characteristics of children with Prader-Willi syndrome. In V.A. Holm, S.J. Sulzbacher, & P.L. Pipes (Eds.), *The Prader-Willi syndrome* (pp. 179–184). Baltimore: University Park Press.

Crary, E. (1979). *Without spanking or spoiling.* Seattle: Parenting Press.

Daniels, L.K. (1974). *The management of childhood behavior problems in school and at home.* Springfield, IL: Charles C. Thomas.

Dreikurs, R., Gould, S., & Corsini, R.J. (1974). *Family council.* Chicago: Contemporary Books.

Dreikurs, R., & Soltz, V. (1964). *Children: The challenge.* New York: Hawthorn Books.

Dunn, H., Tze, W., Alisharan, R. & Schulzer, M. (1981). Clinical experiment with 23 cases of Prader-Willi syndrome. In V.A. Holm, S.J. Sulzbacher, & P.L. Pipes (Eds.), *The Prader-Willi syndrome* (pp. 69–88). Baltimore: University Park Press.

Eyberg, S., & Robinson, E. (1982). Parent-child interaction training: effects on family functioning. *Journal of Clinical Child Psychology*, *11*, 130–137.

Gabel, S., Tartar, R.E., Gavaler, J., Golden, W.L., Hegedus, A.M., & Maier, B. (1986). Neuropsychological capacity of Prader-Willi children: General and specific aspects of impairment. *Applied Research in Mental Retardation*, *7*, 495–466.

Greenswag, L. (1987). Adults with Prader-Willi syndrome: A survey of 232 cases. *Developmental Medicine and Child Neurology*, *29*, 145–152.

Holm, V.A. (1987). *Prader-Willi syndrome parent survey results.* Unpublished manuscript.

Holm, V.A., Sulzbacher, S.J., & Pipes, P.L. (Eds.) (1981). *The Prader-Willi syndrome.* Baltimore: University Park Press.

Krotkiewski, M., Fagerberg, B., Bjorntrop, P., & Terenius, L. (1983). Endorphines in genetic human obesity. *International Journal of Obesity*, *7*, 597–598.

Kyriakides, M., Silverstone, T., Jeffcoate, W., & Laurence, B. (1980). Effect of naloxone on hyperphagia in Prader-Willi syndrome. *Lancet*, *1*(8173), 876–877.

Leconte, J.M. (1981). Social work intervention strategies for families with children with Prader-Willi syndrome. In V.A Holm, S.J. Sulzbacher, & P.L. Pipes

(Eds.), *The Prader-Willi syndrome* (pp. 245–257). Baltimore: University Park Press.

Lovitt, T.C. (1984). *Tactics for teaching*. New York: Merrill.

McMahon, R.J., & Sulzbacher, S. (1980). Relaxation training as an adjunct to treatment in a hyperactive boy. *Clinical Pediatrics*, *19*, 497–498.

Nielsen, S.L., & Sulzbacher, S.J. (1981). Relaxation training with youngsters with Prader-Willi syndrome. In V.A. Holm, S.J. Sulzbacher, & P.L. Pipes (Eds.), *The Prader-Willi syndrome* (pp. 219–227). Baltimore: University Park Press.

Reitan, R.M., & Boll, T.J. (1973). Neuropsychological correlates of minimal brain dysfunction. *Annals of the New York Academy of Sciences*, *205*, 65–88.

Slater, M.A. (1986). Modification of mother-child interaction processes in families with children at-risk for mental retardation. *American Journal of Mental Deficiency*, *91*, 257–267.

Sulzbacher, S., Crnic, K.A., & Snow, J. (1981). Behavioral and cognitive disabilities in Prader-Willi syndrome. In V.A. Holm, S.J. Sulzbacher, & P.L. Pipes (Eds.), *The Prader-Willi syndrome* (pp. 147–160). Baltimore: University Park Press.

Sulzbacher, S., & Holm, V.A. (1977). *Medication and reinforcement techniques in the classroom for PWS*. Unpublished manuscript.

Thompson, D. (1985). *Behavioral management programs for people with Prader-Willi syndrome*. Unpublished manuscript.

Turner, R., & Ruvalcaba, R.H.A. (1981). A retrospective study of the behavior of Prader-Willi syndrome versus other institutionalized retarded persons. In V.A. Holm, S.J. Sulzbacher, & P.L. Pipes (Eds.), *The Prader-Willi syndrome* (pp. 215–218). Baltimore: University Park Press.

11
Education of the Child with Prader-Willi Syndrome

MARSHA H. LUPI

Since the passage of PL 94–142, the Education for All Handicapped Children Act of 1975, education of children with complex care needs and medically related problems has been the responsibility of the public education system. Previous procedures that isolated such children from the mainstream or forced parents to seek private schooling are no longer acceptable by law.

Although placement of school-age children remains somewhat of an issue between proponents of residential schools and those who advocate public school placement, children with Prader-Willi syndrome (PWS) are guaranteed a free, appropriate public education and must be provided with those special education and related services necessary to meet goals and objectives written into the child's individualized education program (IEP). Furthermore, because PL 94–142 acknowledges that any assessment and/or evaluation of the child must be multidisciplinary, children with PWS are entitled to an ongoing team approach to determine their educational, related services, and special education needs.

Defining the scope of related services as they have an impact on the school experience is of particular interest to those involved in the education of the child with complex care needs and medically related problems such as PWS. A recent Supreme Court decision (*Tatro v. State of Texas*, 1979) upholding the right of a young girl with spina bifida to have clean intermittent catheterization as a related service to allow her to participate fully in and benefit from special education has expanded the definition of related services significantly (Vitello, 1986). As a consequence of such a ruling, children who were previously excluded from school programming becauses of unique medical needs can no longer be routinely excluded and will be in a good position to seek any related service that will enable them to fully profit from attending school.

The implication of this expansion of related services for the education of students with PWS is great. It may mean, in many cases, the difference between a program that successfully manages the student's hyperphagia and accompanying behavioral problems and one that ignores the implications of the syndrome.

This chapter provides information on the educational characteristics of PWS, focusing on cognitive abilities and deficits, behavioral profiles, and social and emotional behaviors. It will also offer concrete suggestions and examples on how best to accommodate the student with PWS into the classroom.

Typical Findings and Special Considerations of the PWS Child

Almost all PWS individuals have some degree of mental retardation, although IQs of 100 have been reported. Typically one finds the PWS student to be borderline or mildly retarded or to have learning disabilities (Cassidy, 1984; Lupi, 1986; Seltzer, 1985). In many ways the PWS child more closely resembles a learning-disabled child in test and school performance because of a tendency to have some inconsistent and surprising strengths as well as weakness in just one or two areas (Sulzbacher, Crnic, & Snow, 1981). There is evidence that very selective learning ability is characteristic of PWS children, which is an indication of a learning disability. For example, they may tend to be good readers but may be very poor in mathematical concepts (Cassidy, 1984).

Warren and Hunt (1981) found that PWS students had great difficulty with short-term memory (STM) processing. Others (Inwood, 1986; Lupi & Porcella, 1987) have noted a short attention span if too much information is presented. Long-term memory does not, however, tend to be a problem. In fact, many PWS students have incredible memories for activities and events that far surpass their anticipated capabilities. Strategies for recalling information such as rehearsal techniques seem to be effective when working with PWS students in strengthening memory. Weaknesses in arithmetic skills and reasoning have been noted by Holm (1981). This may be attributed to the STM deficit postulated by Warren and Hunt (1981) as a consistent characteristic, since arithmetic skills are often sequential and depend on prior learning.

Generally speaking, students with PWS may have delays in achieving developmental motor milestones and motor coordination, which may contribute to their resistance to participation in physical activities. Educators should be aware that evaluation of body scheme is always preceded by progress through a normal sequence of developmental movement patterns. Ayres (1979) indicates that "both motor planning and motor skills require a perception of how the body is designed and functions as a mechanical unit" (p. 95).

However, educators should encourage a well-rounded program of physical activity and exercise once a doctor's permission has been obtained (see Chapter 13).

Other findings about the cognitive and educational characteristics of the

PWS student include strengths in activities such as puzzles and needlecrafts.

Children with PWS also exhibit distinct behavioral abnormalities linked to the frustrations associated with the syndrome. They may manifest a variety of deviant eating behaviors such as foraging for food, eating uncooked meats, consuming 10 pies at one sitting, and even eating dog food (Otto, Sulzbacher, & Worthington-Roberts, 1982). Other behavior problems include verbally and physically aggressive behaviors such as lying, stealing, scratching, and kicking. Tantrums are very common among PWS students and are discussed in the behavior management portion of this chapter. Self-mutilating behaviors such as skin picking and self-biting have been reported by parents and teachers.

Students with PWS also have a poor social profile, with an inability to pick up social cues, poor peer interactions, and generalized immaturity as key characteristics. Given the fact that many children with PWS have low self-esteem because of their obesity and negative response toward them from others in their environment, it is understandable that they may consider themselves outcasts and assume such a role.

As this chapter indicates, the child with PWS presents a unique set of characteristics that must be handled with special consideration in the school setting. Because their test profiles indicate a lowered IQ and/or learning disabilities, they are likely be placed in special classes or programs.

Educational Programming

The design of IEPs for PWS students in special education classes and programs varies according to the students' individual learning needs. It is not so much that their academic strengths and weaknesses need to be challenged in ways very different from non-PWS children who have similar test profiles, but rather that the issues arising from the syndrome (e.g., hyperphagia) may have an impact upon the structure and techniques utilized in the classroom and school setting.

Parental concern that the school environment be a "safe" one (free of opportunity for indiscriminate eating) requires the school's recognition that the attendance of a child with PWS means the extension of the school's responsibility beyond the classroom door to the entire school community. It is critical that all people who come in contact with the child (e.g., bus drivers, matrons, lunchroom aides) be instructed not to provide the child with food or money (Lupi & Porcella, 1987).

The teacher who is primarily responsible for the education of the PWS child must be instructed on the nature, characteristics, and demands made by the syndrome. Literature such as *Prader-Willi Syndrome: A Fact Sheet for Teachers and Other School Personnel* (Lupi & Porcella, 1985), *Prader-*

Willi Syndrome: A Handbook for Parents (Neason, 1978), and "A New Kind of Learning Disorder" (Lupi, 1986) can assist teachers in gaining a better understanding of the syndrome.

For example, if a teacher does not fully comprehend the effect of snacking on the student's health and dietary maintenance, the child may be at risk the entire school day, week, month, and year. In fact, the teacher must be directed to adjust the classroom and curriculum to facilitate the best interests of the child. Adjustment of the classroom environment on the elementary level must focus on the following areas: 1) modification of classroom routines and milieu, 2) evaluation of existing systems of reward and behavior management techniques, and 3) ongoing communication with parents and school personnel working with the child.

Modification of Classroom Routines and Milieu

The school calendar provides many opportunities for children to eat. Free breakfast programs, semi-supervised lunchrooms, and birthday and holiday parties, if not thought about and planned for in advance, can create dangerous situations for the child with PWS. Lupi and Porcella (1985) have suggested the following "Do's" and "Don'ts" for the teacher of the student with PWS. They provide guidelines for structuring the classroom environment and various aspects of the school day that may need special consideration in light of the reported difficulties and issues surrounding the management of the child with PWS.

DO'S

Do check to see that all children in the class are free from snack food during school hours.

Do request that parents provide you with the child's daily menu so that you can prepare yourself for any special change in program or food-related events.

Do cut child's portions in half (e.g., pizza slice) to make it appear like a larger portion.

Do lock up all food items, including pet food.

Do assess each child's strengths and weaknesses, individually providing him or her with remediation specific to his or her needs.

Do plan lessons that are high interest, age appropriate, and of shorter duration.

Do include physical education and physical activities as a part of your daily program. The child should be encouraged to participate to the maximum extent appropriate.

Do provide the child with every opportunity to work together with other children by sharing classroom responsibilities and encouraging interaction whenever possible.

Do provide the child with successful school experiences, providing immediate feedback and positive reinforcement.

Do compliment the child on weight loss or the maintenance of an appropriate weight.

DON'TS

Don't leave a child with PWS alone or in a situation where food is easily attainable.

Don't provide the child with access to money or small objects that can be used to buy or trade for food.

Don't emphasize curricular material that is food oriented unless it presents material that focuses on good nutrition and the positive aspects of weight control.

Don't prevent the child from attending birthday parties or holiday parties. Consult instead with parents and the child's physician to work out a suitable substitute for birthday cake.

Don't send the child anywhere in the school unescorted. The escort should be someone who understands the problem and will not be easily manipulated by the PWS child.

Don't accuse parents of feeding their child too much food. Remember, the parents need support and encouragement too.

Inwood (1986) has offered the following suggestions concerning food and the PWS child in school:

1. Food should be a constant in the student's schedule. It should be served at specific times and unavailable the rest of the time. (This helps to alleviate the obsessive thinking about food.)
2. Punishment for taking food should be minimal due to the involuntary nature of their eating behavior. Students should not be made to feel that they are "bad people."
3. Food should *never* be taken away as a punishment. This could lead to increasing stress and accompanying behavioral problems.
4. If possible, lunch time should be structured so the PWS student leaves the food area as soon as lunch has been eaten. (p. 2)

Teachers should also make every attempt possible to provide students with classroom experiences that enhance their self-image. Students should be encouraged to take part in success-oriented activities (determined by their individual strengths and weaknesses) and group activities wherever possible. Age-appropriate activities such as aerobic dancing, Ping-Pong, shuffle board, bingo, and crafts are examples of forms of recreation that may serve to create a sense of socialization for the student with PWS.

The use of these suggestions paired with an increased awareness of the food-related issues should provide a structured environment within which learning can occur.

Evaluation of Existing Systems of Rewards and Reinforcement

Food has traditionally been used as a very effective reinforcer for good classroom behavior and work. It has also been the mainstay of many behavior modification programs within special education settings. With the possible exceptions of sugarless gum and diet soda, the use of food (e.g., M&M's) as a reinforcer or reward for PWS children in learning situations may seem inappropriate (Caldwell & Taylor, 1983).

Heiman (1978) and Inwood (1986) strongly believe that the base of any structured environment for the PWS student is the removal of all food cues. Inwood (1986) believes that using food as a reward affects the PWS student in at least two ways:

1. It reinforces the obsession with food.
2. It begins a behavioral pattern in which food is emotionally rewarding.

Since the availability of other, less harmful reinforcers is feasible, it is suggested that the teacher utilize a hierarchy of reinforcers to select others that are less harmful to the health of the PWS child, no matter how judiciously the food would be used.

Rotatori, Fox, and Switzky (1979) have developed a comprehensive reinforcement hierarchy based on those reinforcers used in public and private school programs for severely and profoundly mentally retarded individuals ages 3–50 and also on those reinforcers used with young children. A summary of their findings is given in Table 11.1, with the omission of food items. The comprehensiveness of this hierarchy should serve to assist the teacher in selecting a developmentally and age-appropriate reinforcer for his or her PWS student. Rotatori et al. pointed out that it is essential to avoid a mismatch between the child's motivational preferences and the reinforcement preferences provided by the educational program. They believe that a mismatch may interfere with learning. An unpublished study by Lupi and O'Neill (1985) supports the fact that PWS students can and do have an interest in reinforcers other than food. When asked to select their preference from a pair of reinforcers, which consisted of one food item and one age/sex-appropriate item (e.g., potato chips and nail polish), a group of adolescent PWS females always selected the nonfood item with the exception of diet soda. This same group of females also chose a nonfood activity over food when the two were paired (e.g., cookie and calling your friend).

These findings, although done on a limited sample ($N = 12$), do point out that PWS students can have age/sex-appropriate preferences that may supercede the need to use food as a reinforcer for learning.

Behavior Management

The PWS child is likely to display a variety of inappropriate and even antisocial behaviors. The literature indicates that many of the behaviors are

TABLE 11.1. A summary of a reinforcement hierarchy (omitting food items).

Category	Examples
Drinking	Water, milk, diet soda, coffee, tea, lemonade
Listening to	Radio, television, tape, records, instruments
Looking at	Shiny objects, films, magazines, cards, slides
Playing with/in/on	Puzzles, sandbox, puppets, blocks, clay, soap suds, toys, balloons
Academic activities	Coloring book, running errands, painting, reading, writing
Home living chore activities	Watering plants, wiping tables, washing board, sweeping floor
Touching/feeling of	Wet sponges, pet animals, fur, squeeze toys, moisture cream, pat on back
Social	Verbal praise, hug, tickling, kiss, smiling, shaking hands, applause
Smelling of	Perfume, aftershave, lotion

Note: From "An Indirect Technique for Establishing Preferences for Categories for Reinforcement for Severely and Profoundly Retarded Individuals" by A. Rotatori et al., 1979, *Perceptual and Motor Skills*, *48*, 1307–1313. Adapted by permission.

food related (Cassidy, 1984). Although the relationship between food acquisition and undesirable behavior has not been empirically demonstrated, any teacher of a PWS child will certainly encounter tantrums and outbursts. These are likely to be short but intense (Lupi & Porcella, 1987). Behaviors such as biting, scratching, and the throwing of classroom objects necessitate the teacher taking decisive action to protect both the involved student and others. The teacher may be forced by the intensity of the outburst to intervene physically, presenting the obvious need for training in humane, effective intervention strategies. It has been observed that these behaviors tend to be of short duration, supporting the contention that the PWS student must be encouraged to continue with the class routine immediately following an outburst.

It is believed that tantrums often begin because the PWS student has difficulty in expressing fears, confusion, and frustration. Inwood (1986) suggested working on the affective domain of the student, that is, helping the student to identify what makes him or her sad, mad, happy, frustrated, and so on. It might be helpful if the teacher provides the student with some constructive coping strategies such as progressive relaxation or talking over problems. Also suggested are walking, an activity the student enjoys, or a quiet influence such as a soft record.

Management of the PWS child's tendency toward somnolence (sleepiness) beginning during the middle years also requires the teacher's attention and planning. The teacher should attempt to plan activities that do not require the youngster to remain seated for long periods. By varying the classroom schedule to include both in-seat and out-of-seat activities, this

TABLE 11.2. Two examples of consequences for inappropriate behaviors displayed by a 13-year-old PWS male.

Inappropriate behavior	Consequence
Foraging for food	Each time he is found looking in garbage pails for food, D will be asked to empty pail, bag garbage, and scrub can with disinfectant. (*overcorrection*)
Lying	Each time D is caught in a lie, he will lose 2 points from the token economy system. (*response cost*)

may be accomplished easily. In more severe cases, the child should be allowed to get up occasionally and stretch (Lupi & Porcella, 1987).

Some of the more severe behaviors associated with the syndrome, such as skin picking and scratching as reported by Holm (1981) and well supported by classroom observation (Lupi & Porcella, 1987), can be reduced by utilizing a variety of behavior intervention strategies. Techniques of increasing behavior such as behavior shaping, behavior chaining, prompts, contingency contracting, and token economy systems are all recommended as effective behavior modification strategies (Alberto & Troutman, 1985) (See Table 11.2). In addition, techniques to decrease behavior (i.e., skin picking) may be needed to help manage classroom behavior. Alberto and Troutman (1985) provided a detailed guide of such strategies in their textbook. Strategies discussed include differential reinforcement (DRO, DRL, DRI), extinction, removal of desirable stimuli (response cost, time-outs), and principles of overcorrection.

Behavior management of the student with PWS should be viewed by the teacher as part of the child's IEP. Annual goals and short-term objectives should be written into the IEP document to assist the teacher in planning appropriately for the child. Techniques to decrease behavior need constant monitoring and should be done in conjunction with a clinical team.

Ongoing Communication with Parents and Other School Personnel

Because so little has been written or is available to teachers and school personnel on PWS, the parents' role in assisting the school to accommodate their child is valuable. Parents should be viewed as a resource and support system. Teachers should understand, however, that raising a child with PWS is an arduous task that places an enormous strain on the family.

It is recommended that teachers and other school personnel make every effort to develop a positive family-professional relationship. Since most parents appreciate receiving information about their child's progress, the

Date: Nov. 3

Time: 2:20 PM

Purpose:

Just wanted to let you know that Marla worked on a "nutrition tree" with her classmates today. She planned a "school menu" within her calorie allowance. I am very pleased!

Yours truly,

Ms. J. Bennett

FIGURE 11.1. Sample occasional message to parents.

TO: ______ Mr. Smith, Art Teacher

______ Dr. Sandler, Psychologist

✓ Mrs. Murphy, Lunchroom

FROM: Ms. Jenkins

RE: Sally Rogus

Please be advised that Sally is allowed to bring the following foods into the classroom daily:

carrot sticks
lettuce
diet soda

FIGURE 11.2. Sample in-school occasional message.

teacher should make every attempt to communicate with parents and/or family members.

A variety of methods exist to accomplish this goal. They include handouts, newsletters, telephone calls, daily/weekly progress reports and letters, notes, logbooks and messages (Turnbull & Turnbull, 1986). Figure 11.1 presents a sample occasional message to parents. Whichever way a teacher chooses, ongoing communication is critical if the PWS child's weight and general health are to be maintained.

Other school personnel also need to be contacted on a regular basis. For example, psychologists, the school nurse, unit teachers, and cafeteria monitors need to be constantly apprised of the PWS student's academic, social, emotional, and medical status. Figure 11.2 presents a sample of an in-school occasional message.

Communication between all those responsible for the education and life of the PWS student can thus be seen as an important role for the teacher. Effective communication will be of great assistance in the daily management of the child with PWS.

Summary

The education of the child with PWS in the public school setting is guaranteed by PL 94–142 and must be viewed by educators as both a challenge and a responsibility. Although students with PWS can be warm and friendly, they also present unique problems associated with the syndrome. These behaviors may require that teachers and school personnel consistently plan to effectively structure the classroom and school environment to maximize learning. The opportunity for both teacher and PWS student to enjoy the school experience rests on the school's ability to manipulate the environment to provide a safe educational milieu.

References

Alberto, P., & Troutman, A.C. (1985). *Applied behavioral analysis for teachers*. Columbus, OH: Charles E. Merrill.

Ayres, H.J. (1979). *Sensory integration and the child* (p. 95). Los Angeles: Western Psychological Services.

Caldwell, M.L., & Tayler, R.L. (1983). A clinical note on food preference of individuals with Prader-Willi syndrome: The need for empirical research. *Journal of Mental Deficiency Research*, *27*, 45–49.

Cassidy, S.B. (1984). Prader Willi syndrome. *Current Problems in Pediatrics*, *15*, 1–53.

Education for all handicapped Children Act of 1975, 20 U.S.C. §1400–1420 (1983).

Heiman, M.F. (1978). The management of obesity in the post adolescent developmentally disabled client with Prader-Willi syndrome. *Adolescence*, *13*, 291–296.

Holm, V.A. (1981). The diagnosis of Prader-Willi syndrome. In V.A. Holm, S.J. Sulzbacher, & P.L. Pipes (Eds.), *The Prader-Willi syndrome* (pp. 27–44). Baltimore: University Park Press.

Inwood, S. (1986). *Food and the Prader-Willi child in school.* Unpublished manuscript.

Lupi, M. (1986). A new kind of learning disorder. *Academic Therapy*, *21*(3), 353–355.

Lupi, M., & O'Neill (1985). Food items vs. age-appropriate non-food items as preferred reinforcers in Prader-Willi students. Unpublished manuscript.

Lupi, M., & Porcella, J. (1985). *Prader-Willi syndrome: A fact sheet for teachers and other school personnel.* (Available from Dr. M.H. Lupi, Hunter College, 695 Park Avenue, New York, NY 10021.)

Lupi, M., & Porcella, J. (1987). Some considerations in the education and management of the child with Prader-Willi syndrome in the special education classroom. *Techniques*, *3*, 230–235.

Neason, S. (1978). *Prader-Willi syndrome: A handbook for parents.* Longlake, MN: Prader-Willi Syndrome Association.

Otto, P.L., Sulzbacher, S.J., & Worthington-Roberts, B.S. (1982). Sucrose-induced behavior changes of persons with Prader-Willi syndrome. *American Journal of Mental Deficiency*, *86*, 335–341.

Rotatori, A., Fox, B., & Switzky, H. (1979). An indirect technique for establishing preferences for categories for reinforcement for severely and profoundly retarded individuals. *Perceptual and Motor Skills*, *48*, 1307–1313.

Seltzer, E. (1985). *Prader-Willi syndrome: A plea for policy.* Research report prepared for Assemblyman R.A. Straniere. Albany, NY: Author.

Sulzbacher, S., Crnic, KA., & Snow, J. (1981). Behavioral and cognitive disabilities in Prader-Willi syndrome. In V.A. Holm, S.J. Sulzbacher, & P.L. Pipes (Eds.), *The Prader-Willi syndrome* (pp. 147–160). Baltimore: University Park Press.

Turnbull, A., & Turnbull, H.R. (1986). *Families, professionals and exceptionality: A special partnership* (pp. 155–164). Columbus: Merrill Publishing Co.

Vitello, S.J. (1986). The Tatro case: Who gets what and why. *Exceptional Children*, *52*(4), 353–356.

Warren, H.L., & Hunt, E. (1981). Cognitive processing is children with Prader-Willi Syndrome. In V.A. Holm, S.J. Sulzbacher, & P.L. Pipes (Eds.), *The Prader-Willi syndrome* (pp. 161–178). Baltimore: University Park Press.

12
Speech and Language Development

JOYCE A. MUNSON-DAVIS

Communication development is the specific domain of the speech-language pathologist on the interdisciplinary team. However, communication is essential in all areas of an individual's daily life. Therefore, the speech-language pathologist works closely with other members of the team to determine functional communication needs, develop an appropriate habilitation program, and incorporate speech and language goals into daily activities. In working with the child with Prader-Willi syndrome (PWS), consultation with team members, such as the occupational therapist, audiologist, pediatric nurse-practitioner, and psychologist, is particularly important. Visual-motor abilities, hearing sensitivity, auditory processing, visual acuity, and cognitive limitations can all affect communication development, as well as the child's test performance.

Although the diagnosis of PWS has usually been made prior to the child's first being evaluated by a speech-language pathologist, the effects of the disorder may have direct impact upon the child's communication development. In infancy, the severe hypotonia characteristic of PWS babies results in feeding and respiratory problems. This same hypotonic musculature is needed for speech production—a task that requires precise coordination of movements of the articulators, oral-nasal resonance cavities, larynx (voice box), and lungs. In addition to problems affecting speech acquisition, visual-motor difficulties, auditory processing problems, and cognitive limitations may be present, affecting language comprehension and expression. Each of these factors must be considered, singly and in combination, in order to accurately evaluate the individual's current communication status, and to set appropriate goals for speech and language development.

A baseline evaluation of all aspects of communication abilities is important, with periodic reevaluation of rate and pattern of speech and language development. Reevaluation of the preschool and elementary-age child is essential. Oral-facial anomalies and neuromotor impairment affecting speech may become more apparent over time, despite general improvement in overall body tone. Because the PWS infant has difficulty reaching out to his or her environment and those in it, he or she may initially appear to be more intellectually limited than is the case. More comprehensive evaluation of cognitive and receptive language skills may be possible as hypotonia decreases and the child can better explore his or her environment and exhibit developmental readiness for objective testing.

Speech Concerns

When most persons think of speech, articulation skills (speech sound production accuracy) probably first come to mind. Articulation problems are still those most commonly associated with speech-language services in the schools. Misarticulations are, in fact, the most frequently encountered problem in children with PWS (Bransen, 1981; Siegel-Sadewitz & Shprintzen, 1982), and may persist into adulthood (Kolar & Johnson, 1984). Articulation development normally follows a general sequence in children, with sounds such as /p/ and /b/, for example, occurring much earlier than sounds such as /r/, /l/, and /s/. These patterns occur because /p/ and /b/ are physically easier to produce. As oral-motor control develops, the more difficult /r/, /l/, and /s/ are possible. Because hypotonia is generally more severe in the very young child with PWS, delays in speech development are common. In addition to articulation, the low muscle tone seen throughout the body may affect other aspects of speech production, including voice quality and usage, and resonance patterns.

Articulation Problems

A narrow overjet and a high, narrow, arched palate are part of the midline central nervous system anomalies that commonly occur in PWS. These anomalies may contribute to problems in speech sound acquisition and development of intelligible connected speech. Movement of the articulators—lips, jaw, soft palate, and tongue—is also slow and frequently imprecise as a result of hypotonia of the oral musculature. With the combination of oral anomalies and hypotonia, the child may have difficulty building sufficient intraoral pressure to adequately produce many of the consonant sounds.

The most classic oral features in PWS are a bow-shaped mouth, micrognathia (small lower jaw), and high, narrow palate (Dyken & Miller, 1980). The short upper lip and recessive jaw may impede lip closure, resulting in the child's producing sounds such as /p/, /b/, and /m/ with his or her upper teeth on the bottom lip. This pattern may become quite pronounced over time, exacerbating the narrow overbite. Tongue-tip movements may be performed with the entire tongue blade, and difficulties in executing tongue movements commonly persist into adulthood (Kolar & Johnson, 1984). The narrow arching of the palate and failure of the palate and pharyngeal walls to function properly can also interfere with articulation as well as other aspects of speech production.

Analyzing the child's articulation can provide important information as to whether normal, delayed, or deviant patterns of speech sound development are occurring. Occasionally, other factors may be suspected if speech sound development is severely impaired and oral structural and neuromotor impairment do not seem sufficient to account for the extent of dysfunction. For example, developmental apraxia of speech (a motor-planning problem) may result in severely limited consonant and vowel variety and inconsistent sound usage. Bransen (1981) reported apraxia in two of three children with PWS who exhibited severe articulation deficits.

In addition to evaluating the child's ability to produce sounds in isolation, in syllables, and in single words, *connected* speech should be assessed whenever possible since intelligibility in connected speech may be quite different from articulation accuracy in single words. Because of increased demands for coordinated movements among the respiratory, laryngeal, resonance, and articulatory systems, problems may become more evident as the child attempts to combine words into phrases and short sentences.

Voice and Resonance Deviations

Problems in voice quality and usage may include weak speaking volume, high pitch usage, breathy and/or hoarse vocal quality, faulty phrasing and timing, and problems in stress and inflection of running speech. Constant or intermittent nasal emission on pressure sounds and an overall quality of hypernasality may be particularly noticeable. Improved voice characteristics may be obvious when the child is seated in a stable, upright position, with good foot, upper extremity, and trunk support. More noticeable problems in voice and connected speech may be apparent during ambulation efforts or when the child is engaged in other competing motor tasks. These problems are directly related to the child's hypotonia, and can be expected to be more pronounced when oral-facial anomalies are present. Difficulties in lip closure and a high, arched palate may prevent adequate velopharyngeal closure (contact of the soft palate with the lateral and posterior pharyngeal walls of the mouth), particularly when muscle tone is low and slows movement. Results will be greater problems with excessive nasal resonance and difficulty in maintaining an adequate breath stream for speech because of loss of air through the nose.

As in other syndromes and neuromotor disorders causing oral structural and mobility problems, the child with PWS is at risk for increased problems with nasal resonance if the adenoids are removed. For that reason, further evaluation of palatal function by an experienced otolaryngologist is recommended if an adenoidectomy is ever considered in conjunction with a tonsillectomy or tympanostomy tube placement for middle ear problems. Because lateral still X-rays reveal velar length but do not demonstrate function, fluoroscopy (running X-rays during speech) may be advised. However, fluoroscopy of the anterior-posterior dimension alone is also limited, since information is not provided regarding mesial movement of the lateral pharyngeal walls. With a very narrow palate and hypotonia of the musculature, adequate contact may occur in the anterior-posterior plane with leakage still occurring at the sides of the velum.

Management

For the child with marginal speech, therapy may be successful in developing acceptable oral communication skills. Initial goals should include working on sounds easiest for the child to produce in functional words. The whole-word approach is usually emphasized since it helps the child to develop a vocabulary base that will be useful in the classroom, at play, and in the home, and may help to motivate him or her to work harder at communication. Incorporating techniques from physical and/or occupational therapy goals for improving overall muscle tone may also assist in improving speech in the child with marginal skills (see Chapter 13).

In cases of severe articulation limitations accompanied by marked nasal emission and hypernasal resonance, traditional habilitation methods may not be sufficient to achieve adequate speech production. Referral to an oral surgeon and/or prosthodontist is indicated when palatal dysfunction appears to be the primary deterrent to speech development. Pharyngeal flap surgery or construction of a palatal prosthesis may be recommended, depending on evaluation findings and preferences of the professionals involved. Because of possibilities of tissue breakdown and continued nasal emission laterally, pharyngeal flap surgery may have disappointing results in the child with PWS. Although wearing of a palatal prosthesis involves periodic enlargement or replacement, motivation on the part of the child to consistently wear the appliance, and the ability to care for it properly, it usually will be the method of choice.

A multi-modality approach may be particularly helpful with the child suspected of having Developmental Apraxia of Speech (DAS). Because the child is thought to experience problems in sensory input, difficulties occur in processing, organizing and planning the motor movements necessary for intelligible speech production (Edwards, 1973). Multi-modality habilitation provides input via all sensory channels to compensate for deficits that may be present, particularly in auditory discrimination and proprioceptive feedback. Visual and tactile cues, such as mirror work and the clinician's manually manipulating the articulators, may lead to establishing the motor patterns necessary to develop a variety of speech sounds and sound combinations that can be shaped into functional expressive vocabulary (Lohr, 1978). Graphic representations, such as comparisons of "*b*oy" and "*t*oy," have also been successful in developing awareness of speech sound differences in words, even with young non-reading children.

In cases when intelligible speech does not develop adequately, even with concentrated habilitation efforts, alternative forms of communication will need to be considered.

Language Problems

Simply put, language involves the ability to understand ideas expressed by others and to express oneself. Most communication takes place through listening and speaking, although nonverbal cues also play an important role in communication. In individuals with PWS, a wide range of language abilities are found, related to a variety of factors.

Language Comprehension

In general, understanding of language is closely related to one's cognitive abilities. Because mental retardation is frequently associated with PWS, language comprehension will usually be impaired to a certain degree. Cognitive abilities in the individual with PWS vary markedly, however, with IQs ranging from severe retardation to normal skills (Smith, 1983). Language skills in the PWS population are much more heterogeneous than speech abilities, both in children and in adults (Bransen, 1981; Kolar & Johnson, 1984). Bransen found receptive language abilities commensurate with cognition in approximately half of a group of 11 children with PWS, with a comprehension-production discrepancy in 3 of the children. In the adult group tested by Kolar and Johnson, intelligence appeared to be more of "a regulating factor in language performance" than it was for a comparison group of children.

Caution is important in assuming an automatic degree of delay in understanding, particularly with the young child who initially may appear much more cognitively limited than is actually the case. Severe hypotonia contributes to a somewhat "flat" affect in the child with PWS, and facial expressions may be quite depressed, leading to an impression of dullness. Motor delays secondary to the hypotonia also prevent the young child from exploring and learning from the environment in the same manner that the normal infant does. Therefore, special efforts may be needed to provide appropriate stimulation for learning, as is suggested with other children with severe hypotonia (Blackman, 1984).

Hypotonia and motor deficits may also interfere with the preschool-age child's carrying out directions, either in a play environment or objective testing situation. Of course, knowledge of the child's visual acuity and auditory sensitivity are critical prior to testing. Because of the incidence of visual-motor deficits in the PWS population, consultation with the occupational therapist is particularly important. It will frequently be necessary to find alternative ways for the child to respond and to adapt test materials to compensate for poor body posture and balance and fine motor difficulties in order to achieve optimal results.

Expressive Language

The child with PWS may have difficulty in expressing ideas for several reasons. For many children, expressive language may be delayed to the same degree as cognitive skills and receptive abilities. However, expressive language may be significantly more impaired than might be expected for a given developmental level if marked oral-facial anomalies and hypotonicity are present, severely affecting speech abilities. As muscle tone improves, which is the general case, articulation accuracy and normal voice and reasonance patterns may be possible, allowing expressive language to grow concurrently. In cases in which oral structures become more deviant with growth and hypotonicity continues to affect the speech musculature, an increasing discrepancy between language comprehension and expressive abilities will usually become apparent. Specific habilitation to develop compensatory techniques in speech production may be required.

In addition to expressive problems related to speech difficulties, deficits in word retention and recall, grammatical errors, and poor sentence structure may occur and continue into adulthood (Kolar & Johnson, 1984). These problems may be related to short-term memory limitations, which are frequently encountered in persons with PWS (Warren & Hunt, 1981). Deficits in pragmatics—awareness of socially appropriate behavior in communication interactions—may also be a problem, particularly in the older child and adolescent. Learning about turn-taking and topic maintenance may be needed to assist in both classroom performance and social interactions. Knowing when it is appropriate to say something and how to say it may become increasingly greater needs, and may become goals in a program jointly managed by teacher, psychologist, speech-language pathologist, and/or social worker (see Chapter 16).

For the child whose speech problem is so severe that it prohibits adequate oral expressive language, an augmentative communication system may be needed to aid communication in the classroom, family discussions, and peer interactions. Many parents and professionals fear that pursual of communication modalities other than speech will interfere with further oral communication development. However, in developing augmentative communication techniques, goals for speech improvement are not set aside, but maintained to the extent possible as a part of the individual's communication system. Rather than precluding further speech development, provision of a "backup" to oral communication frequently results in renewed efforts on the individual's part to speak.

Two types of augmentative communication are most frequently pursued: a "total communication" approach involving the use of manual sign language and speech, and the "language board" or "communication board."

Although either may enhance the child's communicative potential, problems are inherent in both approaches, particularly for the child with PWS.

Use of total communication involves the child's being able to execute manual signs clearly enough that they can be interpreted by others. Because of the hypotonia and accompanying fine motor delays common in PWS, the child may not be able to produce differentiated signs for many vocabulary words. However, if sign approximations are consistently produced, and especially if they are more intelligible than the child's speech efforts, total communication may be a viable option.

Communication boards containing photographs or colored drawings along with the printed word have a clear advantage in being easily understood by both the child's peers and adults. The need to have these augmentative materials always available can be a particular problem, however, for the child with PWS, who is struggling to be ambulatory and cannot easily transport excessive baggage. This problem can be alleviated somewhat in the home and school setting by having vocabulary available in the specific environments in which it is needed. "Miniboards" for clothing, toys, foods, colors, and the like can be developed and placed in strategic locations that the child can easily reach and/or brought out during specific classroom and home activities. Other adaptations may include small vocabulary cards on rings easily hooked to the child's belt, or a communication notebook.

For the older elementary-age child, adolescent, or adult with marginal oral communication abilities, a portable electronic augmentative communication device may be appropriate. Typing and computer use may also be important for academic and social written expression if handwriting is not sufficient.

Case Studies

The following cases are offered to depict the broad range of speech and language abilities and potential that occur among children with PWS.

AA (Birthdate 9/5/74)

All developmental milestones were markedly delayed, with AA first producing single words at 18 months. Optic hypoplasia was noted at an early age, but despite corrective lenses usable vision was limited to color discrimination and general shape perception. By age 6, articulation skills were normal for age, with misarticulations developmental rather than deviant in nature. Hypotonia was minimal by this age and did not impair articulation or voice in connected speech. Expressive language was also within normal limits by the time AA entered kindergarten, although some deficits were apparent in her comprehension of language, and she made inappropriate responses and comments. Further testing indicated that problems in visual perception, secondary to her limited visual acuity, were responsible for these deficits.

Recommendations were made for developing other modalities to compensate for AA's visual limitations, including capitalizing on her excellent auditory memory skills and developing increased tactile awareness. Individual work with a teacher for the visually impaired was begun in her local school program, with consultation to the regular classroom teacher for ideas in adapting tests and classroom materials. AA continues in a regular school program where she uses taped books for reading assignments and a tape recorder in place of written assignments and tests.

MM (Birthdate 5/1/80)

MM's language skills were at the 16-month level when she was first evaluated at 33 months of age. Speech sound development was judged commensurate with her language abilities at that time, and delays in communication were thought to be part of an overall developmental delay including cognitive, gross motor, and fine motor deficits.

Over the next several years, MM's language and speech development was closely monitored. Although language comprehension skills continued to develop at a rate of about one half of chronological age expectations, and MM was obviously trying to communicate in short sentences, speech intelligibility was relatively poor. Therapy was begun prior to her beginning school, with a total communication approach initiated. This communication system was encouraged both at home and at school, with MM's parents and sister learning signs as she acquired them.

A change in school placement last year also resulted in MM's being assigned to a new speech-language pathologist. This clinician believed that MM was relying too much on signs and gestures, and that oral communication should be more heavily emphasized. At her last visit to the PWS clinic, MM's parents were pleased with the gains in oral communication they perceived her to be making. Difficulties arose throughout the evaluation day, however, in the examiners' frequently being unable to understand her responses. In addition to continued misarticulation of consonants, vowel errors were frequent and inconsistencies in sound usage suggested an apraxic component to MM's speech problem. Interpretation by the parents was often necessary and sometimes unsuccessful, and MM showed little awareness of those times when she was not understood.

KK (Birthdate 2/10/76)

KK showed severe hypotonia at birth and had significant feeding problems for the first several months of life. When first evaluated at 9 months of age, his language age equivalency was only 3 months. KK was closely monitored in all developmental areas, and although progress was apparent on return visits to the PWS clinic, functioning remained at half or less of chronological age expectations in speech and language through age 3. Inconsistent attention and cooperation were frequent problems in trying to estimate progress, with reliance on parents' reporting usually necessary.

By age 3½, KK was able to cooperate for objective evaluation of language skills using a test instrument that separated comprehension abilities from verbal skills. Comprehension with this measure was found to be close to the 3-year level, whereas speech abilities remained severely limited and expressive language attempts were almost totally unintelligible. Words consisted of initial consonant sounds with nasalized vowels, and consonant variety was extremely limited. Connected speech attempts were markedly hypernasal with audible nasal emission, and KK could not consistently close his lips to produce bilabial sounds, had a narrow overbite, and a very high, vaulted palate. It was obvious that previous behavioral problems and KK's severe hypotonia had masked a large discrepancy between his receptive language abilities and his expressive skills.

Neither a palatal lift nor a pharyngeal flap was judged appropriate bacause of the marked impairment throughout the remainder of KK's oral mechanism. Because KK and his parents were beginning to experience frustration in trying to communicate, and because of the large gap between comprehension and verbal abilities, recommendations were made to begin a manual sign system in his preschool program to supplement his verbal attempts.

Despite consistent receptive language scores in the borderline to low-average range throughout the past several years, KK has been diagnosed as mildly mentally retarded by local school personnel. He has remained in a classroom for the trainable mentally retarded in order to receive the total communication program and individual attention that he needs. Although KK has made adequate gains in oral communication, frustration regarding his speech continues and personal-social interactions have become a primary problem. An augmentative communication notebook has been recommended in order that he may communicate with persons who do not understand his speech or manual sign. The hope is that KK can then be mainstreamed for certain classes with children at his level of understanding while continuing to receive the special services he needs.

Summary

Whatever the particular communication problem of a child with PWS, close consultation and cooperation by all members of the interdisciplinary team is essential for maximal skill development. Involving parents, siblings, and the child in developing goals is an important aspect of the interdisciplinary team process, and is especially critical for communication. By providing the child with PWS with as effective a communication system as possible, frustration may be potentially reduced and negative behavior replaced by more socially appropriate means of expression.

References

Blackman, J. (1984). The floppy infant. In Blackman, J. (Ed.), *Medical aspects of developmental disabilities in children birth to three* (pp. 111–114). Rockville: Aspen Publishers Inc.

Bransen, C. (1981). Speech and language characteristics of children with Prader-Willi syndrome. In V.A. Holm, S.J. Sulzbacher, & P.L. Pipes (Eds.), *The Prader Willi syndrome* (pp. 179–183) Baltimore: University Park Press.

Dyken, P.R., & Miller, M.D. (1980). *Facial features of neurologic syndromes* (pp. 138–154) St. Louis: C.V. Mosby.

Edwards, M. (1973). Developmental verbal dyspraxia. *British Journal of Disorders of Communication*, *8*, 64–70.

Kolar, E., & Johnson, M.G. (1984). *The speech and language characteristics of Prader-Willi adults.* Unpublished manuscript, Speech-Language-Hearing Clinic, Minneapolis, MN.

Lohr, F. (1978). The nonverbal apraxic child: Definition, evaluation, therapy. *Western Michigan University Journal of Speech, Language and Hearing, 15,* 3–6.

Siegel-Sadewitz, V., & Shprintzen, R.J. (1982). The relationship of communication disorders to syndrome indentification. *Journal of Speech and Hearing Disorders, 47*(4), 338–354.

Smith, D.W. (1983). *Recognizable patterns of human malformation* (3rd ed.) Philadelphia: W.B. Saunders.

Warren, J.L., & Hunt, E. (1981). Cognitive processing in children with Prader-Willi syndrome. In V.A. Holm, S.J. Sulzbacher, & P.L. Pipes (Eds.), *The Prader-Willi syndrome* (pp. 167–178). Baltimore: University Park Press.

13 Physical and Occupational Therapy for Prader-Willi Syndrome

MARY ALICE DUESTERHAUS MINOR and TRUE CARR

Professional physical therapists and occupational therapists are significant members of interdisciplinary teams who work with the developmentally disabled. Each retains his or her professional responsibility to evaluate clients and recommend therapeutic interventions unique to his or her discipline and at the same time contributes to the team process by collaborating with other professionals to establish diagnoses and plan and implement appropriate management strategies. The "interrelatedness" of the role of both the physical and occupational therapist is reflected in the goals and concerns they share. These include recognizing that children change over time; promoting gross and fine motor development; fostering interest in activities that promote weight management, optimum health, and work potential; achieving independence in daily living by encouraging pursuits that enhance self-esteem and creativity; and training and supporting parents/care providers.

Individuals with Prader-Willi syndrome (PWS) require physical and occupational therapeutic interventions beginning early in life; the efforts of these professionals to promote optimal motor development throughout these children's growth and development is essential. It should be pointed out that it is not unusual for physical and/or occupational therapists to provide services to unidentifed cases of PWS. The potential for these professionals to identify undiagnosed individuals should not be underestimated and, in many instances, they may be responsible for an initial referral for diagnostic clarification.

Typical Findings Associated with Physical Activity in PWS

Children with PWS typically are hypotonic. This low muscle tone interferes with normal progression through the developmental sequence of gross and fine motor skills. PWS children, although delayed in acquisition of normal motor milestones, may achieve independent ambulation, dressing, and self-care skills. In the infant and toddler stage, feeding difficulties due to the hypotonia and oral motor involvement may present significant problems. Affected children are prone to develop significant scoliosis, even at a very young age. School performance is influenced by sensorimotor integration or perceptual problems such as difficulties in motor planning, integrating the two sides of the body, and developing visual-perceptual skills. Poor overall gross motor performance and a preference for fine motor repetitive play is characteristic.

Therapeutic Interventions

Implications for Physical Therapists

Selection of physical therapy interventions for a PWS child is affected by the age of child and the presenting symptoms. Assessment should take into account cognitive and motor development, skeletal integrity, general and aerobic fitness, and sensory and perceptual function.

A variety of standardized assessments are available to evaluate and monitor development of gross and fine motor skills. At least until skeletal maturity is achieved, postural-skeletal assessment is very important. Muscle tone and range of motion are monitored using traditional methods. Such tests as the revised Gesell (Knobloch, Stevens, & Malone, 1980) and the Bayley (1969) are appropriate for the younger child. The Bruininks-Oseretsky Test of Motor Proficiency (Bruininks, 1978) can be used with older children. Necessary information can be obtained using observations of the child during free and directed play. Where appropriate, a step test or stress test can be included. The child must be able to follow directions and attend to the task in order to yield meaningful data. Consideration must be given to the child's cognitive capacity, his or her behavioral adjustment in the testing setting, and observations and impressions of how care providers handle the child.

An infant or young child who has feeding difficulties, low tone, and developmental delay requires a developmental evaluation. Such assessment determines:

1. Level of gross motor development
2. Status of feeding skills
3. Level of muscle tone
4. Status of skeletal system
5. Activity level of the child
6. Equipment needs for positioning and mobility

This information can be used to direct and instruct parents/care providers in how best to facilitate gross motor development, feeding skills, and activity levels. Feeding of infants in the hypotonic stage of PWS can be enhanced by varying sensory stimulation, type of equipment used, and the consistency of the food. However, *eating and food-related issues must be carefully considered in light of the PWS child's predictable development of an insatiable hunger drive.* Monitoring the skeletal system for indication of the development of scoliosis or other orthopedic problems is essential. Suggestions about the use of baby equipment such as baby walkers and strollers for mobility as well as proper positioning and handling of the child are part of the teaching process (Harris, 1984).

In addition to standardized tests that are used to indicate level and rate of motor development, motor control and movement patterns must be monitored. Hypotonia prevents development of good stability/co-contraction. Hypermobility of the joints may accompany low muscle tone. Hypermobile joints also make attainment of stability/co-contraction difficult. When stability/co-contraction is delayed, abnormal movement patterns often develop to compensate. The child needs to develop stability/co-contraction of the trunk, shoulder girdle, and pelvic girdle followed by weight-shifting and truck rotation in order to progress through the developmental sequences of gross and fine motor skills (Sullivan, Markos, & Minor, 1982). Motor control and movement patterns are assessed by observation and manipulation of the child to elicit stability/co-contraction, weight shifting, trunk rotation, and skilled activity (Minor & Minor, 1985).

Physical therapy assessment of preadolescents with PWS is important not only for parents/care providers but also to provide essential information to school personnel. Determination of the status of the skeletal system, girth measurements, aerobic and general fitness, activity levels, and gross motor development is critical to establishment of activities, goals, and expectations for performance. The PWS child who has any associated sensorimotor integration or perceptual problems such as difficulties in depth perception or kinesthesia requires careful management. If a child spends most free time in fine motor play, such as coloring, reading, or writing, decreased integration of the two sides of the body may prevent crossing of the midline. Care providers and teachers should encourage involvement in gross motor activities such as tricycle riding or playing with a ball. The child with perceptual motor problems may need more supervision when engaged in gross motor play and may have more difficulty with associated tasks. For example, depth perception difficulties may cause him or her to trip frequently. Negotiating playground equipment and/or games may be frustrating.

The school-age child with PWS should not be excluded from participation in physical education classes unless a valid health concern exists. In fact, physical education classes can reinforce the use of gross motor play for the development of skills, weight management, and wellness. The therapist is a resource person for the physical education and classroom teachers regarding activities that promote motor skills and wellness. Games and sports that encourage motor and perceptual skill development are generally more beneficial than strengthening through progressive resistive exercise.

Suggestions for modification in the classroom include chairs that provide back support and are of appropriate height (hip and knee angle of 90° with feet resting on the floor). Desk or table tops should be at elbow height, keeping in mind that PWS children are typically very short. Often an easeled work surface is an easier and less fatiguing work space.

By late childhood regular exercise should be included in the child's weekly routine for general fitness and weight management (Carmen, 1981). Walking, tricycle or stationary bike riding, swimming, and low-impact aerobics classes are appropriate. It has been reported that the knee joints of individuals with PWS are not protected well enough to allow jumping or twisting exercises, jogging, or any other high-impact activities (M. Wett, personal communication, the Prader-Willi Syndrome Association, Edina, MN, 1987). Supervision is usually necessary, but with encouragement, PWS children can learn to take their own pulse readings.

Evaluation of adolescents and young adults with PWS is essentially the same as for preadolescents. The older individual may be able to complete the stress test and may be capable of assuming responsibility for selecting and carrying out exercise and activity programs. One important consideration in all such assessment is the cognitive capacity of the individual.

Implications for Occupational Therapists

Typical assessment and intervention procedures for occupational therapy for children with PWS are compiled on the basis of the degree of developmental delay evidenced. In initial evaluation, the subjective and objective tests used are determined by the child's age, developmental history, and presenting problems. Children with PWS might be expected to have difficulties in sensoimotor areas that include:

1. Low muscle tone
2. Diminished balance
3. Low energy postures and movement patterns
4. Depressed use of arms for postural support
5. Depressed endurance in antigravity postures
6. Poor trunk rotation and weight shifting with lack of differentiation of shoulder and hip girdles
7. Weak proximal musculature
8. Predominance of external rotation and abduction
9. Scoliosis
10. Visual-motor defects
11. Diminished fine motor dexterity and proficiency
12. Postural insecurity
13. Poor bilateral integration

Several standardized and nonstandardized developmental tools are used to establish age-equivalent scores and functional levels. (The Beery Developmental Test of Visual-Motor Integration [1967], Goodenough Draw-A-Person [1927], and Motor Free Visual Perception [Colarusso & Hamill, 1972] tests are easily administered and reliable; an annotated list of these evaluation tools can be found in Appendix D, Section 1.) Such tests also indicate strengths and problems, knowledge of which is invaluable when planning activities for the individual child. For example, when the PWS child indicates interest, or is developmentally ready, strategies can be offered that promote independence in self-care, such as dressing. Expecting a child to master donning and removing all clothing simultaneously may be unrealistic, but he or she may be able to learn to remove one piece at a time. Fastenings on apparel can be difficult to manage, and initially pull-on pants may be easier than those with zippers, buttons, or snaps. Use of large buttons before small ones is best; snaps make take a very long time to master because of the strength required (PWS children tend to have muscle weakness). Pull-on tops can be very difficult for children with perceptual problems.

Recommendations for school activities are based on evaluation of fine, sensory, and perceptual motor skills, hand/arm function, and visual motor perception. Appropriate activities are suggested that will help the child adapt in the work-play environment. The focus of these activities is two-fold: first, to improve postural tone, co-contractions of trunk, shoulder girdle, and pelvic girdle, and joint stability; and second, to incorporate activities that call for bilateral hand use. The school-age child's perceptual abilities influence educational progress. School physical activities should focus on development of weight shifting and trunk rotation in a variety of postures such as prone, hands-knees, kneeling, sitting, and standing. Movement into and out of a variety of postures should be encouraged. These activities also can enhance perceptual-motor integration and can be achieved through noncompetitive activities such as Follow-The-Leader.

Parents and teachers should be aware of the PWS child's tendency to gravitate to preferred fine motor tasks, which, in turn, encourages low-energy postures, the potential for perseveration, and rote repetition. Fine motor play using puzzles and board games can be modified by varying the location of the board in space, having the child reach for pieces with alternating hands, and varying the location of the game pieces as well. Movement-based interventions are essential and require ongoing supervision and monitoring by the occupational therapist. Teachers who carry out motor programs need to be aware of the importance of quality of posture and control in order to facilitate normal movement patterns and avoid compensated postures. Several activity protocols are identified in Appendix D, Sections 2–6.

Prevocational Assessment and Planning

When the child with PWS reaches high school age, prevocational assessment can provide the foundation for vocational training for employment once the formal educational process is completed. A good resource for such an assessment is the occupational therapist, whose previous working relationship, experience, and familiarity with PWS will be very beneficial. Areas to consider in assessment of prevocational skills include posture and movement, hand/arm use (strength, speed, precision, coordination, and dexterity), positioning, and work habits.

Children with PWS have the postural and movement characteristics typical of children diagnosed as hypotonic. Low trunk tone with poor stability of the pelvic and shoulder girdles is noted, as well as diminished co-contractions of the trunk musculature and lack of weight shift and trunk rotation on a stable pelvis. When assessing endurance for static activities, the presence of low trunk tone with poor postural stability may contribute to early fatigue.

As with other types of hypotonia, individuals with PWS generally utilize low-energy postures and developmentally immature movement patterns of arms and hands. This underlying hypotonia and delay in developing good trunk, hip, and shoulder stability as well as diminished trunk rotation mean a lack of a solid base of support for precise hand and arm use. PWS children tend to utilize immature, less efficient movement patterns that are neither well differentiated nor well localized. They prefer whole hand/arm patterns, which tends to decrease the speed, precision, and dexterity necessary for fine motor manipulation tasks. Correct positioning for fine motor tasks is an important aspect of prevocational and vocational programming. For tasks that involve sitting, chair height should permit feet to rest flat on the floor with hips to the back of the chair. A chair with a low back might be preferred and the work surface should be at elbow height to permit ease of hand/arm movement. When standing, work surfaces should also be at elbow (waist) height. Proper attention to positioning will promote better posture and potentially decrease postural fatigue.

Specific prevocational evaluations recommended include: 1) upper extremity range of motion, especially shoulder girdle rotation and forearm supination; 2) upper extremity strength, including strength of gross grasp (this can be accurately measured by a dynamometer); and 3) speed, precision, and hand dexterity, as well as bilateral hand/arm use. The recommended test to assess these areas is the Jebsen Developmental Test of Hand Function (Jebsen, Taylor, Treishmann, Trotter, & Howard, 1969), which evaluates broad aspects of functions commonly used in everyday activities. The tasks are standardized and normed for ages 6 through 19 years and may be administered in a short period of time using readily available materials.

Earlier in this chapter, it was suggested that physical therapy assessment include the Bruininks-Oseretsky Test of Motor Proficiency (BOMP). This evaluation instrument is also recommended for use by occupational therapists, particularly for fine motor assessment. Three subtests evaluate speed of response to a moving visual stimulus, visual motor control, and upper limb speed and dexterity. Although not as quick or as easily administered as the Jebsen, the BOMP does yield a composite score and percentile rank as well as age-equivalent scores. Both tests may be used to identify specific areas of strength and weakness.

Clinical observations that can be made during testing include:

1. Sitting posture
2. Ability to understand and follow instructions
3. Work habits
4. Developmental movement patterns, including trunk rotation and weight shift
5. Precision of hand-arm use
6. Ability to cross the body midline
7. Control and grading of movement
8. Postural control and stability during movement

In helping with work-study planning, the occupational therapist can provide invaluable assistance to teachers and vocational training personnel by evaluating the above motor functions, by developing work simplification techniques based on knowledge of fine motor strengths and weaknesses, and by consulting about optimal positioning and use of proper body mechanics.

Conclusions

Physical and occupational therapists may see children with PWS prior to their having been diagnosed. In these instances, they may be responsible for the initial referral for diagnostic clarification. Focus of concern about newborns and young children with PWS is on feeding problems and lack of progress through the normal developmental milestones. Therapeutic interventions incorporate strategies that promote motor development within the everyday routine of the child and his or her family (strategies are the same as those used with all hypotonic children). For older children, emphasis is placed on encouraging gross motor activity and independence in daily living. Individual therapeutic strategies and collaborative efforts can maximize the physical potential of individuals with PWS and enhance their capacity for integration into vocational programs.

References

Bayley, N. (1969). *Bayley Scales of Infant Development*. New York: Psychological Corporation.

Beery, K.E. (1967). *Developmental Test of Visual-Motor Integration: Administration and scoring manual*. Chicago: Follett Publishing Company.

Bruininks, R.H. (1978). *Bruininks-Oseretsky Test of Motor Proficiency*. Circle Pines, MN: American Guidance Service, Inc.

Carmen, P. (1981). Physical exercise for children and adults with Prader-Willi syndrome. In V.A. Holm, S.J. Sulzbacher, & P.L. Pipes (Eds.), *The Prader-Willi Syndrome* (pp. 299-311). University Park Press, Baltimore.

Colarusso, R., & Hamill, D. (1972). *Motor Free Visual Perception Test*. Los Angeles: Western Psychological Service.

Goodenough, F. (1926). *Children's drawings (measurement of intelligence by drawings)*. Downey, CA: Rancho Los Amigos Hospital.

Harris, S. (1984). Down syndrome (clinics in physical therapy). In S. Campbell (Ed.), *Pediatric neurological physical therapy* (pp. 169–204). New York: Churchill Livingstone.

Jebsen, R., Taylor, N., Trieshmann, R., Trotter, M., & Howard, L. (1969). Objective and standardized test of hand function. *Archives of Physical Medicine and Rehabilitation*, *50*, 311–319.

Knobloch, H., Stevens, F., & Malone, A. (1980). *Manual of developmental diagnosis: The administration and interpretation of the Revised Gesell and Armtruda Developmental and Neurological Examination*. Hagerstown, MD: Harper & Row.

Minor, M., & Minor, S.D. (1985). *Patient evaluation methods for the health professional*. Reston, VA: Reston Publishing Co.

Sullivan, P., Markos, P., Minor, M.A. (1982). *An integrated approach to therapeutic exercise theory and clinical application*. Reston, VA: Reston Publishing Co.

14 Vocational Concepts in Prader-Willi Syndrome

JAMES TIMOTHY INWOOD

Vocational training and rehabilitation is an area of service that has increasing relevance as the Prader-Willi syndrome (PWS) population grows older. In the past most PWS individuals were not expected to reach adulthood, so the concept of vocational rehabilitation (e.g., preparation for the world of work) seemed a remote consideration. However, advances in effective nutritional management have led to an extended life span. Now, once formal education is over, the process of vocational counseling, evaluation of skill levels, vocational education, work adjustment training, and appropriate work placement is of paramount concern.

General Considerations

It is not the intent of this discussion to review concepts of rehabilitation in depth, but rather to explore briefly those areas that directly affect the PWS population, specifically, vocational services.

Rehabilitation means implementing realistic methods of coping while understanding that the presence of one or more problems in the same person usually compounds the task of adjustment. If rehabilitation is to be a reality, the concept "cannot be separated from the environmental factors associated with the needs of these adults past, present, or future" (Andrew, 1981, p. 225). The rehabilitation process helps disabled adults meet the demands of life, and it is essential that the general public understand the scope of physical and psychosocial problems posed by the handicapping condition.

Significant Legislation

It is abundantly clear that laws exist to serve and protect the disabled population. Briefly, federal legislation passed between 1943 and 1978 focused on: 1) developing services for mildly retarded adults in their home communities; 2) improving the delivery of services by funding workshops, research, and development grants; and 3) providing guidelines for enhancing the role of the professional. The Vocational Rehabilitation Act of 1943 (PL 78–113) acknowledged that mentally disabled persons were entitled to funds and services. The next 10 years saw the expansion of humanistic, sociocultural aspects of care. By 1966, the act had been amended (PL 89-333) to enlarge the target population and at the same time eliminated economic need as a criterion for federal funding. Two terms used in the legislation are particularly important: eligibility and feasibility. *Eligibility* for services requires: 1) the presence of a physical or mental disability that can be documented by a physician, 2) that the disability must represent a substantial handicap to employment, and 3), that there must be reasonable expectation that services will render the client employable. *Feasibility* refers to the fact that employment should be available in the area for which the person has been vocationally prepared (R. Roberts, Lecture and class discussion, 1982), and that the individual is able and willing to cooperate with an established program. The Rehabilitation Act of 1973 (PL 93-112) mandated the use of individualized written rehabilitation plans (IWRPs) to set realistic, contractual goals and encourage the accountability of service providers.

Unfortunately, there is still quite a discrepancy between what has been legislated and the conscientious delivery of these services within the individual states and local communities. Enactment of laws is not an end in itself, and too often the individual family entitled to care remains uninformed and underserved.

Vocational Concepts

Although the term "rehabilitation" broadly addresses the effects of a disability on the total person, vocational rehabilitation speaks specifically to "the relationship between the world of work and people who have a physical or mental handicap" (Daniels, 1981, p. 169). The goals of vocational rehabilitation are to evaluate and assist in planning services with the individual, to work closely with families (since they too are affected), to coordinate community resources, and to act as liaison between the disabled person and the community.

It appears that most mentally disabled adults are employed or being trained in a sheltered workshop (SW) where there is a twofold goal of: 1) providing remunerative employment together with training for work outside the SW environment, and 2) providing permanent jobs for those who will never be able to function in the everyday work world. Sheltered workshops are not competitive; administrative and supervisory personnel are clinically trained and service, rather than profit, oriented (Kolstoe & Frey, 1965). "Working is a vital element in the lives of people with mental retardation, and the daily experience of working, producing, and being compensated may increase feelings of self worth and dignity as a contributing member of society" (Chinn, Drew, & Logan, 1979, p. 305).

Vocational Services for PWS Individuals

As a disability, PWS fits well within the eligibility guideliness mandated by law. Regrettably, vocational services for this syndrome are few and far between. Too often, affected people are funneled into existing services despite hard evidence that such programs are simply not suitable. The importance of providing appropriate programs becomes increasingly clear. Vocational services become a special challenge because PWS individuals face life with physical *and* mental problems, both of which interact with and have a servere impact on their ability to function. Questions arise: What vocational planning is currently available for individuals with PWS? How successful are such programs? What can enhance existing services and ensure the effectiveness of new ones?

Finding answers to the above queries is not easy since PWS is such a rare, low-incidence condition; many vocational service providers may never see a case in the entire course of their professional career. In response to a increasing need identified by its membership, the Prader-Willi Syndrome Association conducted a survey. The organization's newsletter, *The Gathered View*, reported that few individualized vocational programs exist for PWS individuals who live at home and, in most instances, these programs have been instituted only when parents have been able to exert tremendous pressure on the agency involved. Successful vocational training programs depend on how well informed the professional staff are about PWS and the extent to which they are willing to individualize the training process (Wett, 1986).

As identified previously, in most vocational settings, client adjustment and adaptation are measured by established standards based on productivity, compliance, and the ability to function in a competitive job enviroment. For individuals with PWS, the presence of an uncontrollable craving for food and emotional lability make such criteria for successful adaptation unrealistic. Vocational programs for the mildly retarded indicate that most are clearly capable of performing at very high levels in a typical workshop setting; the majority of PWS individuals function in this retardation category and are sporadically very capable and productive. However, enhancing existing programs and ensuring the effectiveness of future ones requires sensitive counseling, vocational assessment, education, adjustment training, and work opportunities that offer this population a challenge *without* the pressure of competition in a setting where food is not available. Healthy self-esteem, frequently a problem for individuals with PWS, can be enhanced where vocational services focus on their natural and learned abilities—in particular, their fine motor skills, vocal aptitudes, gift for relating to younger children, somewhat sedentary nature, need for structure, and perseverance on task.

Counseling

PWS presents an unusual combination of problems that require thoughtful intervention by a vocational counselor. Such counseling is needed because PWS individuals and their families must confront personal acceptance of the syndrome and its impact on the entire family system, the reaction of outsiders to the condition, a lowering of self-esteem, and the significance of having to function in a restricted environment (Thomas & Butler, 1981). Specifically, those individuals who have been sheltered by their families and other social institutions will require extensive ongoing support. In addition, it is to be expected that the unique characteristics of PWS will have considerable impact on the overall effectiveness of the counseling process and choice of counseling strategies. Most of the successful PWS vocational programs report counseling that focuses on behavioral change as most effective.

Vocational Evaluation

There is a clear correlation between vocational evaluations and practical prescriptions for vocational programming. At best, such assessment is a difficult and complex task, but it is fundamental to the development of individualized services. When evaluating individuals with PWS, the key issue is to acknowledge the presence of mild mental retardation. This is especially perplexing since the verbal skills and artful maneuvering of this population mask their true capacity to function. Prevocational assessment and training are discussed elsewhere within the context of occupational activities (Chapter 13); however, it is important to recognize that most PWS individuals level off in cognitive achievement somewhere between the second and fifth grades. This means that in areas of adaptive behavior, these individuals can take personal care of themselves and may be self-directed. Were it not for the presence of constant hunger and emotional instability, they would be very capable of considerable social independence.

In general, evaluation calls for analysis or assessment of three types of skills: adaptive, functional, and work skills (Mund, 1978). Adaptive skills include self-management, impulse control, taking direction, responding appropriately to authority, adjusting to change, staying on task, conforming, and learning new things. Anyone familiar with PWS will see immediately that developing adaptive skills will be a major issue, particularly adjusting to new situations and cultivating impulse control. Functional skills evolve from natural aptitudes such as mechanical ability, artistic talent, use of tools, and, to a degree, sociability. These skills are likely to be better in one sphere than another. PWS exhibits a complex combination of functional abilities, the strongest being fine motor skills and the weakest appropriate sociability. Work skills accumulate through actual training and experience and are job specific. This is particularly relevant for individuals with PWS, who, if given instruction in appropriate tasks, will function well with supervision.

Definitive assessment of motor skills in PWS often begins at an early age during physical and occupational therapy activities. This is important since the natural capacity for fine motor skills provides a firm basis for hands-on vocational training. One recommended resource for evaluation perceptual motor performance is the Developmental Test of Visual-Motor Integration (Beery, 1967). This tool assesses how well motor behavior and visual perception meld and indicates individual potential for performing various fine motor tasks. Behavioral assessment is equally important. Vocational services must take into account the presence (or absence) of adaptive behaviors. It is suggested that the strengths and weaknesses of individuals with PWS be evaluated by use of the following assessment tools (Halpern, Lehmann, Irvine, & Heiry, 1982):

1. *The Vocational Behavioral Checklist* (Walls, Zane, & Werner, 1978). This checklist evaluates individual skills, provides input for program planning, specifies curriculum/training objectives, and offers a tool to measure program effectiveness. Although not designed for any specific disability, it is of value in assessing PWS prevocational skills, areas of sensory development, attending and responding to simple discriminations, and utilization of visual, auditory, and tactile modalities.
2. *The Adaptive Behavior Scale* (ABS) (Nihira, Foster, Shellhaas, & Leland, 1974). This scale was designed to provide an objective description of the abilities of retarded individuals to cope with normal environmental demands. It measures personal independence in daily living and social competence. Intended for use not only with the retarded population but also with emotionally maladjusted and developmentally delayed persons, it should be viewed in light of input from other types of associated information sources. The ABS is particularly relevant for individuals with PWS, in whom assessment of physical development, social skills, self-direction and math and time concepts affects vocational programming. Moreover, this tool can also identify the degree to which maladaptive psychosocial behaviors (violence, destruction, antisocial acts, or rebellion) are present.

Vocational Training Programs

It has been documented that for many mentally retarded people, their school years are the most difficult time of their lives, primarily because by adolescence, abstract skills have such a high priority (Robinson & Robinson, 1976). Parents of PWS individuals consistently report that as their children progress through special education programs during their teen years, their behaviors visibly deteriorate (Greenswag, 1984). Therefore, it seems appropriate that postschool vocational settings can be a place for acquisition of reasonable work and coping skills for a population who, despite their limitations, are entitled to opportunities to reach their potential. Of note is the fact that in recent years the term "training" in vocational literature, almost without exception, refers to exposure rather than treatment, or refers to placing clients in a job situation where it is hoped that training occurs (Gold, 1972).

PWS individuals require a cohesive, supportive vocational education/training environment that takes into account counselor assessment and detailed vocational evaluation, and focuses on what PWS people do best. Where professionals are ill prepared, written plans poorly conceived, and supervision lacking, failure follows.

Chausow (1986) reported that many affected persons have excellent fine motor coordination in their hands and fingers, reasonable spelling skills, a great deal of patience, and an inclination to sit in one place for long periods of time. She suggested that vocational training programs should be directed to developing office skills, performing simple laboratory tasks, and doing piece work on a sewing machine. All the aforementioned work opportunities are potentially safe settings because: first, food is not usually available, thus the temptation is removed; second, desks can be locked, reducing the opportunities to steal money; and third, most office or lab personnel are more likely to be sensitive and less likely to tease or ridicule.

Basic office skills include sorting, filing, stuffiing envelopes for mailing, and use of equipment such as copiers, adding machines, and simple calculators. In some instances where individuals have enough finger dexterity, typing and some simple computer skills can be taught. By nature, PWS trainees are precise and exacting in task performance (when they want to be) and therefore they can work in a library, recording book titles and cataloging numbers. In the same vein, laboratory work that requires precise titration is another option that fits the PWS characteristic of persistence.

Another suggested work environment is supervised child care (Chausow, 1986). Parents of PWS adolescents and adults indicate that among the characteristics their offspring demonstrate are two that, under ordinary circumstances, might not be very congruent: trouble with authority figures and strong parenting instincts. In actuality, PWS individuals do very well as assistant child care aides. As a group, they relate well to children and can control situations without fear of rejection.

Office, labs, and child care are not the only settings in which PWS individuals can work. Again, natural talents for fine motor activity makes the development of carpentry skills a realistic option; this includes operating simple power machinery.

Horticulture presents excellent opportunities for vocational training and placement. Nurseries and greenhouses deal in garden equipment, sod, seed, plants, plant supplies, floral goods, and services such as ground maintenance, care, and planning (Richmond, 1983). This industry offers a rare combination of physical and cognitive activities for individuals with PWS: a continuum of simple to complex tasks; possibilities for problem solving, communication, and decision making; and the potential to teach responsibility, productivity, and specific job skills. Although not normally "outdoor" people, outside maintenance provides opportunities for PWS individuals to exercise muscles in activities such as digging, planting, pruning, and land clearing. Greenhouse tasks include potting, seeding, floral arranging, and perhaps plant sales.

Another reason horticulture is a viable vocational option is because PWS people need a chance to increase their self-esteem. This setting provides almost endless opportunities to "show and tell," ranging from participation in seasonal community events to highlighting on-the-job projects. It offers what Lewis and Gallison (1976) call "people-plant value." Each person needs to feel needed, and a living plant is almost totally dependent on personal care. A care-providing role reverses the usual dependency of the disabled, engenders competence and personal growth, and enhances self-esteem (Copus, 1980).

At this time, SW programs offer the best environment for the PWS population. Within the framework of vocational serivces, these workshops are a very positive phenomenon. They exist to provide remunerative employment and training, and, where necessary, permanent job placement for individuals unable to function independently in a competitive work setting. Individual interests, abilities, and potential are evaluated in an ongoing manner, as are social and behavioral patterns, and training emphasizes personal and social adjustment (Chinn et al., 1979). Admittedly, PWS individuals usually have higher functional and cognitive skills than may other SW clients. However, their limited adaptive abilities make this setting a realistic option. Successful SW programs exist where staff are willing to "go the extra mile" in supervising and understand that the presence of emotional lability is part of the syndrome. Clearly, when the functional, adaptive, and work skills of PWS persons are constantly evaluated against the backdrop of the syndrome's characteristic behaviors, chances for vocational adaptation increase.

Three sample workshop evaluation forms that address individual goals and objectives appear as Figures 14.1 through 14.3. Figure 14.1 outlines a sample set of expectations for improving adaptive behaviors for a PWS client in a vocational program. Figure 14.2 is a sample daily workshop check-in sheet to accompany the adaptive behavior plan. Figure 14.3 is a sample take-home slip that indicates hour-by-hour and day-by-day progress in a training center. Other workshop checklists for task completion for carpentry, use of power machinery, and horticulture appear in Appendix E.

Client: *Jane Doe* Case Manager: *G. W.*

Date of IWRP: ________ Staff: *trainer; laundry/shop area*

Starting date: ________

Target date: ________

Completion date: ________

I. Long-term Goal: *J. will increase production rate from 55% to 70% of community standards in laundry and shop area*

II. Objective:

A. Condition behavior/skill: *Given clear instructions on task; encouragement and no more than one warning* each a.m. and p.m. and check-in slip*

B. Desired behavior/skill: *J. will keep hands and feet moving on task*

C. Desired level of performance: *at rate which is acceptable** to supervisor: 90% for 18 out of 20 days*

III. Method (include what will be done, where, by whom, and any special techniques or materials to be used):

1. information about acceptable work rates (yes/no) will be on check-in slips

*2. at end of each a.m. and p.m. work supervisor will circle yes/no re: acceptable***

3. if "yes", J. may sit with peers in dining room from 3:30–4:00 p.m.

4. if "no", J. must stay in freetime area from 3:30–4:00 p.m.

**warning = staff will simply say "J., you have had your first warning."*

***acceptable = means no more than one warning per a.m. or p.m. for the following behaviors: 1) standing or sitting for more than one minute not working, 2) not sticking to her own program (bossing others), 3) raising voice to nonconversational tone to staff or other clients.*

IV. Collection/monitoring procedures: *Performance will be monitored through daily check-in slips*

V. Attached data collection graphs, charts, logs, etc: ____ Yes ____ No

Signature: ________ Title: ________ Date: ________

FIGURE 14.1. Sample objective plan for workshop programs for PWS individuals. (Reprinted by permission of Hope Haven, IKnc., Rock Valley, IA.)

Name ________ Date ________

Punctuality

1. Work on time @ 8:30 ________
2. Lite Club @ 9:30 ________
3. Work/free time @ 10:15 ________
4. Work at 12:000 ________
5. Finish task by 12:45 ________
6. Work @ 2:45 ________
7. Other ________
8. Other ________

*Acceptable Work**

a.m. ________ Yes ________ No
p.m. ________ Yes ________ No

*Acceptable means no more than one warning per a.m. or p.m. for the following behaviors

1. Standing or sitting for more than one minute not working.**
2. Bossing others.
3. Raising voice to nonconversational tone toward staff or clients.

***Note:* These times are to the minute. If J. is one or more minutes late, she is late. If on time, initial the blank. If late, do *not* initial the blank. Instead, put "late" on the blank and in parenthesis indicate the number of minutes late.

FIGURE 14.2. Sample daily performance card. (Reprinted by permission of Hope Haven, Inc., Rock Valley, IA.)

Discussion of vocational services would not be complete without including words of caution about some training programs that, on the surface, may seem to be very realistic options. Particular reference is made to training for motel housekeeping or janitorial work. Two important features of PWS must be considered when planning for this type of employment. First, many individuals with PWS have a decreased sensitivity to pain and delicate skin; they can easily incur serious burns from use of water that is too hot or chemical cleansers. Second, the penchant for scavenging both food and money requires constant supervision.

Careful consideration should also be given to teaching money skills to people with PWS. Few seem to be able to handle anything beyond simple math concepts well enough to manage money. However, they are very talented when it comes to understanding the value of money for buying food or manipulating others.

In one or two instances, vocational programs have reported PWS clients successfully functioning in food settings (dishwashing and kitchen tasks). Long-term assessment of these programs is not yet available, but it is suggested that maintenance of a reasonable weight will be the best measure of success in this environment. Consideration should also be given to the emotional well-being of any PWS individual working in an environment in which food is always in view; such a setting may be a constant source of frustration even for those individuals who are able to maintain a reason-

Name *Jane Doe* Date ______

	8:45–10:45 a.m.	10:30–12:00 a.m.	12:45–2:45 p.m.
Back to work on time	*X*	*No*	*No*
Follows directions promptly	*X*	*X*	*No*
Pays attention to task	*X*	*X*	*X*
Uses appropriate voice tone	*X*	*No*	*X*
Does not take items without asking	*X*	*X*	*X*
Follows all workshop rules	*X*	*X*	*X*

Daily Comments:

Overall, J. had a very positive day

______

Supervisory Staff

FIGURE 14.3 Sample take-home slip for reporting daily workshop adjustment for PWS individual's daily progress note. (From Goldstein, A., & Carr, L. [1985]. *Daily progress note*. Evanston, IL: Shore Training Center, Shore Community Services for Retarded Citizens. Reprinted by permission.)

able weight. As pointed out in other discussion in this text, PWS people seem to be less upset when food is available only at specific times.

Vocational Adjustment Concerns

Under ordinary circumstances, vocational training and adjustment would be considered complete when the trainee is able to work independently and be self-sufficient. This is not the case for individuals with PWS. In actuality, vocational adjustment for this population is a rather elusive, continuing process of encouraging appropriate behaviors, some sense of social propriety, and satisfactory interpersonal relationships that may enhance self-worth. Difficulties arise early in evaluation and training when neither the affected person nor his or her family readily acknowledge the limitations of the syndrome. Accepting PWS offspring as functionally retarded is a long, painful process. For example, many parents are very tuned in to their child's extensive vocabulary and verbal skills; they feel that the child is "too bright" for a sheltered workshop environment and wish to avoid the stigma of such a setting. Yet, few PWS clients adjust beyond this point without dangerous weight gain and trouble with authorities. Certainly, any social adaptation is seriously hampered where PWS people work alone, and their stubbornness and lack of ability to adjust to new situations are major barriers to adaptation.

Vocational adjustment entails reaching beyond "pay for work done"; goals should include increased feelings of self-worth and dignity, which emerge from being a contributing member of a community. Participation in productive work and social interactions go hand in hand, and social responsibility, supposedly a product of maturity, will always be a long-range objective of vocational services.

Work Options

Earlier discussion of potential work settings for individuals with PWS takes into consideration their natural functional talents, personality characteristics, food-seeking behaviors, and need for structure. Vocational planners are wise to pay close attention to these issues, and reassessment of program goals should be ongoing. Those vocational professionals who follow PWS cases should be advised that educating potential employers and direct care aides about the syndrome should be a top priority. Also, there is evidence that some residential group homes for PWS who originally contracted with local vocational providers have developed their own programs out of desperation when PWS clients were perceived as not able to function in a traditional workshop program. It is hoped that in the future vocational service providers will be more sensitive to the needs of the PWS population and separate programs will not be required.

Summary

Vocational programs should become an integral part of the life of adults with PWS. Services for this population are mandated under law and opportunities for vocational options are expanding. Sensitive counseling, careful assessment, and realistic vocational training are essential. At present, sheltered workshops are the best source of services since it is not clear whether individuals with this syndrome can function in a competitive work setting with unsupervised proximity to food.

References

Andrew, J.W. (1981). Evaluation of rehabilitation potencial. In R. Parker, C. Hansen (Eds.) *Rehabilitation counseling* pp. 205–225, Boston: Allyn and Bacon.

Beery, K. (1967). *Developmental Test of Visual-Motor Integration: administration and scoring manual*. Chicago: Follett.

Chausow, R. (1986). *Position paper on vocational and recreational skills for Prader-Willi syndrome clients*. Unpublished manuscript.

Chinn, P.C., Drew, C.J., &, Logan, D.R. (1979). *Mental retardation, a life cycle approach*. St. Louis: C.V. Mosby.

Copus, E. (1980). *The Melwood manual*. Menomonie, WI: University of Wisconsin–Stout, Materials Development Center.

Daniels, J. (1981). The world of work and disabling conditions. In R. Parker & C. Hansen (Eds.), *Rehabilitation counseling* (pp. 169–97). Boston: Allyn and Bacon.

Gold, M.W. (1972). Stimulus factors in skill training of the retarded in complex assembly tasks: Acquisition, transfer, and retention. *American Journal of Mental Deficiency*, *76*, 517–526.

Greenswag, L.R. (1984, May). *The adult with Prader-Willi syndrome: A descriptive investigation*. Unpublished doctoral thesis, University of Iowa. (DA 056952, University Microfilms International, Ann Arbor, MI.)

Halpern, A.S., Lehman, J.P., Irvin, L.K., and Heiry, T.J, (1982). *Contemporary assessment for mentally retarded adolescents and adults*. Baltimore: University Park Press.

Kolstoe, O. & Frey, R. (1965). *A high school work study program for the mentally subnormal student*. Carbondale, IL: Southern Illinois University Press.

Lewis, C., & Gallison, S. (1976). *Plants for people*. Paper presented at a conference of the National Council for Therapy and Rehabilitation through Horticulture, Gaithersburg, MD.

Mund, S. (1978). Vocational rehabilitation: Employment; self employment; a vocational rehabilitation process. In R. Goldenson (Ed.), *Disability and rehabilitation handbook* (pp. 67–87). New York: McGraw-Hill.

Nihira, K., Foster, R., Shellhaas, M., & Leland, H. (1974). *Adaptive Behavior Scale*. Washington, DC: American Association on Mental Deficiency.

Rehabilitation Act of 1973, 29 U.S.C. § 701–794. (1973).

Richmond, C. (1983). *Horticulture: Hiring the disabled*. American Rehabilitation, Vol. 9, No. 1 Jan-Feb-March. Washington DC: U.S. Department of Education, Office of Special Education and Rehabilitation Services.

Robinson, N., & Robinson, H. (1976). *The mentally retarded child*. New York: McGraw-Hill.

Thomas, K., & Butler, A. (1981). Counseling for personal adjustment. In R. Parker & C. Hansen (Eds.), *Rehabilitation counseling*. Boston: Allyn and Bacon.

Vocational Rehabilitation Act of 1943, 29 U.S.C. § 31–41. (1943).

Vocational Rehabilitation Amendments of 1966, 29 U.S.C. § 31–42 (1965).

Walls, R., Zane, T., & Werner, T. (1978). *Vocational Behavioral Checklist*. Dunbar, VW: West Virginia Rehabilitation Research and Training Center.

Wett, M. (1986, July–August). *Vocational Placement, The Gathered View*, p. 3. (Edina, MN: The Prader-Willi Syndrome Association.)

15
The Role of the Social Worker

JAMES F. PORTER

The role of the social worker is to identify and work with the frustrations, demands, and conflicts encountered by families of individuals with Prader-Willi syndrome (PWS). Children with PWS present unique needs to their families and communities. Poor muscle tone, difficulty in feeding, and nonresponsiveness are major concerns during infancy. Early in childhood, the presence of developmental delay and mental retardation is compounded by the emergence of an insatiable drive for food and the potential for morbid obesity. Over time, behavioral problems intensify, and by adolescence the combination of emotional lability and lack of secondary sexual growth seriously hinders adaptation. As the child with PWS approaches adulthood, decisions need to be made regarding future vocational and living environments in the community.

Social Work Practice

Respect for human dignity and the individual's right to self-determination is the foundation upon which social work practice is built (Minahan, 1987). Historically, as a profession, social work has focused on working with people and their social environment to improve quality of life, to act as advocates in helping people to help themselves, and to obtain the resources necessary to function in society. It has only been in the last 15 years that social workers have increased their involvement in working with people with developmental disabilities (Wikler & Berkowitz, 1983). With the movement toward deinstitutionalization and normalization, there is a greater need for community-based services for this population. Social workers are called on to link the developmentally disabled population to their social environment; they function as coordinators of community-based services designed to meet individualized needs and clarify and interpret the results and recommendations made by community resource persons to the family. As advocates, social workers strive to provide for: the rights of the disabled to live and work in their home communities when possible, financial assistance from federal and state resources, education and functional self-help skills, and recreational services and transportation (Gelman, 1983). As a resource for the family and affected child, social workers frequently help to obtain vocational training and residential job placement. At times when services cannot be met by local providers, the social worker must look elsewhere, or attempt to create these services by using pre-existing resources in innovative ways. For example, a local agency serving a non-PWS population may be encouraged to establish a PWS group home.

The Social Systems Model

The social systems model is used effectively for the developmentally disabled and their families. This model asserts that the family is composed of interacting units, each with its own set of functioning parts, each unit being part of a larger whole (Anderson & Carter, 1974). All aspects of individual and family functioning must be addressed to optimize growth and development. For example, failure to consider recreation and respite care services may lead to an accumulation of family stresses resulting in divorce, abuses, or noncompliance with management strategies. Figure 15.1 illustrates the family and community systems and their respective subsystems, which interact with and have an impact on each other. Application of this "systems" perspective can assist in determining how family and community units interact, and ensures that family "issues" are incorporated into interdisciplinary team interventions in a clinical, school, or social setting. Interdisciplinary teams that serve the developmentally disabled population are most effective when there has been an accurate assessment of family dynamics, subsystems, financial status, community resources, stress levels, coping mechanisms, and the family's ability to plan for the future. As a team member, the social worker is an important resource for information about these issues.

The Family System

The social worker is in an ideal position to identify many of the needs of a family with a child with PWS, assess stress levels in the family system, and provide assistance in helping to alleviate that stress. An understanding of the family's subsystems is important.

Parental Adjustment

All parents have certain expectations and dreams for their unborn children, and when a child is born with a disability, parents experience a

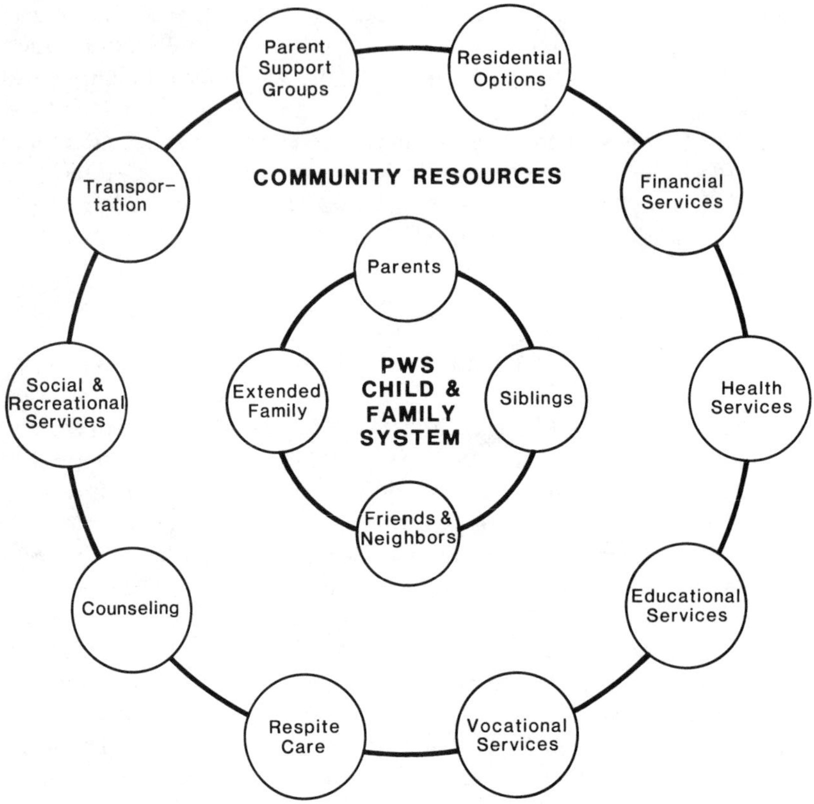

FIGURE 15.1. A social work perspective that illustrates how a PWS family fits within the framework of services from community resources.

natural grieving process similar to that which occurs when a "loved one" dies. Kubler-Ross (1969) identified this grieving as a five-stage process of denial and isolation, anger, bargaining, depression, and acceptance. Sieffert (1975) discussed parental reaction to having a disabled child as occurring in three stages: nonacceptance (shock, anger, denial); acceptance (accepting the reality of the child, depression, sadness, and relinquishing attachment to the fantasy child); and acceptance of the child (beginning activity to meet the needs of the real child). It is important to emphasize that grieving is a normal, nonlinear process. People rarely move through the stages in a predictable sequence or time frame and may exhibit characteristics of several stages at once or even "regress" in some circumstances. Parents of children with developmental disabilities indicate their belief that they rarely ever "accept" their childrens' disabilities, but rather constantly keep "adjusting." In other words, the grieving process does not end as their affected child grows older. Anniversaries such as birthdays or Christmas may elicit unexpected sadness and depression. Olshansky (1962) described this as "chronic sorrow," the repeated episodes of parental sadness and disappointment that occur as the affected child grows without achieving normal developmental milestones. Powell and Ogle (1985) identified the transitional periods of stress for the parents of a child with a disability: the birth of the child, when the child starts school, when the child completes school and faces the decisions associated with where to work and live, and when the parents age and/or can no longer assume the responsibility of caring for the child. It is during these transitional periods that parents experience more intense grief reactions. Periodic grief counseling may be necessary as an integral part of any ongoing support service, and every effort should be made to reassure parents that episodes of increased sorrow are normal and to be expected. Unfortunately, parents of children with PWS are often placed in a very difficult position of having to delay their efforts to adjust because most affected children are not clearly identified at birth. Despite the fact that parents are well aware that something is wrong early in the child's life, diagnosis frequently is not made until the child begins to gain weight (Zellweger, 1981). Parents often remain confused and frustrated. Furthermore, even though the eventual diagnosis of PWS may offer parents some measure of relief about "what's wrong with our child," they will need considerable help and understanding in adjusting to the long-term implications of PWS. The correct diagnosis effectively "closes the door" on any hope the parents may have that their child will prove to be "normal." This may exacerbate dormant grief.

Once the early stage of PWS is over, families face years of caring for a somewhat mentally retarded, sexually underdeveloped, stubborn, aggressive child with an uncontrollable appetite, bizarre behaviors, and the potential for morbid obesity (Greenswag, 1984). Parents must institute low-calorie diets, control all sources of food, and deal with ever-increasing behavior problems. Management becomes even more difficult when the child gains access to food at school and in the neighborhood. Children with PWS have been known to go to a neighbor and say they are hungry because their parents will not feed them. (In one such case, a neighbor filed a child neglect report with the Department of Human Services.) Children with PWS have been known to eat dog food, forage in garbage, rob refrigerators, and steal money in an attempt to obtain food. Such behaviors may isolate a family; they may be reluctant to go out in public or ask friends over to visit. Coping with normal family issues is complex enough; the additional demand of caring for a child with PWS are a challenge for which few families are prepared. When parents are forced to constantly focus on their affected child's needs, the rest of the family inevitably suffers.

Because a single community is not likely to have more than one family with a child with PWS, support groups related to children with other developmental disabilities may be of considerable help. All too often, the needs of the family are overshadowed by services that focus primarily on management of the child with PWS. Support groups may encourage parents to express their feelings and needs, exchange ideas and share common issues, and develop a feeling of trust, and may clarify information and answer questions about available resources. Additional aid can be given by specific PWS support groups in areas of the country where they exist. Whether or not community options exist, many care providers find the national Prader-Willi Syndrome Association[1] to be an excellent source of information and moral support (see Chapter 21).

Marital Relationships

The stability of the marital relationship is particularly vulnerable in families where there is a child with PWS. It is not unusual for a husband and wife to be at different stages of adjustment to their child's disability, and one spouse may not be able to respond to the emotional needs of the other. One source of stress between husband and wife may result if one parent feels the child with PWS is entitled to be "fat and happy" while the other feels compelled to restrict food for health reasons (LeConte, 1981). Both parents may feel ambivalent or hostile toward the child, whose cravings trap the rest of the family system. Even finding a babysitter for a child with PWS is difficult because of behavioral problems; this leaves little or no time for parents to be away from their child and interact as a couple. The social worker should provide counseling to improve communication between parents and help them to better understand and express their feelings. The social worker also needs to be aware of community resources that provide more intensive marital and/or family counseling, respite care, or babysitting if necessary. Single parents face even greater stresses, frequently trying to balance commitments to other children and a career. The care of the child with PWS may make outside employment a virtual impossibility. Respite care, medical coverage, and other sources of support may be even more critical in these instances. By anticipating these needs before they arise, the burden to the parent, child, and other family members may be minimized.

Siblings

Siblings are an integral part of a family system but may be neglected when one child in the family has a disability. Most siblings describe both positive and negative feelings about having a brother or sister with a disability. Feelings of bitterness and resentment may be present if it is perceived that extra attention is given to the affected sibling. Some normal siblings report feeling guilty because they are healthy, others are given additional respon-

[1] Located at 5515 Malibu Drive, Edina, MN 55436; (612) 933-0113.

sibilities at home, and some are pressured to mature too quickly. On the positive side, some adult normal siblings feel that their tolerance for individual differences is increased because of their experiences of growing up with a disabled brother or sister (Powell & Ogle, 1985). Many variables affect the adjustment of normal siblings to the situation; parental attitudes toward the disabled child play a large role in how healthy children relate to both their parents and the disabled sibling (Powell & Ogle, 1985). In medical and educational settings, it is common for one or both parents to accompany the child with PWS for evaluation while the healthy siblings are frequently left at home, or sent to family or friends. In some instances, normal children have had behavior problems at school that parents attribute to the stress of having a sibling with PWS. Their normal offspring may be reluctant to bring friends home to see locked kitchens and/or an exhibition of bizarre behavior. Normal brothers and sisters who met as a group discussed being embarrassed by the eating habits and temper tantrums of their affected sibling at school, how stressful life is at home because of diet restrictions, the need for food control, and stealing behaviors (LeConte, 1981).

At every opportunity, parents need to be reminded to be sensitive to how their normal children view the sibling with PWS. Parents should be encouraged to be open and honest with their children regarding the affected sibling; listen to and accept the children's feelings without making them feel guilty; schedule individual time with the children; avoid or limit assignment of care-providing responsibilities; provide opportunities for normal family activities and involvement such as scouting, 4H, and sports; and include their normal children when attending school meetings, medical appointments, and discussions of future plans for the PWS brother or sister (Powell & Ogle, 1985). Older siblings will benefit from a thorough review of PWS to avoid misconceptions. Genetics counseling is particularly important for teenage siblings beginning to consider a future that could include children of their own (Chapter 4). The social worker should also be active in establishing support groups so that siblings can meet other PWS siblings and discuss common concerns.

Extended Family Members

Most families have subsystems of grandparents, aunts, uncles, and cousins, all of whom may be sources of support (through child care and financial and/or emotional help). However, extended family members also need time to adjust, to understand, and to ask questions. Siblings of the parents (maternal and paternal aunts and uncles) may voice concerns about recurrence risk factors for their own offspring. Grandparents, in particular, may be very sensitive to having a disabled grandchild; adjusting their expectations may take a long time. Helping extended family members to understand the need for consistent food control is critical if they participate in the primary care of the PWS child. Social workers should be aware of the role that extended family members play; sensitivity to their needs can preserve or restore an important resource for family support.

Community Resources

Many services are needed to help children with PWS and their families. Assessment of community resources is a major area in which social workers are particularly effective. Before individuals with PWS finish school, plans must be made for their future. Older adolescents and adults will require a living environment that provides 24-hour supervision, complete control of food intake, and a structured program to promote social adaptation. Location and implementation of these community resources are essential. Decision-making about alternative living arrangements is one of the most difficult "transitional periods" that parents must face. They frequently need considerable time to discuss their feelings concerning the delicate issue of out-of-home placement versus continuing management at home. Arranging for respite care maybe a vital service. Such care may be overnight or may involve a structured recreational program that encourages child participation in community activities while offering relief to parents and family. Home Health Care agencies can be of assistance, particularly when unusual medical problems occur.

Compliance with weight management programs is a problem noted by health care providers. In the tertiary setting, failure to show for scheduled appointments increases concerns for the child, the family, and the proper utilization of limited clinical resources. In some cases, compliance with clinic appointments is similar to that seen in exogenous obesity clinics, suggesting that weight management is a frustrating burden to parents or other care providers. In contrast to slowly increasing weight, behavior problems may increase clinic compliance because they are less able to be ignored in the home setting. Perhaps the best method to increase compliance with weight management programs and clinic appointments is the creation of support groups for parents (and siblings), particularly on clinic days. The social worker is often instrumental in initiating and facilitating such groups. Thus the clinic visit can become the "family visit."

Summary

Individuals with PWS and their families have unique needs that require special services. By viewing the families using a social systems model, social workers can be a valuable resource by providing assessment information to interdisciplinary team members and helping families obtain services necessary to function in their social environment. Social workers' knowledge about PWS can be most effective in assisting affected children and their families to adjust, cope, and plan for the future.

References

Anderson, R.E., & Carter, I.E. (1974). *Human behavior in the social environment: A social systems approach*. Chicago: Aldine Publishing Co.

Gelman, S.R. (1983). The developmentally disabled: A social work challenge. In L. Wikler & M.P. Keenan (Eds.), *Developmental disabilities: No longer a private tragedy* (pp. 12–14). Silver Spring, MD: National Association of Social Workers; and Washington, DC: American Association on Mental Deficiency.

Greenswag, L.R. (1984, May). *The adult with Prader-Willi syndrome: A descriptive investigation*. Unpublished doctoral thesis, University of Iowa. (DA 056952, University Microfilms International, Ann Arbor, MI)

Kubler-Ross, E. (1969). *On death and dying*. New York: Macmillan Publishing Co.

Leconte, J.M. (1981). Social work intervention for families with children with Prader-Willi-syndrome. In V.A. Holm, S.J. Sulzbacher, & P.L. Pipes (Eds.), *The Prader-Willi syndrome* (pp. 245–257). Baltimore: University Park Press.

Minahan, A. (Ed.-in-Chief.). (1987). *Encyclopedia of social work: Volumes I and II*. Silver Spring, MD: National Association of Social Workers.

Olshansky, S. (1962). Chronic sorrow: A response to having a mentally defective child. *Social Casework*, *43*, 190–193.

Powell, T.H., & Ogle, P.A. *Brothers and sisters: A special part of exceptional families*. Baltimore: Paul H. Brookes Publishing Co.

Sieffert, A. (1975, April). *Normal parental reaction process to having a defective child*. Unpublished manuscript, Topeka, Kansas.

Wikler, L., & Berkowitz, N.N. Social work, social problems, and the mentally retarded. In L. Wikler & M.P. Keenan (Eds.), *Developmental disabilities: No longer a private tragedy* (pp. 8–11). Silver Spring, MD: National Association of Social Workers; and Washington, DC: American Association on Mental Deficiency.

Zellweger, H. (1981). Diagnosis and therapy in the first phase of Prader-Willi Syndrome. In V.A. Holm, S.J. Sulzbacher, & P.L. Pipes (Eds.), *The Prader-Willi syndrome* (pp. 55–69). Baltimore: University Park Press.

Part IV The Socialization Process

He has no friends outside school, does not like to do anything physical except dance to records. Watches TV and plays games with his sister. Has taken physical and verbal abuses from children in school but does not complain because he is starved for peer relationships. When visitors come to our house, which is very rare, their kids are always snacking and totally ignore [the] PWS, which is very hard on him.

I think young retarded men and women should be allowed to live together provided they cannot produce children. . . . it could be much less expensive than housing two of them separately. They have the same emotional needs as normal people. And with the same supervision provided as individuals, they could make it as couples.

It has been difficult coping with this problem, trying to understand it and have patience. It was difficult for the other children growing up . . . it took so much of my time that I should have devoted to the other children. The worst part was the staring and whispering of people when we were out, . . . I would never go through this again—to raise another child with this disorder.

16
Social Skills Training for Prader-Willi Syndrome

William Mitchell

Although the incidence of Prader-Willi syndrome (PWS) is relatively rare in the general population, those who are affected by the disorder demonstrate significant lifelong needs that include medical care, specialized educational and vocational programming, psychotherapeutic intervention, and family support services. However, traditional remedial academic strategies and behavioral management techniques have failed to meet the needs of individuals with PWS. A strict dietary regimen with food kept inaccessible (including locked kitchens) in conjunction with a highly structured behavior-shaping program is required to manage these clients. Even in programs that focus on overeating and inappropriate behavior through environmental and behavioral controls, these clients often experience significant difficulty because of their impulsivity and poor social judgment.

The Developmental Evaluation Clinic (DEC) at Children's Hospital, Boston, piloted a social skills training program specifically for individuals with PWS. It was designed to teach staff who work in a family-style residential facility to help this population improve their social skills. The development of the project's assessment materials and training procedures are described here. Some of the program's teaching tools were adapted from existing curricula, and others were designed especially for the PWS clients. This teaching project, conducted in a workshop format, was based on the staff's evaluation of PWS client social skills deficits and the need for staff training.

Social Skills Training: An Overview

Social skills are behaviors that enable people to interact with one another effectively, and poor social skills interfere with job performance and daily function. Although effective skills require the complex coordination of several cognitive processes and motor or performance skills, the acquisition of such skills has been left largely to chance by modern educators.

Recently, a number of social skills training curricula and training programs have been developed. Researchers at the University of Massachusetts in Boston created materials for elementary school teachers (Nezer, Nezer, & Siperstein, 1986), and the American Guidance Service (Circle Pines, MN) publishes a number of packaged social skills and affective development training materials for several age groups and populations (e.g., "Transitions," "Toward Affective Development," and "DUSO"). Roffman (1981) developed a social skills training curriculum and course materials for use in a program for learning-disabled young adults called *Threshold.* Ellis and Whittington (1981) designed an inclusive listing of social skills subdivided by means of theoretical constructs into four dimensions that they believe can guide trainers in identifying those skills most needed by the client. Other researchers and practitioners have targeted parents as trainers. Baker, Brightman, Heifitz, and Murphy (1976) created specific parent-training materials to help parents learn to teach their developmentally disabled children and/or children with behavior problems appropriate social skills.

The trend toward providing social skills training to various client groups has done much to address a long-urgent need. Classroom teachers have welcomed aids to teaching what has been referred to as the "hidden curriculum." Parents, previously frustrated in their attempts to establish control of their children's behavior, now have a means of working with even the most problematic behaviors. However, despite advances in social skills training, some developmentally disabled groups with very special needs have not been served; one such group consists of people with PWS.

Social Skills Training for Clients with PWS

Numerous investigators have detected behavioral abnormalities associated with PWS that range from mild social transgressions to major psychiatric disorders (Bray et al., 1983; Greenswag, 1984; Hall & Smith, 1972; Sulzbacher, Crnic, & Snow, 1981; Zellweger & Schneider, 1968). It is believed that behavioral difficulties, notably unprecipitated acting out, mood lability, decreased social-interactive skills, and depression, become more pronounced with age and cause social isolation and poor academic and vocational achievement. In this respect, PWS clients represent an exaggeration of a statement from the *University Affiliated Facilities Adult Services Networking Initiative Technical Report on Learning and Adjustment* (1986) that "more jobs are lost among developmentally disabled populations because of social behavior problems and deficits than because of lack of job skills."

PWS clients not only lose jobs because of social skills deficits, but also are often precluded from consideration for work placement. The basic components of social interaction, such as eye contact, appropriate interpersonal distance, listening, turn-taking, and shaking hands are frequently missing from the repertoire of social behaviors of PWS clients. Even in supported work environments such as those run by the DEC, social behavior deficits associated with PWS create problems for supervisors and coworkers accustomed to interacting with clients with other developmental disabilities. Special behavior-shaping contracts have been established for the PWS population in order to limit some social transgressions in controlled and closely supervised settings. It is evident, however, that direct training in prosocial skills may more effectively help these clients develop the requisites for improved interaction and less isolation in their social environment.

The Pilot Staff-Training Program

The pilot social skills training was conducted in two types of workshop formats, one of which was a series of four workshops offered over a 2-month period. Conceptual material was given in brief talks with maximum time spent in discussion and demonstration (Appendix F, Sections 1–4). The second format was a single workshop that was more didactic and less experiential (Appendix F, Section 9). Before conducting the workshops, assessment procedures were designed and training materials gathered.

Assessment

Because this was a pilot staff-training project specifically for the PWS population, assessment procedures were created "from scratch" and were administered to staff in two residential settings where workshops were conducted. The assessment tools consisted of the *Rating of Client Social Skills Deficits* (Appendix F, Section 5), the *Rating of Effective Techniques and Activities* (Appendix F, Section 6), the *Staff Questionnaire* (Apendix F, Section 7), and the *Curriculum Test* (Appendix F, Section 8). The first two rating forms completed by staff gave a reasonably accurate view of the needs of the clients.

There were four categories of deficits in social skills on the *Rating of Client Social Skills Deficits:* conversational skills, nonverbal communication skills, assertiveness, and inappropriate behaviors. Staff indicated that clients were most in need of training in conversational skills and, within this category, the greatest deficits were in turn-taking and in learning to listen. The category of inappropriate behaviors had the second highest priority, with emotional outbursts, verbal assaultiveness, and noncompliance rated as the three most troublesome. Interestingly, theft of food and property and stereotypies were given lower priorities. It was speculated that these behaviors, common among PWS clients, were already under good control compared to other behavioral issues. Deficits in assertive behaviors were ranked as a third priority, with nonverbal communication deficits ranked as the lowest category. Assertive behavior deficits requiring the most attention were a relatively poor ability to express annoyance, presence of irritability, and refusal to interact appropriately. Failure to maintain appropriate distance was the most problematic issue in nonverbal communication.

Responses by staff to the *Rating of Effective Techniques and Activities* indicated that role-playing and modeling were considered to be the most effective. Games were rated second, followed by coaching, labeling feelings, and finally relaxation and biofeedback. Answers to the *Staff Questionnaire* given to 13 residential staff trainees indicated that all levels of personnel were involved. All had some direct care duties with PWS clients and all but one had experience with other mentally retarded clients. Most were in their first year of experience working with PWS clients and high staff turnover was reported. At one facility two parents also participated.

Although in-service training was frequently budgeted in both residential settings, only four staff in both facilities had received specific education about PWS and only two had participated in a social skills training program of any kind. All expressed a desire for more information, techniques, and materials that might be helpful in their work with this population.

Materials

Each workshop trainee received a notebook containing conceptual materials with definitions of relevant terms and procedures, descriptions of prosocial skills, and a list of the goals of a social skills training project. Techniques such as modeling, role-playing, labeling of emotions, coaching, timing, biofeedback and relaxation, and activities and games were described.

Because conversational skills were identified as the highest training priority, more elaborate materials were developed in this category. Several activities from Roffman's social skills curriculum were adapted and made into games, as noted below.

The Timing Game consists of social situations, printed in large letters on cards that can be read aloud in turn. Each player (client) has a response card that is used to indicate whether the situation read by the leader presents a good or bad time to initiate a conversation. The goal is to improve the timing skills of clients and to encourage group discussions on this topic.

The Open/Closed Questions Game is similar in format to the Timing Game. Questions printed in large letters are read aloud, one at a time. Clients hold up cards indicating whether each person thinks the question is open-ended (requiring more than a one- or two-word answer and thus stimulating further conversation) or closed-ended (requiring a very brief answer, and presenting an awkward silence thereafter). The goal is to teach clients how to begin and maintain coversations.

The Assertive Game provides clients with definitions of assertive, aggressive, and nonassertive behaviors. The leader (staff member) then reads the descriptions of behavior and each participant decides whether that behavior is assertive, aggressive, or nonassertive. The goal is to help increase understanding and use of assertive behaviors.

The Book Method teaches clients how to give criticism tactfully. Originally called the Sandwich Recipe by Roffman, the name was changed because of the sensitivity of clients with PWS to food-related themes. This method encourages initiating criticism with a positive statement (front cover of book). This is followed by the criticism itself, along with a rationale (the contents), and finally by a request for a change (back cover). Clients are asked to write a book. The goal is to encourage constructive, assertive criticism.

Another effective activity is *The Ungame*, a commercially available board game (The Ungame Company, 1984). It was adapted by preparing directions relevant for individuals with PWS as a structured way to encourage turn-taking and listening.

Conclusion

The efficacy of teaching residential care staff to provide social skills training for individuals with PWS can be fully assessed only after controlled studies of staff training programs are conducted in other facilities that serve this population and only if staff training is of sufficient duration and consistency. As an in-service project, social skills training can be done on a very small budget and, certainly, the single workshop format is most cost-effective.

The *Curriculum Test* used in the pilot project as a pre- and posttest measure of staff knowledge indicated that staff awareness and comprehension of PWS and the special needs of affected individuals clearly improved. However, whether this knowledge will be used to train PWS clients and whether such training will be successful is not yet known. Because social skills training has been effective, in many other settings, there is reason to be optimistic that the concept will gain wide use in the future for individuals with PWS.

References

Baker, B.L., Brightman, A.J., Heifetz, L.J., & Murphy, D.M. (1976). *Behavior problems*. Champaign, IL: Research Press.

Bray G.A., Dahms, W.T., Swerdloff, R.S., Fisher, R.H., Atkinson, R.L., & Carrel, R.E. (1983). The Prader-Willi syndrome: A study of 40 patients and a review of the literature. *Medicine*, *62*, 59–80.

Ellis, R., & Whittington, D. (1981). *A guide to social skill training*. Cambridge, MA: Brookline Books.

Greenswag, L.R. (1984, May). *The adult with Prader-Willi syndrome: A descriptive investigation*. Unpublished doctoral thesis, University of Iowa. (DA 056952, University Microfilms International, Ann Arbor, MI)

Hall, B.D., & Smith, D.W. (1972). Prader-Willi syndrome. A resume of 32 cases including an instance of affected first cousins, one of whom is of normal stature and intelligence. *The Journal of Pediatrics*, *81*, 286–293.

Nezer, H., Nezer, B., & Siperstein, G. (1986). *Improving children's social skills*. Boston: Center for the Study of Social Acceptance, University of Massachusetts.

Roffman, A. (1981). The effects of social skills training on the attitudes and behaviors of adolescent CETA trainees. Unpublised doctoral dissertation, Boston College.

Sulzbacher, S., Crnic, K.A., & Snow, J. (1981). Behavioral and cognitive disabilities in Prader-Willi syndrome. In V.A. Holm, S.J. Sulzbacher, & P.L. Pipes (Eds.), *The Prader-Willi syndrome* (pp. 147–160). Baltimore: University Park Press.

University Affiliated Facilities Adult Services Networking Initiative Technical Report on Learning and Adjustment. (1986). Administration on Developmental Disabilities.

Zellweger, H., & Schneider, H. (1968). Syndrome of hypotonia-hypomentia-hypogonadism-obesity (HHHO) or Prader-Willi syndrome. *American Journal of Diseases of Children*, *115*, 558–598.

17
Understanding Psychosexuality

LOUISE R. GREENSWAG

As the life span of the Prader-Willi syndrome (PWS) population lengthens, psychosexual growth, development, and education become legitimate concerns for parents and other care providers. Adolescents and adults with PWS verbalize their sexual thinking and a desire for sexual expression. Their parents, acutely aware of the social dimensions and implications of this sexual "awakening," often are at a loss as to what to expect and how to manage their offspring. Recently, enlightened attitudes toward sexually have opened the door to a more frank discussion of this very "human" subject. Such openness is important because if guiding sexual growth and behavior in normal children is not easy, helping a short, overweight, cognitively impaired, permanently sexually immature child is an even greater challenge. In addition, parents and care providers are now more willing to play an active role in channeling the natural tendencies of affected individuals in appropriate directions.

This discussion offers information that may help individuals with PWS and their families adapt to the sexual limitations imposed by the presence of the syndrome. It includes a commentary on human sexuality and sexual expression in the mentally retarded population, guidelines for management from a developmental perspective, and suggested roles for parents and professionals. It should be acknowledged at this juncture that human sexuality is a very sensitive issue and one that is profoundly influenced by personal value systems. At no point does this discussion endeavor to substitute knowledge or mechanical information for morality.

Human Sexuality and PWS

For parents and other care providers, sexual activity in the PWS population may seem almost a contradiction in terms. The first question that comes to mind might well be, "Why discuss sexuality in a population where males are impotent and have very small external genitalia, where females rarely menstruate, where neither sex develops more than rudimentary secondary sex characteristics, and none are known to reproduce?" (Zellweger & Schneider, 1968). Such a query indicates a lack of understanding of sexuality as a multidimensional concept. An enduring part of each person, sexuality has been described as the sum of one's feelings about being male or female, which arises from cultural attitudes and value system and relates to the assignment of sex roles (Hogan, 1985; Mims & Swenson, 1980). It encompasses many subtleties that coexist in social/sexual relationships where discreet behaviors need not be overtly genital or associated only with physical acts and, as a means of expression, it cannot be isolated from other aspects of life. Although few PWS adolescents and adults are physically prepared to participate in intimate sexual activities, their capacity for sexual expression should be viewed as an important aspect of their psychosocial development and they should be offered guidance about appropriate sexual behaviors.

Although there are reports of lack of strong sexual drives in individuals with PWS (D. Thompson & M. Wett, personal communication, 1985), these individuals tend to verbalize identifiable, albeit unrealistic, expectations about marriage and parenting that give some indication of their awareness of sociosexual conventions. Parental descriptions of adolescent and adult offspring document these persons' potential for social/emotional dimensions of sexual expression (Greenswag, 1985). One parent commented:

He is a very affectionate boy and likes girls very much and they like him. He likes to dance and put his arm around them and even kisses them, but he has never given any indication of anything more.

Males with PWS have been teased about their small genitalia and their obesity, which produces the appearance of having breasts. Another parent said:

We haven't discussed the typical differences from other boys except when he was small and was made fun of beacuse of his breast. We just try to comfort him by downplaying the whole thing. We found it was very difficult to explain without confusing him.

A third parent stated:

He knows the basics, he has a girlfriend, but their relationship, because of her condition and his, is an occasional kiss. Talk about marriage is limited because neither realizes or copes with the process of children. Actually, not being able to reproduce is one blessing we see for our Prader-Willi son.

Parents of females with PWS observe that their daughters desire to be like normal girls and fantasize about boyfriends, marriage, and having babies. One parent wrote:

She seems preoccupied with wanting a baby, seems to understand where they come from, but doesn't know how they are made. She accepts the fact that mothers and fathers produce babies with their love. She has always been fond of babies and works as a volunteer one day a week in a daycare center.

Another indicated:

It was difficult for our daughter to understand and accept the fact that she will never have children. This fact was presented to her as gently as possible. She internalized sexual information and occasionally would play out sexual roles, acting out fantasies and romantic ideas. When the doctor told her she would never have any children it was a great psychological shock. She wants to be normal, to marry, and to have children.

It is apparent from these comments that the human dimension of sexuality should not be downplayed or ignored.

Sexuality and Mental Retardation

Historically, overt sexual activities by the mentally retarded evoked fear, which in turn fostered laws that segregated "defectives," encouraged sterilization, and prohibited marriage (Craft & Craft, 1984). Even now, in an enlightened era that purports to acknowledge that sexual expression is appropriate for mentally retarded individuals, public attitudes and acceptance lag far behind. Undocumented myths still place the mentally retarded at one of two extremes on the continum of sexual expression: mentally retarded people are either oversexed and sexually irresponsible or totally lacking any drive at all. In fact, "the sex drive of the mildly retarded is no different than the nonretarded" (Simonds, 1980, p. 173) and most mild to moderately impaired (non-PWS) individuals to develop normal reproductive function (Salerno Park, & Giannini, 1975). However, although mating, marrying, and having children is a normal sociosexual model, when retarded persons express or act out these desires, their behavior is likely to be considered inappropriate (Hall, 1975). Despite research that indicates that individuals with lower IQs show delayed sexual maturation and lowered drive, these persons do express sexual awareness (Hall, 1975; Salerno et al., 1975; Watson & Rogers, 1980; Wolfensberger, 1972). Evidence of this awareness in PWS individuals is described previously.

Although the presence of at least mild mental retardation in most individuals with PWS affects their capacity for psychosocial adaptation, they are no less impressed by seductive, sexually suggestive television advertising than is the normal population. They watch their normal siblings grow up and participate in family life cycle events where sexual expression of some sort is at least an implied activity. In school, PWS children are often mainstreamed into physical education classes where budding sexuality is highly visible. Unfortunately, the discrepancies between normal adolescents and the rather clumsy, socially immature, emotionally labile, sexually underdeveloped PWS teenagers are quite evident. And, although few will develop the cognitive ability necessary for further maturity, their sensitivity to being "different" does not diminish. Wolfe (1987) indicates a need for "opposite sex friends even if sexual feelings were minimal" (p. 719). Mental limitations and a healthy self-esteem should not be considered mutually exclusive concepts. Clearly, psychosexual adaptation for the PWS population is a difficult, painful process.

Psychosexual Growth and Development as a Developmental Process

Understanding sexual expression requires an appreciation of interrelatedness of cognitive, social, and psychosexual development. Social development and sexual behavior generally go hand-in-hand, and it usually takes several years even for normal teenagers to be comfortable with pubertal body changes. Evolution of a "sexual self" begins very early in life and progresses through fairly predictable stages of psychosexual development that should be clearly understood when assessing/evaluating sexual behavior in individuals with PWS. For instance, in the normal population, masturbation as a common self-stimulating activity beings early in life and continues thereafter in one form or another. The issue is not whether such behavior is appropriate, but rather how and when it is expressed at different points along the developmental continum. What is socially acceptable in toddlerhood changes as the child grows older. Another example of how sexual development evolves is the way in which children express their curiosity about body functions and explore one another by playing "doctor." This behavior, common in 5- to 7-year-olds, is usually accompanied by giggling about bathroom activities and discussion of breasts and genitalia. By preadolescence, bathroom humor shifts to use of more explicit terms, to jokes with sexual implications, and to budding attraction to the opposite sex.

Developmental tasks associated with normal intellectual, psychological, social, and sexual maturity, which have implications for individuals with PWS, are identified in Table 17.1 and may be a useful guide to expected behavior and appropriate management. (Note that the chronological age range identified in the table ends with early adolescence [13–15 years] because most individuals with PWS rarely reach this developmental stage physically, cognitively, or emotionally.

Parental Roles

The role parents play in helping their children achieve sexual maturity cannot be underestimated. In a real sense they orchestrate their children's future and should be aware not only of their offspring's developmental processes, but also the extent to which they influence their child's sexual identity. This awareness is fundamental to the promotion of appropriate sociosexual interactions, whatever their child's developmental level. The onset of puberty for normal offspring is a particularly stressful time. Parents tend to become anxious when questions arise about hygiene, menstruation, masturbation, nocturnal emissions, dating, homosexuality, sexual interactions, intercourse, and potential sexual abuse. Craft and Craft (1985) pointed out the fact that "many normal children mature in spite of, rather than because of, parents" (p. 495). Furthermore, although many parents feel they should have a good "woman-to-woman" or "man-to-man" talk and discuss sex and reproduction, few actually do (Farrell, 1978).

If many parents are ill-at-ease in discussing sexuality with their normal offspring, what happens in families in which a child is developmentally disabled? Certainly, in families with a PWS child, parental roles are more complicated and discussion of sex may be very disconcerting and awkward. In some instances, parents, believing their child is asexual, ignore evidence of sexual thoughts and attempt to suppress sexual expression. Others feel that purposeful talk about sex will only stir up "bad ideas" and that provision of information and/or sex education is to be discouraged. Some hold the view that sex should remain simple, uncomplicated, and available only for procreation within the sanctity of marriage, and since they expect the PWS child will neither marry or reproduce, they see no need to discuss sex at all. In some instances parents unwittingly transmit mixed messages; they admit their child's need for healthy social interactions, but are fearful of encouraging "closeness." Concerned that simple hand-holding may lead to overt sexual activity, they overprotect to eliminate hurt and disappointment. A major concern is that if the child lives away from the family, sexual expression may not be appropriately supervised or prevented.

How well individuals with PWS adapt psychosexually depends to a great extent on parental coping mechanisms and their perception of their child's needs (Buscala, 1983). Parents should be encouraged to discuss their own attitudes about sexual expression as well as how they feel about sexuality as a social dimension of PWS. Some will need help in developing realistic responses to the questions put to them by their PWS children about getting married and having children. Perhaps the current sociological phenomenon of "voluntary childlessness" may serve as an example that not everyone need be a parent.

The question that remains is, "Can an individual with PWS be whole if the potential for sexual expression is repressed?" Perhaps the healthiest response will be for parents to acknowledge that their children are entitled to human relationships and have needs for gratification and emotional closeness. Since most affected individuals are capable of learning to express their feelings and engage in appropriate interactions, their sociosexual relationships should be encouraged.

TABLE 17.1. Stages and tasks in normal sexual development that are relevant for individuals with Prader-Willi Syndrome.[a]

Physical	Emotional	Social
Embryo		
Sex determination chromosomes: male, XY; female, XX		
Fetus		
Male: develop testes at 6–7 weeks. Female: ovaries at 12 weeks.		
Birth		
Gender assignment		
Infancy: 0–1 year		
Oral pleasure. Physical response to genital stimulation by self or others. Erective capacity. Touch response. Able to tell self from others.	Self-centered. Self love, sense of feeling of pleasure and displeasure. Trust/mistrust.	Interacts with primary family. 6–12 months = fear of strangers. Likes an audience.
Toddler: 1–3 years		
Total body exploring. Learns muscle control and toilet training. Masturbation to pleasure self. Learns about physical sex differences.	Needs to achieve. Anxious about being accepted. Developing self-control. Senses "goodness or badness" of body. Core gender identity and sex differences evolve.	Uses force to get own way. Likes getting affection. Less fear of strangers. Explores sex differences of others.
4–6 year-olds		
Genital manipulation to explore self, to feel pleasure, to relieve mysterious "tension." Sex play and exploration with playmates.	Awareness of genital differences leads to a sense of guilt. Internal controls increase as conscience develops. Attachment to parental figures.	Time for learning basic skills of interpersonal relationships. Development of appropriate social behavior. Identification with parent of same sex. Begins to assert self and reinforce sex identity and gender role.
Early school years: 6–10 years (latency)		
Gradual build-up of hormones triggered by the pituitary gland at about age 8 (adrenarche). Accurate knowledge of genital anatomy. Physical change is not evident until late in this "latency stage."	Begins sexual daydreaming. Repression of sexual expression increases as understanding of significance of sexual activity develops. Freudian concept of "latency" does not mean that "sexual thinking" is not present, but rather that it is low-keyed.	Child learns that sex is not "discussed" in everyday conversation. Social identification with parent of same sex. Sex role rehearsal increases. Sex awareness increases along with increased self-consciousness. Plays with peers of same sex. Ambivalence toward opposite sex. Give-and-take in social interactions; sharing fears and fantasies with friends of same sex, but rarely with parent. Expects to select a non-family member as a partner but not sure why.
Preadolescence: 10–12 years		
Onset of menses. Secondary sex characteristics: pubic and axillary hair. Beginning of seminal emissions, continued self-exploration and stimulation.	Concern over body image increases. Self-concept tied to signs of sexual growth. Guilt over sexual ideation causes confusion. Worries about onset of puberty if lacking information. Lack of positive experience leads to poor self-concept.	Learning about self-control. Testing of behavioral limits incorporates sexual identity. Same-sex relationships are "safe" but ready to shift.
Early adolescence: 13–15 years		
Masturbation common. Capacity for erection. Pubic and axillary hair prominent. Breast development. Broad variation in height and growth. Nocturnal emissions in normal individuals.	Sexual thoughts and fantasies common. Need for recognition as male or female. Much anxiety over appearance of sexual growth. Fear of being different from peers. Loneliness if not accepted. Feelings of inadequacy if not like others.	Desire for opposite-sex relationships. Puppy love. Awkward heterosexual interactions. Social attempts create worries about acceptance by peers.

Note: From *Comprehensive Psychiatric Nursing* (pp. 176–178) by J. Haber, A. Leach, S. Schudy, and B. Sideleau, 1982, New York: McGraw Hill; and *Sexuality: A Nursing Perspective* (pp. 62–70) by F. Mims and M. Swensen, 1980, New York: McGraw-Hill. Adapted by permission.

[a]These stages and tasks of development are listed only through very early adolescence as research indicates that individuals with PWS rarely develop secondary sex characteristics or reach this era cognitively or emotionally.

Intellectual	Cultural	Examples of behavior
Imitates others.	Parental influence is supreme.	Warm physical relationship with nurturing person stimulates sensory perceptions. Likes to cuddle for warmth and safety. Wants to be held.
Sense of success and failure begins. Reassures self about own genitalia. Learns sex role expectations. Vocabulary related to genital anatomy, elimination, reproduction. Begins to understand right and wrong.	General acceptance of limited nudity in public.	Impulsivity channeled into socially acceptable behavior. Lack of awareness of sexual significance of masturbation; just "does it." Sensual/erotic activities such as hugging, kissing, rhythmic motions reflect desire for pleasuring self.
Vocabulary of "dirty" words increases. Differential thinking leads to understanding how sexes differ. Interactions with opposite sex begin to be overtly structured. The concept of a relationship with the opposite sex is noted (i.e. marriage). Asks questions about "where babies come from." Can learn to use proper terms such as "penis" or "vagina."	Social customs beginning to have impact, but parental influence still paramount. Responsive to sanctions to activities such as masturbation. The idea of "not nice," "nasty," or "don't touch" has impact. Feelings about being male or female culturally integrated.	Giggles and uses "dirty" words. Fascination with bathrooms and bathroom activity. Curious about sex differences and different postures for urinating. Wants to marry parent of opposite sex. Begins to develop childhood romance. Pretends to be "in love" by sitting close and giving gifts. Purposefully explores own body. Play "doctor" games.
Understands the social significance of sexual behavior. Much curiosity and questions are very specific. Moral attitudes and values are intellectually integrated. Appropriate behavior is understood. Verbal "banter" now has significance.	Parental influence still predominates but peer pressure, media influence, and school begin to have impact. Close observation of non-family members' sexual behavior noted and questioned. Heterosexual interactions still limited. This is a critical time for integrating male/female sexual cultural attitudes. Parents tend to worry about child being "appropriate." Same-sex association to learn "good" role model encouraged. This is the one stage of sexual development when homosexual relationships are encouraged.	As interest in bathroom activities decreases, curiosity about more subtle overt sex differences increases (beards, breasts, pregnancy, etc.). Ages 5–7: play house, doctor, pretend having a baby. Much sex play with same sex but it is more covert. Inspection of genitals of same sex. Ages 8–10: Less role playing but verbal discussion and interest increases. Females curious about menses. Males want details of fertilization and pregnancy. Refuse to be seen nude by parent of opposite sex. Begin to rate self for attractiveness. Sex jokes rather crude, based on primitive knowledge base. Normal voyeurism. Dirty words for shock value. When sexes are mixed, teasing increases and kissing games are common.
Able to make cognitive connection between anatomy and use, but self-conscious about asking about specifics. Will seek a nonparent figure for information.	Parental values strong but peer values being integrated in secret. Cultural norms very influential. Rigid parental values will cause conflict and merely delay development of internal value system. Parental level of sexual comfort has impact on adaptation.	Interest in sex demonstrated through preoccupation with body changes and sex-related jokes. Interested and awed by changes in self and others. Conflicted ideas based on biases against opposite sex along with a defined but limited romantic interest. Tries to copy older role model. Heterosexual activity begins with teasing and roughhousing with the opposite sex as an excuse for physical contact. Boys report homosexual experiences between ages 11–13, girls usually a year or so earlier. Dressing to look "older" begins. Girls want to buy "bras," boys "supporters."
Testing self as a source of self-control. Awareness of sex differentiation from a cognitive level. Demands independence.	Peer pressure overcomes parent value system. Conflicts over limits and controls and decision making. Parental concerns over less control and desire for appropriate behavior.	Compulsive, mechanical masturbation as a relief. Groupie behavior. "Dress alikes." Flirtation. Seeks out opposite sex for interactions. Jealousies cause conflicts. Arguments with authority figures common.

The Role of the Professional

Professionals, aware that sexual expression is a relevant aspect of life for the developmentally disabled, are now giving considerable thought to managing these issues. Interventions (counseling, teaching, group facilitating, etc.) require them to be comfortable in their own sexuality, at ease with the topic, and skilled in communication concepts.

The professional role in assisting PWS individuals to adapt pyschosexually has four major dimensions, the first of which is understanding the syndrome's characteristics and acknowledging that this population has the potential for sociosexual activity within the constraints of the condition. Second, parents and primary care providers should be incorporated into any counseling/learning process since their attitudes and acceptance play a major role in how, when, and where sexuality is expressed. When parents collaborate with professionals to nurture sexual awareness in PWS children the process becomes legitimized. The very fact that they "know their child best" aids in developing individualized approaches. First-hand knowledge about what their child understands may deescalate parental anxieties about this sensitive issue.

The third dimension of professional support of psychosexuality in PWS individuals concerns the need for honest, uncomplicated sex education programs that incorporate discussion of sexual issues appropriate for this population. Optimally, parents provide sex education during day-to-day interactions. However, where gaps exist in this teaching process, carefully structured, formalized programs are available that can be adapted to the special needs of PWS. The Sex Information and Educational Counsel of the United States (SIECUS) is an excellent resource that recognizes the importance of human sexuality in the developmentally disabled and the need for interactions with the opposite sex. SIECUS also supports the premise that appropriate behavior can be learned with guidance. Its curriculum focuses on awareness of self, awareness of physical sex differences and body changes, development of healthy interpersonal relationships that can progress from self-respect to respect for privacy, and the importance of responsibility to society as males and females participating in a variety of life-styles (single, married, etc.) (Spurr, 1976).

Healthy psychosexual adaptation can also be strengthened and enhanced through interdisciplinary collaboration. For example, the social worker's assessment of the family unit may offer special insights into family dynamics, living arrangements, and vocational expectations; a marital counselor may have a better view of parental strengths and limitations; and educators may be in the best position to evaluate how PWS individuals relate to their peers (of both sexes).

Finally, the role of the professional in understanding psychosexuality in individuals with PWS would not be complete without addressing the issue of potential sexual abuse in this population. Several accounts of abuse of children with PWS have been reported (where the children were bribed with candy). However, there are no data to suggest that these children are sexually abused more than comparably handicapped children. Heinemann (1983) identified the PWS population as being at risk because they are generally cognitively limited, more dependent and vulnerable to anyone who befriends them, in need of physical attention, likely to be in a setting where "adults" are in control, and more easily bribed with food.

Prevention of sexual abuse in PWS is no small task. It should be emphasized to the child that there is a difference between "good touch" and "bad touch"; cognitive limitations require that this lesson be periodically reinforced. The child needs to be taught that it is all right to say "no" to an adult, and that there are physical and emotional limits to be enforced. Reduction of sex role stereotyping, particularly submissiveness or passivity, is also important. Letting the child know that any concerns or fears they may have will be carefully heard, and that "secret" behavior is to be avoided, is essential.

How to discuss the topic of sexual abuse is a challenge and is best addressed within the larger context of body safety. It is best to initiate this discussion of body safety when the children are very young. Be specific, ask "what if" questions, be nonjudgmental, and believe the child. Recognize that it is not the child's duty (nor always within his or her capability) to recognize and terminate inappropriate sexual advances, but that the ultimate responsibility of inappropriate behavior is with the perpetrator.

Conclusion

Understanding the concepts of human sexuality from a developmental perspective offers parents, care providers, and professionals the opportunity to develop realistic attitudes and feelings about sociosexual behavior in the PWS population. A list of facts about sexuality that have significance for persons who serve individuals with PWS follows. It has been adapted from Perski (1981), Mims and Swenson (1980), Robinault (1978), Gordon (1974), and de la Cruz and LaVeck (1973).

1. Individuals with PWS are not asexual; they have drives and interests and, most significantly, will develop strong gender role identification. Individual family, religious, and social values play a major part in how their sexuality is expressed.
2. Psychosexual maturation occurs at a later chronological age as compared to person of normal intelligence. However, sexual interest tends to remain lower where intellectual functioning is lower.
3. Although the average age at which most developmentally disabled individuals reach physical maturity is essentially the same as normal pubescence, PWS sexual maturation is usually indefinitely delayed.

4. Difficulties in motor coordination in PWS often result in a lack of participation in those group activities that normally encourage social exposure and may contribute to the delay in acknowledgment of sex roles.
5. The sexual activity of most individuals with PWS is basically exploratory and innocent in nature. Genital manipulation and masturbation are most often fostered by boredom, lack of activities, and a failure to understand what is acceptable public social conduct.
6. Many individuals with PWS have difficulty expressing their feelings appropriately, no matter how verbal they appear, possibly because they do not perceive themselves as receiving either symbolic or concrete evidence of affection.
7. Affected adolescents have been known to express a desire for companionship and dating, and either ask or infer sex-related questions and thinking. They have the same needs for intimacy, privacy, and relationships as anyone else.
8. Ongoing support and understanding is needed as individuals with PWS become aware of how different they really are from their normal peers. When encouraged to deal with the realities of their psychosexual limitations early in life, most can learn to adapt. These realities include:
   a. understanding that most PWS individuals "know that they are" different. This "differentness" produces increased stress in adolescence and needs to be addressed.
   b. the fact that many individuals with PWS have the capacity for some measure of sexual expression.
   c. a society that currently accepts females in nonmateral roles and families in general as voluntarily childless.
   d. teaching people with PWS to be responsible for their public and private sexual activities.

In the final analysis, it should be emphasized that the inability to develop a traditional sex life does not mean that individuals with PWS are less male or less female; their capacity to be sociosexual beings is not diminished.

References

Craft, A.N., & Craft, M. (1985). Sexuality and mental handicap: A review. *British Journal of Psychiatry*, *139*, 495–505.

Buscala, L. (1983). *The disabled and their parents.* Tornoto: Holt, Rinehart, and Winston.

de la Cruz, F., & La Veck, C. (Eds.). (1973). *Human sexuality and the mentally retarded.* New York: Brunner-Mazel.

Farrell, C. (1978). *My mother said. . .*, London: Routledge and Kegan Paul.

Gordon, S. (1974). *Sex rights for people who happen to be handicapped* (Monograph Number 6, pp. 351–381). Syracuse, NY: Center on Human Policy, Syracuse University.

Greenswag, L.R. (1985, June). *Sexuality for people with Prader-Willi syndrome: Is ignorance bliss?* Proceedings of National Conference of Prader-Willi Syndrome Assocation, Windsor Locks, CT.

Hall, J. (1975). Sexuality and the mentally retarded. In R. Green (Ed.), *Human sexuality: A health practitioner's text* (pp. 181–195). Baltimore, MD: Williams and Wilkins.

Heinemann, J.T. (1983). *Caution, children at risk; dealing with sexual abuse in developmentally disabled children.* The Missouri View, Prader-Willi Syndrome Association, St. Louis, MO.

Hogan, R. (1985). *Human sexuality, a nursing perspective.* Norwalk, CT: Appleton-Century-Crofts.

Mims, F., & Swenson, M. (1980). *Sexuality: A nursing perspective.* New York: McGraw Hill Book Company.

Perski, R. (1981). *Hope for families.* Nashville: Abington Press.

Robinault, I. (1978). *Sex, society and the disabled: A developmental inquiry into roles, reactions and responsibilities.* New York: Harper Row.

Salerno, J., Park J., & Giannini, M. (1975). Reproductive capacity of the mentally retarded. *Journal of Reproductive Medicine, 14*, 123–129.

Simons, J. (1980). Sexual behavior in retarded children and adolescents. *Developmental and Behavioral Pediatrics, 1*, (4), 173–179.

Spurr, G. (1976). Sex education and the handicapped. *Journal of Sex Education Therapy, 2*, (2) 23–26.

Watson, G., & Rogers, R.S. (1980). Sexual instruction for the mildly retarded and normal adolescent: A comparison of educational approaches, parental expectations, and pupil knowledge and attitude. *Health Education Journal, 39*, 88–95.

Wolfensberger, W. (1972). *Normalization: The principal of normalization in human services.* Toronto: National Institute of Mental Retardation.

Wolff, O. (1987). Prader-Willi syndrome—psychiatric aspects. *Journal of the Royal Society of Medicine, 80*, 718–720

Zellweger, H., & Schneider, H. (1968). Syndrome of hypotonia-hypomentia-hypogonadism-obesity (HHHO) or Prader-Willi syndrome. *American Journal of Diseases of Children, 115*, 558–598.

18
A Parent's Point of View

Janalee Tomaseski-Heinemann

"Prader-Willi syndrome—what's that?" I asked, as most people do, when I first met my husband, Al. At that time he was raising his 6-year-old daughter Sarah and 7-year-old son Matt, who has the syndrome. As a social worker who raised three children of my own, I thought I knew a lot about child rearing. However, as my relationship with Al grew, I decided to research PWS before making a commitment to marriage. Although I read some articles dealing with the syndrome's diagnosis and physical aspects, I discovered that the realities and impact of Prader-Willi syndrome (PWS) could not be comprehended until I actually lived with it. Seven years have gone by and we have survived as individuals and as a family despite the frustrations and tears associated with Matt's diet restrictions and behavior problems. In fact, we have done more than survive; we have loved and laughed and grown a lot. How have we endured? What have we done? Well, our solutions will not guarantee complete success nor do they "follow the book" on discipline, but they represent our point of view about living with a child with PWS. If some of the commentary seems disjointed, it's probably because, from time to time, so are our lives.

PWS Diet Secrets (For Adults Only)

Heading a long list of concerns that parents of children with PWS must confront are the issues of food and eating. When Al was raising the kids alone, he attempted many diets with Matt with no success. There was always an angry struggle because Matt had to eat differently than the rest of the family and never had his favorite foods. "Giving in," plus the fine art of sneaking food, made eating all his lettuce salads a futile effort at weight control. We recognize that Matt constantly lives in an unfair situation and, although our policy with the kids is to be honest, we do what we can to make Matt feel that he is being treated more fairly. Our trick is always to be a little smarter, more alert, and occasionally more devious than he is. Anyone who has lived with a child with PWS knows that when it comes to food, this can be a challenge and one that we don't always win. But, the fact is, Matt did lose 32 pounds in a year.

Although I agree that the dietary guidelines from nutritionists and doctors are clinically correct, it is another issue completely to live with the recommended restrictions. Here is some offbeat advice that reduced some of the grief and aggrevation associated with food-related problems.

Lock Away Temptation

It would have been hard to convince me before, but the pain of putting locks on the refrigerator and cupboards was our headache—not Matt's. He not only seemed to understand, but seemed relieved that the responsibility for not sneaking food had been taken from him since he had no control. As he said to us, "I try not to sneak but my hand reaches in the refrigerator and I can't stop it."

The Fine Art of Sneaking

Even if children with PWS have to live in an unfair world, why rub their noses in this inequity? I was appalled when I read an article about behavior management of adolescents with PWS who were forced to sit with half a plate of food in front of them and punished if they touched it. (Perhaps we should also try electric prods on the refrigerator!) Since we are fortunate enough to be able to eat more than Matt, the least we can do is to be discreet. Sneaky is another word for it. Matt's sister, Sarah, is allowed snacks and extra treats, but *only* if she asks when out of sight and sound of Matt. This allows her to have the same privileges as other kids and Matt is no worse off. Perhaps when Sarah grows up, her husband will have a difficult time understanding why she prefers to eat behind the bedroom door. As for Al and me, we have a "stash drawer" and lock ourselves in the bedroom—for more than sex.

The Hand Is Quicker than the Eye

Matt is not allowed to fix his own food, dish out his own plate, or hover in the kitchen while meals are being prepared. At first he was unhappy at not being able to "help out" in the kitchen (after all, his goal in life is to be a chef), but he finally accepted this rule. Now, he isn't as aware of when we skimp on his food and we don't have to worry whether *his* hand is quicker than *our* eyes.

Dinner Time Drama

Serving food can be a fine art. We quit kidding ourselves long ago about emulating the ideal American family at the dinner table. Matt and Sarah are allowed to eat in front of the TV and their food is set up on trays, which solves several problems. Matt is less aware of who gets what portion, watching TV reduces his obsession with keeping his eye on the food, and food is served out of pans directly onto plates, reducing dirty dishes (an extra bonus). Al and I have a chance to sit down to a peaceful meal and conversation and don't have to guard the dinner table.

Garnishing the Garnish

Food preparation requires visual skills along with the usual nutritionist's advice. Matt gets the same food we do, but his portions are smaller. A smaller plate and cup are used and his food is spread out on the dish. Extra, nonfattening foods items such as carrots, dill pickles or diet jello are added to make the amount on the plate look larger. Since he may only get one-half a banana or apple, it is cut up into slices and served in a bowl to make it less obvious that it's only half. Less visible foods are skipped (i.e., butter or mayonnaise on sandwiches, and potatoes). The finishing touch is to serve Matt a little bit smaller portion than we plan on him eating, so that he can come back for "one more spoonful."

Surviving the Cafeteria

Packing a diet lunch for school is an unrewarding chore we have learned to avoid. Matt is allowed to buy the hot lunch and skip one fattening item on the menu (e.g., the potatoes or the dessert). The item skipped is his choice, providing it's not the salad. He receives great praise from his teacher, who monitors his choice. Of course, this means nothing if he sneaks leftovers or snacks from other students. We keep in close touch with the school, his teacher, and the cooks, to see that Matt is closely watched in the lunchroom, constantly reminding them that although he may appear to have control over his diet, *his* hand may also be quicker than *all* of their eyes. The teacher has explained to Matt's classmates why it is so important for Matt's health not to give him any of their food.

The Payoff—Self-Pride

Children with PWS vary in terms of how much they can eat and not gain weight. Furthermore, it is hard to monitor every calorie. Our solution is to have a daily weigh-in that we record on a chart on the refrigerator. At first, when Matt lost 2 pounds, he was rewarded with a small toy. Now we have been able to eliminate the reward because Matt seems to get enough self-satisfaction from his weight loss to want to continue. With a total lack of modesty, and beaming with pride, he says "I think I world's champion weight loser!"

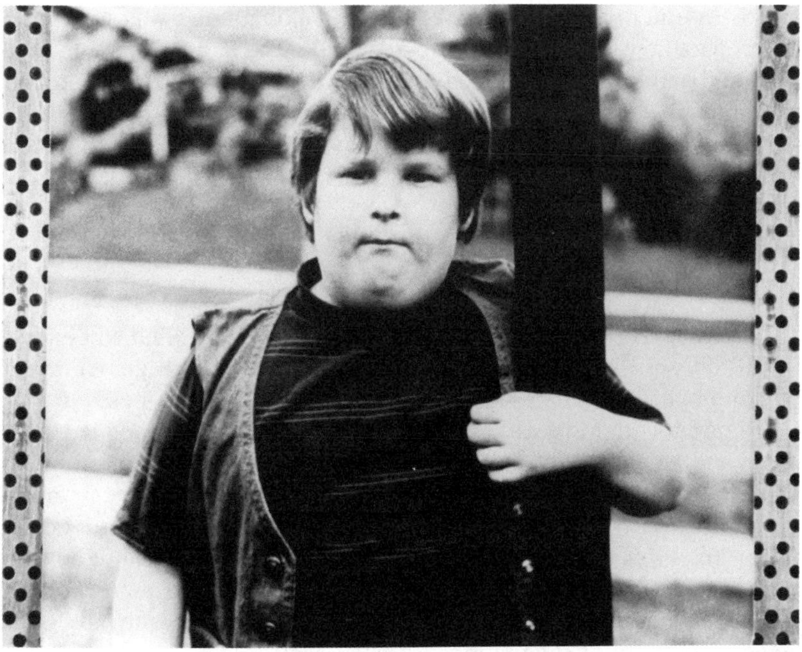

FIGURE 18.1. Matt at age 7, before his weight loss.

Love Means Saying "No"

All of the hard work of weight control will be to no avail if relatives, friends, or babysitters are feeding your child behind your back. People who really care about you and your child will not sabotage your efforts. Parents do not have to apologize when requesting that no treats be given. In fairness to others, though, education is necessary. This may mean swallowing one's pride and explaining PWS in detail, with all its "do's and don'ts." At first it was hard for Al to admit to the extent of Matt's problems. Also, it's confusing for the child with PWS when Grandma (or heaven forbid, Daddy!) slips him a treat while Mommy always says "No!" When the child is treated with consistency, there won't be any "good guys" and "bad guys." We try to help Matt understand that we are truly sorry that he is always hungry and frustrated and it seems that he is learning that "no" can still be a loving word.

Behavior and Your Child with PWS

When it comes to dealing with behaviors, rule number one is "Don't wait for experts, you may be it." There is no magic person out there with all the answers. In other words, when your boat is sinking, don't wait around for "the professionals" to tell you how to handle the situation, just grab a bucket and bail. Educate yourself about PWS, the effects of brain impairment, and behavior modification. Don't close your ears to the professionals, just sift through and weigh what they say and see how it fits your needs. (That goes for all this advice as well.) The following guidelines may help.

Set the Rules, Explain the Options, and Rehearse

Let your child know exactly what the limitations are and what will happen when he does well or if he "blows it." Spell out expected guidelines for eating and behavior *before* going anywhere. It used to be impossible to go to a restaurant with Matt without having him push for more food than he is allowed and having a tantrum if he didn't get his way. Now, before we go he is told exactly what he can order and cautioned that he'll get no more. He used to have to be reminded (this is no longer necessary) that if he gets upset or pressures us, one of us will leave immediately with him, he'll get no bedtime treat, and he will not be allowed to go the next time. This system not only spells out the rules for Matt but also helps us avoid getting trapped in an emotional situation. Recently Matt was even able to handle a Thanksgiving visit with all the relatives with no upsets or pushing for extra food—a feat beyond our dreams a few years ago.

Consistency (That Evil Word) and Vigilance

You've heard of the importance of being consistent time and time again. Unfortunately, I need to give you the bad news—it works! PWS is similar to other brain-impaired conditions in which affected individuals have difficulty with abstract reasoning; rarely can they think in terms of "exceptions." They thrive on routines and knowing exactly what the guidelines are. One day of extra food privileges creates days of grief before we get Matt back to proper behavior. The real challenge is getting *both* parents to be consistent, since behavior management is not just a part-time job.

Rewards (There Are "Good Days")

There is conflicting advice on whether to use food as a reinforcement. One concern is that the use of food as a reward may encourage even more of an obsession. Tell me, how can a child with PWS become even *more* obsessed about food than he already is? Matt thinks, talks, and dreams food 24 hours a day. We can be driving on a long trip and talking continuously with Matt sound asleep in the back seat. Mention the word "pizza" and he will immediately sit straight up with his eyes wide open and say "Pizza? Who say that?" The fact is that for us, using food as a reward works. Of course, the food reward is minimal. If Matt is good all day, he gets a small piece of candy as a bedtime treat but supper must have fewer calories to compensate. A nonfood reward system was used to deal with Matt's "crying behavior" at school. We arranged for his teacher to send us daily "good day" or "bad day" reports. When he collected 5 "good days" in a row, or 10 cumulatively, he could buy a small toy. Gradually, as he gained more control, the reward was reduced and then eliminated.

Punishments (Time Out for Both Sides)

Since Al and I are heavily into talking problems out with the kids, it took a while for us to learn to keep our mouths shut. Talking things out with a child with PWS *DOES NOT WORK!* This makes more sense to me as I read more about problems associated with brain dysfunction. I mentioned before that children with PWS don't think abstractly and are rarely able to experience one situation and generalize to others. They also have trouble separating important details from less important ones. *Everything* is critical and they "get stuck" on one concern and cannot go on to the next. Add to this impaired thinking a desperate hunger and emotional "ups and downs" and the stage is set for a large blow-up! I cannot express strongly enough the importance of "defusing" a situation early and not wasting energy on "logic" or "threats." The minute Matt gets upset, he is *immediately* sent to his room. We stay low-keyed and firm. He is allowed to come out as soon as he is "feeling better." At that point the problem is discussed, but only if he can talk calmly. Afterward we don't harp on the issue. Mind you, this tactic didn't come about easily. At first, when Matt was sent to his room, he would kick, scream, and tear it apart. The consequences of this behavior were that anything he wrecked was removed permanently from the room and not repaired, and if the situation became too intense, one of us would go in and calmly say, "You have five minutes to settle down, Matt, and if you haven't done so by then, you will only get a small sandwich for supper." As his room got more barren, Matt got better, and lost a few extra pounds in the process. This tactic has been effective. Although I would never totally eliminate a meal, losing weight helps children with PWS and the expectation of getting less food is a strong incentive. The good news is that we discovered Matt has more control over these tantrums than we thought he could have. They now never go beyond a quiet crying spell (well, most of the time).

Don't Set Yourself Up

I am painfully aware of the difficulties involved with the suggestions for behavioral change just described. Just remember that your other options may be even more painful. While you and your child are in the initial stage of deciding who's boss, try to reduce the number of awkward situations in which you put yourself. For example, attending a buffet dinner is looking for trouble and going to the supermarket isn't much better. Situations are always coming up that others simply will never understand. Once, when I realized that Matt had been alone in the mixed candy aisle at the grocery store, I must have given him "the eye" because he immediately exclaimed "I didn't take any Mom, see!"—and pulled his pockets inside out as proof. Some customers looked with pity at Matt and glared at me. I slunk away.

If you are beginning to feel like a drill sergeant in the Marines, try to remember that caring and loving needs to remain a part of all this. Otherwise any guidelines for changing behavior won't mean a thing.

Use Positive Reinforcement

Although there is plenty to criticize, look hard for opportunities to make positive comments. Matt *thrives* on compliments. *If we can't say anything good, we don't say anything*. Fortunately, his teachers are also good at positive reinforcement. This same young man who can feel so bad about himself can also, at times, be bursting with self-pride. For a long time Matt's behavior and weight seemed to us and to him to be totally out of hand. But now he has learned to have some control. Not too long ago, he came home all excited from school and said, "Your know what? I almost have a bad day. Tears started to come out of my eyes, but I say, 'Stop it! Stop it!'—and the tears stopped!" Later he said, "I'm so proud of me!" That's a whole lot more important than Al and me being proud of him.

Set Rules Out of Love and Set Them Together

Being tough on a child already struggling in life can be painful to watch. Al has said, "when your child can have so few pleasures in life, it's hard to take away what makes him most happy, even when I know in the back of my mind that it's not in his best interest." While Al has struggled with these food and behavior issues, he now can see that Matt is much happier. The fact that Matt's self-concept is improving is our most important reinforcement. No matter how hard it may be to achieve, our ultimate goal is that he will be able to socialize and "fit in" as much as possible, in spite of his special needs. As Matt has said, "When you're fat and mad, you feel sad." An obese, angry, lonely child cannot grow up to be a happy adult. Being "tough" is difficult but the consequences of not being so are even tougher.

Listen Beyond the Tantrum

When a child with PWS is screaming, crying, swearing, swinging his arms, and telling you he hates you, it is hard to listen and to feel anything but anger. It is difficult to understand the speech of a PWS child, and frequently when the child is out of control, he repeats the same words and thoughts

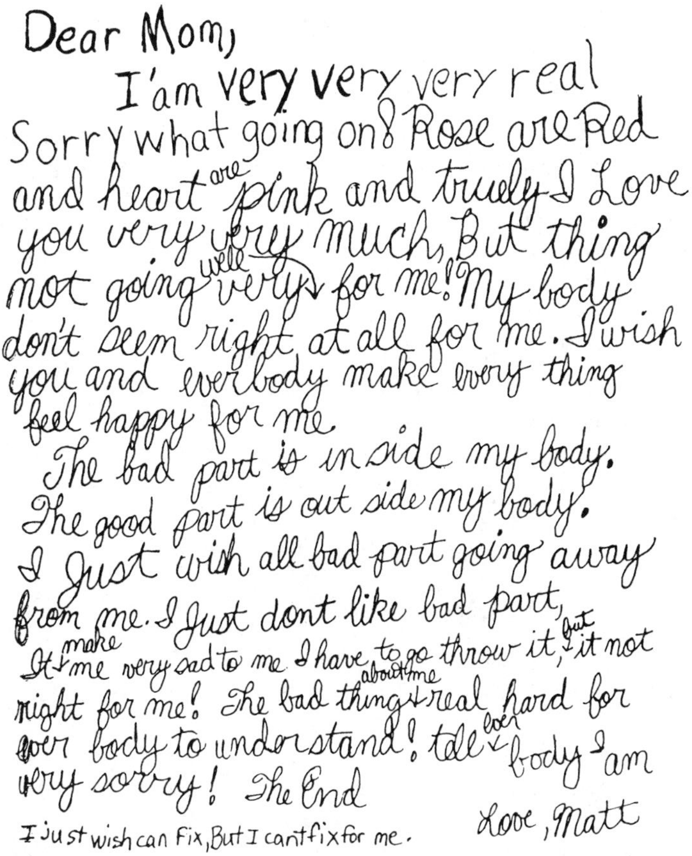
Dear Mom,
I'am very very very real
Sorry what going on? Rose are Red
and heart are pink and truely I Love
you very very much, But thing
not going well very for me! My body
don't seem right at all for me. I wish
you and everbody make every thing
feel happy for me.
The bad part is in side my body.
The good part is out side my body.
I Just wish all bad part going away
from me. I Just dont like bad part,
It make me very sad to me I have to go throw it, but it not
right for me! The bad thing about me real hard for
over body to understand! tale ever body I am
very sorry! The End
I just wish can Fix, But I cant fix for me.
Love, Matt

FIGURE 18.2.

over and over. It is as if his foot were stuck on the accelerator of his rage at 100 mph and he cannot let up until he crashes. At that point, who *wants* to listen to what he is saying? Al has said that during the first moments of a tantrum, it would save a lot of grief if we had a type of spray to squirt in Matt's face which would make him fall asleep instantly. I have included an apologetic note that Matt wrote after a major tantrum (we rate them major, minor, and crying spells). During the tantrum, he said he hated us for "studying about Prader-Willi." He swore, tore the heads off flowers in the yard, then cried and hollered in his bedroom for 2 hours—then fell asleep. When Matt woke up, he was contrite and quiet, played patiently for hours with our 4-year-old grandson and thoroughly enjoyed swimming in the pool with his 20-year-old brother, Tad. The Prader-Willi "demon" has passed and hopefully will stay out of Matt's soul for awhile.

Maybe we don't want to hear "beyond the tantrum" for fear of the pain we might see. In a recent "crying spell" (lowest rating on the tantrum scale) we worked very hard to hear what Matt had to say. Once, after finding an article on PWS, he said that when he sees something written about PWS, it reminds him that he has "it," and:

. . . it goes over and over in my brain. I can't help read about it because I curious. It [the written information] say I always be short and I never have sex. . . . it say I never be normal. It hurt in my heart and in my head. . . . It say about what between my legs [small penis and undescended testicles]. I never have a girlfriend. I be embarrassed she see me. It say I die before I get old. . . . I think about food all the time. [When] I see food I can't have, I feel anxious. I want it real bad and it make me mad. . . . You don't know what it's like. You don't know what I feel!

Matt tends to fixate on an issue for a while, then changes topics, but mostly his thoughts deal with the unfairness of having PWS. I often wonder how much of his rage is a chemical/neurological dysfunction and how much is justified anger at the world. Looking at Matt's tortured mind is sometimes more than we (or he) can bear. You're right Matt, we don't know what it's like. If we let ourselves feel what you feel, we wouldn't be strong enough to lift you up when it was over, give you a hug, and say, "Let's go on from here."

Does a Disabled Child Mean a Disabled Marriage?

"Don't let one tragedy multiply into others!" I heard that remark at a speech at a genetics conference. It helps to cope with our child's disabilities when we can minimize the other stressors in our life and develop a good support system. Too often, though, a "domino effect" begins at birth. Gradually over the years, the tragedy of the child's disability, the personal trauma to each parent, the stress between a husband and wife, and the tension for the entire family leads to a dysfunctional family in which relationships are shattered and the "house comes tumbling down." Al and I have developed our own system for survival.

We have absolved ourselves of guilt. Parents are people and have a right to their own lives. Parents of children with a disability such as PWS deal with more stress than average parents and need to make time to replenish their strength. Notice, I said "make time," not "find time." With five children, two grandchildren, and both of us working full-time plus volunteer work, Al and I have to be conscientious about prioritizing our time. The car may never get waxed, the oven seldom gets cleaned, and the TV never is watched. It also means that occasionally the children are ignored so we can have our personal time together. If we don't nurture ourselves as individuals and as a couple, we cannot joyfully give to our children.

We work hard to avoid taking our relationship for granted because we know it takes time and effort to make it stay good. It's too easy to get wrapped up in Matt and to let everyone and everything take second place.

As couples, most of us put considerable effort into nurturing our relationship when we were dating; we need to continue to do so after marrying. Besides prioritizing our time, we have made a pact never to go to bed angry. This may mean long, late-night discussions, but little hurts can build into major problems if they are not dealt with. Besides, what is the alternative? Being in a bad marriage can be the loneliest place in the world.

We try to keep an eye on our stress factors. It helps to know "where the enemy lies" rather than have a vague feeling of being bombarded from all sides, so periodically we take count. Last year, we had many unforeseen and unavoidable crises. We were able to take count and say, "No wonder we are feeling stressed—we should be!" We decided on survival tactics and reminded ourselves, "this too shall pass." This year, life is going much more smoothly. Now, whenever we feel stressed, we "take count" and usually discover that we are uptight over minor things that just aren't worth it.

Savoring good times is important. It is just too easy to get caught up in an "ain't life awful" frame of mind and not take time to appreciate the "good." We often worry about what will happen next week, next month, or next year and forget to appreciate today. Just how flexible can you be? If it's a beautiful day outside, will you drop your project of cleaning out the garage to take a long walk together with the kids? Are you willing to give up your nightly TV program for an hour together in the bedroom where you can talk about the day over a glass of wine? Sometimes Al and I remind and recite to each other what we are thankful for. Of course, this is easier to do when we are out alone for dinner and the kids, the house, and the bills are at least 10 miles away.

Getting physically active can help. We've all read of how important it is to relieve stress by getting regular exercise. Al works out and I swim at a local health club. We always feel better when we do it on a regular, twice-weekly basis, but I have to admit that sometimes we have difficulty prioritizing this time. (Once it was so long between visits that I forgot my locker combination.) I use swimming as a way to relax and meditate. For Al, swimming isn't relaxing—just a means to keep from drowning. In this era of jogging, I am proud to say I have never run a block in my life. It's all in what turns you on and your tension off. Speaking of what turns you on, "getting physical" also means touching each other a lot, holding hands, kissing, and making love even if it's not Saturday night. It's amazing how many couples feel it's okay to fight in front of the kids, but not okay to snuggle and hold hands in front of them.

Take time to cry a little, laugh a lot, and be a little crazy. There are going to be times when life seems overwhelming and you're hurt—for yourself and for your child. It's even more okay to cry together. But even in the worst of situations you can often find things to laugh about. What's funny about Prader-Willi syndrome? Come to a parent's meeting and find out. The day your child got caught with his pockets full of Brach's mixed candy in the grocery store may not have been funny at the time, but can bring shared humor at a support gathering. Humor is an important survival tactic.

Keeping your life under control is difficult when your child with PWS is often "out of control." But, when life has not been fair, there are choices to be made. You can wallow in self-pity or you can pick yourself up and decide to make the best of your situation. Ask yourself what can you do differently. How can you find some happiness in each day? How can you give some happiness each day? Do you forgive yourself when you have not handled your child as well as you would like? Do you try to break bad patterns? What can you control and what is beyond your control? I don't believe that God has put us on this earth to suffer with our child, but rather has given us a challenge to reach beyond the suffering. Our personal strengths and relationship grow out of difficult situations.

A Word About Siblings

Last week, while going through old mementos, I came across a Christmas card from our daughter, Sarah, written when she was in third grade. Included in the card was a list of jobs she would perform as a gift to us. Between the usual 1) I will clean my room and 3) I will take Lambi for a walk daily was 2) I will help when Matt has a tantrum. What seemed like a normal life to Sarah at age 8 was far from normal for the average 8-year-old. Now that she is 12, she is much more aware of and sensitive to what her peers view as OK or not OK. Furthermore, there is nothing more important to a 12-year-old than to be just like the other kids. When the cupboards and refrigerator are locked, and her brother's behavior is weird and embarrassing at times, it is hard for her to be comfortable with her peers. Sarah recently told me of an incident on the bus, where a Special-Ed school bus went past theirs. The boys on her bus began making fun of the children on the Special-Ed bus and mocking them. Sarah said, "I was mad at them and wanted to say, 'Stop it! How would you feel if someone did that to you?' But, I didn't because I was afraid they would turn on me and make fun of me because of Matt."

Normal siblings of children with PSW are like sibs of children with other developmental disabilities. They feel resentment, guilt, love, jealousy, anger, compassion, embarrassment, and loneliness. They fear isolation, worry that the condition is contagious or inherited, wonder if their parents love their disabled sibling "more," and occasionally desire to get sick too in order to get attention. At the same time they can be protective. When I asked Sarah if I missed identifying any feelings she said, "Sometimes you just feel downright miserable." Remember, the actions and reactions of sibs are usually age-related. I don't mention sibling issues to add more guilt to parents, but rather to emphasize that PWS does have an impact on normal children. Their lives will be partly enriched and partly

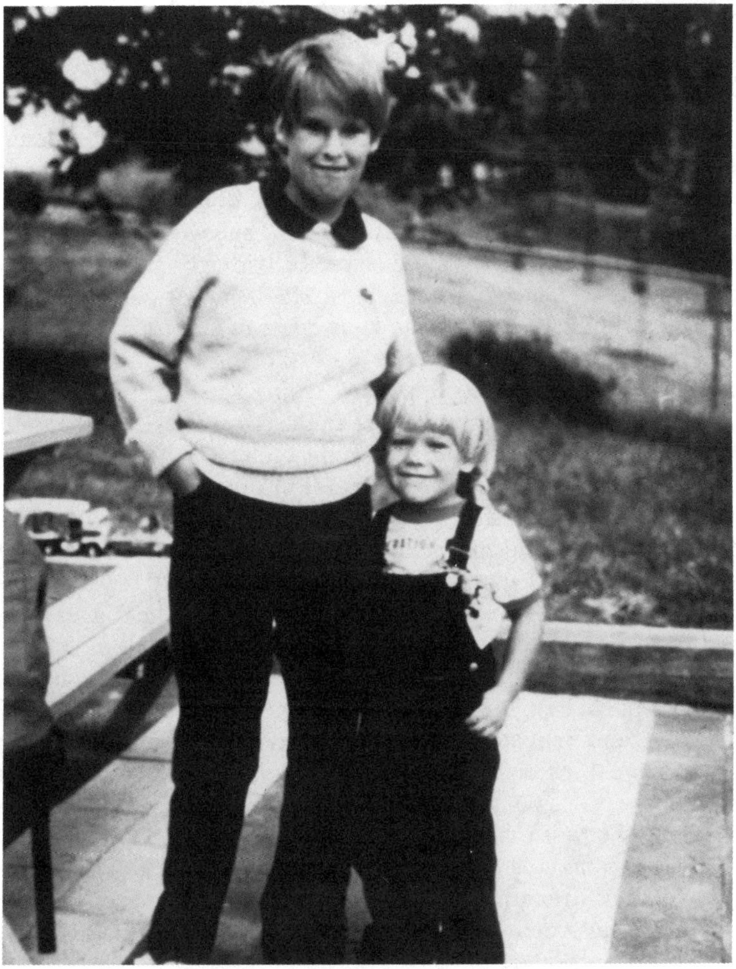

FIGURE 18.3. Matt at age 12, after his weight loss (with him is his nephew, Mikey).

damaged by their sibling's disability. We can nurture the enriched part and minimize the damaged part by accepting them and ourselves with all of the normal faults and feelings that accompany the family of any disabled child.

Coming Out of the Closet

People often say to Al and me, "How do you deal with locks in your kitchen?" I've finally realized that we have lived with PWS so long that we have almost forgotten how bizarre the syndrome must seem to others and what a difference it has made in the way we live. I also think that as parents who deal with PWS, we have hidden our problems behind a well-developed facade and that the true tragedy of PWS, the serious behavior problems, have been kept a secret. But why? Perhaps we're ashamed. Perhaps we are afraid it will appear that the behavior issues reflect an inability to parent.

Al and I have decided to come out of the closet. We aren't ashamed and we don't feel guilty! We know that Matt's behavior problems are not the result of our lack of parenting skills. We have done all the right things. We don't holler, we don't hit, we are consistent, and we use positive reinforcement. There is always a consequence for bad actions and we keep Matt active and encourage social activities. His behavior has improved significantly over the past 4 years and he is down to a normal weight. Basically we are a happy, loving family, but Matt still "loses it" once in a while. Our usually cooperative, loving son starts crying and screaming. We still find that these temper tantrums shake us to the core. These are the times when we feel frustrated and discouraged and wonder, "What else can we do?"

So the pain is still there. We sense it in other parents at local support meetings and on a greater scale at the national conferences. This cry of desperation came loud and clear when I asked one father what he would do if a group home isn't started. He said, "I guess I would buy two guns, hand one to my wife, then hope we have the nerve to pull the trigger at the same time."

Our message is not one of resignation—or we would buy two more guns. We still believe in fighting for every ounce of control we can get over the syndrome, and helping Matt fight for every bit of control he can achieve. Our message to parents is that you have nothing to hide or be ashamed of. It is time we all came out of the closet with our problems. Know that you have done the best job you could have under the circumstances. Remember, that in spite of all our struggles, we families have love, happiness, and a great deal of strengths. Try to forgive yourself at the end of each day for all of the things you wish you had handled differently. Be as patient with yourself as you would like to be with your child.

Part V Delivery of Services

Getting help is so hard . . . it seems like no one believes us, especially R's teacher. Even our social worker said she never heard of PWS and because of her thinking we did not get help for a long time.

Most of the problems are because of our ages and being retired and on a fixed income and being worried about her future. A lot of places tell you right out they will not accept [persons with] PWS.

I am the "end domino" in his life. His sister has her own life. I would like to see him in a group home that is more like a home than an institution.

Being a parent of a PWS person is a very lonely position at times, as I'm positive that being a PWS person must be extremely lonely and upsetting. It is nice to feel that at last some help and support is around [the National Association].

19
Advocacy and Change: A Primer for Parents

Ralph Newbert

Parents and guardians of children with Prader-Willi syndrome (PWS) face an alien world when their children enter school. To the uninitiated, the education bureaucracy generates what seems like a new language and processes that many parents find perplexing. Some parents are shocked to find that most educators have no knowledge of PWS and must be trained "on the job."

Important questions need to be answered about special education due process rights guaranteed by the Education for All Handicapped Children Act (PL 94-142). This discussion is intended to serve as a guide for parents and advocates. Readers are cautioned that laws and regulations vary by jurisdication and change over time.

Historical Perspective

Children and youth with PWS receive special education services because of a series of occurrences that began more than 150 years ago. Legislation in the early 1800s established special schools for children with handicaps, particularly the deaf and the blind. However, education of children with other disabilities did not receive major attention until the 1950s when parents began to persistently request services for their children. In 1963 the federal government expanded the law supporting programs for the deaf and retarded to include all children with handicaps. This marked the start of the current emphasis on the rights of people with disabilities.

Advocacy Legislation

In 1976 the Developmental Disabilities Assistance and Bill of Rights (PL 94-103) gave credibility and official sanction to the advocacy movement by establishing Protection and Advocacy agencies. Under this act, each state and U.S. territory that receives federal funds is required to establish an independent agency to protect and advocate for persons with developmental disabilities. The disabilities originally included under the act were later expanded, and some states passed laws to include certain disabilities not covered by the original legislation.

Although every state and U.S. territory has a Protection and Advocacy agency, services range from involvement in Pupil Evaluation Team meetings in local schools to merely providing information and referral services. In other words, states are given great discretion in the provision of Protection and Advocacy services. A list of state Protection and Advocacy agencies is to be found in Appendix G. It is important to note that those services for individuals with PWS continue when the person becomes an adult.

The Education for all Handicapped Children Act provides the major financial base for the states and guarantees essential educational rights. Although a progression of federal and state laws preceded PL 94-142, this is the centerpiece of public policy in this area. Children with PWS are covered under this law for educational purposes, no matter how severe their physical or learning impairments. Medical services may be covered if they are necessary to help the child benefit from special education, and related services, including speech and language therapy, psychological assistance, physical therapy, occupational therapy, and special individual programs, are provided when deemed appropriate.

PL 94-142 covers children of "school age." This generally means that children with handicaps are entitled to attend school at the same age as nonhandicapped children. Children or young adults who attend federally funded preschool or vocational training programs are also eligible for special education services. Some states choose to serve children and young adults with disabilities who are either too young or too old for school. By law, children and youths with disabilities have the same rights as other children to participate in extra-curricular activities. These activities are a vital part of school programs and may be as essential to a child's development as academic work. Additionally, children and young adults with PWS who reside outside of their natural parents' homes in residential facilities, group homes, correctional facilities, and foster homes are covered by the law.

Most of the PWS population requires specialized day or residential programs. If an appropriate program cannot be provided by the local school, the student may be placed in a private school day program or residential facility, after careful evaluation and with the guardian's permission. The local school district is responsible for paying for all educational, room, board, and nonmedical costs. It is required that children in out-of-home facilities reside as close as possible to their natural home. If parents voluntarily place a child in a private facility, even though the local school district has offered a free *appropriate* education, the local district is *not* required to pay for that placement. However, the child with a disability living in a private setting is still eligible for evaluation by the school district and may take advantage of special education and any related services offered to disabled children in the school district.

PL 94-142 entitles every child with a handicap to a "free appropriate public education," a right that must be defended constantly by parents and advocates. The term "appropriate" does not mean ideal, and what is appropriate for one child may be inadequate for another. The term is subject to interpretation and essentially becomes an item for a multidisciplinary team to define. This team includes the student's guardian, who must be informed of the evaluation in his or her native language and who must give written consent for special education evaluations. If a guardian refuses consent, the school may file for a due process hearing to resolve the conflict.

The concept of "least restrictive environment" presents a special problem for many parents of children with PWS. The intent of "least restrictive environment" is to ensure that students with handicaps are provided with maximum opportunities for education in integrated settings wherever possible. While open, minimally restrictive environments are beneficial for many developmentally disabled children, those with PWS usually require a structured setting for optimal functioning. For them, a most appropriate setting may be very restrictive. The balance between appropriate education and a "least restrictive environment" must be carefully delineated and operationalized in the student's individualized education program (IEP). It is of paramount importance that "least restrictive" not become the "least expensive."

The Evaluation and Planning Process

If children with PWS are to reach their full academic, emotional, social, and intellectual potential, they should be identified as soon as possible and then screened, evaluated, and referred to special education services. Parents should be aware that this process is the precursor to appropriate placement.

Local educational agencies are required to have a screening process to ensure that all children requiring special educational services are identified. Screening provides an indication of potential needs and, where special education is necessary, students are referred to a multidisciplinary team for evaluation.

Evaluation is defined by law as those procedures implemented to determine if a child is handicapped and the nature and extent to which special education and related services are needed. It is the starting point for planning of individual education programs and includes assessing all areas of the suspected disability, such as vision, health, hearing, motor abilities, intelligence, and communication abilities. Many parents of children with PWS who have paid for evaluations are surprised to learn that local education agencies may be responsible for the cost. Most schools are not staffed with personnel qualified to assess a child with PWS and may opt for an outside evaluation. It is wise to determine *beforehand* which tests the school will pay for and which may be "excluded for medical reasons."

Each local education agency is required to provide a multidisciplinary team to develop IEPs. The size and composition of the team may vary. It is essential that a person knowledgeable about PWS be a member of the evaluation team, and guardians have a right to participate as team members. A student cannot be placed in special education without a written IEP. It should contain specific components, including but not limited to sections that:

1. Describe the student's current level of functioning (sometimes referred to as strengths and needs).
2. Outline annual goals, including short-term objectives.
3. Detail the special education and related services to be provided, the extent to which the student will participate in regular educational programs, and the person responsible for providing the programs or services.
4. Identify projected dates for intitiation and duration of services.
5. Describe evaluation procedures and schedules for determining the student's progress toward the stated goals.

IEPs are *not* contracts. Schools cannot promise that any given student will progress at a proscribed rate. However, the services described in the IEPs are legally binding and must be supplied. For example, if an IEP states that a student will receive occupational therapy, the school must deliver that service. Guardians must *write* everything into the plan they consider necessary for their child's education. Guardians should *not* sign blank forms, and if they object to the IEP in whole or part, they should refuse to sign it.

Within 30 days of a finding of special needs and an evaluation, a meeting must be held to develop the IEP. Parents or guardians are entitled to have an advocate present, and the meeting must be scheduled at a mutually agreeable time. It is vitally important for parents to keep anecdotal notes of all phone calls, copies of correspondence, and minutes, as well as a continuous log of the student's behavior; they should ask many questions and review school records, and may be able to provide additional information that can help the team. They should visit the school frequently and talk to other parents about programs and facilities. Frequently the IEP process seems perplexing and threatening; the assistance of another parent or advocate who has been through the process can help immensely. As indicated earlier, parents often are surprisd to learn how little most professionals know about PWS.

The Hearing Process

Parents or guardians may be dissatisfied with the program implemented by the schools. Reasons for dissatisfaction range from inadequate evaluation to overt discrimination to blatant attempts to avoid costly, but necessary services. Most problems are solved by talking to the teacher or director of special education. Accurate memos about these conversations, including names, places, dates, and content, are critical. If identified problems are not resolved after talking with local school personnel, an advocate or attorney should be contacted.

Under the law, there are several avenues available to remedy unsatisfactory situations. These include an independent evaluation, a hearing before an impartial hearing officer, an administrative appeal (at times with mediation), and a complaint to the State Education Agency or federal Office for Civil Rights. Since one course of action may be more effective than another, legal advice is recommended. Outside evaluation may be useful when a diagnosis is questioned or when the parents feel that the school is not responding appropriately to their child's needs. An independent evaluation by an expert in PWS may provide a fresh look at a problem and aid in the solution.

Administrative appeals and mediation vary by state or territory. When a hearing is necessary, all possible sources of support should be enlisted. Parents' groups may be an invaluable resource. Guardians should request copies of all records at this stage of the process. A hearing is initiated when a guardian notifies local school officials and the state director of special education or state commissioner of education *in writing*. The hearing request should include the name of the student and a summary of the rationale for the request. A copy of the hearing process, state special education regulations, and the school district's latest special education program review can add valuable tactical information, and should be available from the state director of special education or local superintendent.

Special education regulations require the state commissioner to appoint the impartial hearing officer in a timely manner. Because hearing officers must be free of conflicts of interest, they cannot be school employees or in any way associated with the school. The appointment of a specific hearing officer may be challenged only on the grounds of conflict of interest. A copy of the appointment is forwarded to both parties along with a list of procedural safeguards. The hearing officer is responsible for establishing a time and place convenient to both parties, and notifying the parties and the commissioner.

Hearings are closed to the public unless guardians request otherwise. Guardians, their representatives, and the student may be present. The superintendent or a designee, the special education director, and the administrative unit's representatives may be present. The hearing opens with statements describing the procedures to be followed. In most cases, witnesses are called one at a time and may listen to each other's testimony only with the consent of both parties. All testimony and evidence presented is recorded either electronically or in written form and becomes part of the record.

In most states, formal rules of evidence do not apply in due process hearings. However, persons presenting testimony are sworn or affirmed and both parties and the hearing officer have the right to cross-examine witnesses. The hearing officer advises the parties that the findings of fact will be made to the state commissioner of education and reviews the timelines when a written decision will be issued. Most decisions can be expected within 45 days. Any party disagreeing with the decision may appeal the matter in court. Appeals should be filed quickly to avoid any problems with the statute of limitations.

The Complaint Process

Whereas hearings are initiated by parties involved in dispute over provision of special education services, complaints can be filed by anyone. Complaints may be useful where there is a violation of law that affects a number of children, such as a refusal to identify or serve children with handicaps or segregation of facilities. In most states and territories, a complaint to a state will be handled more efficiently than a complaint to the federal government.

To file a complaint, a letter must be written to the state department of education outlining the alleged violations. Sending copies of the complaint to the local superintendent of schools, state legislators, and other important politicians is helpful. Once the complaint is filed, the state department of education will assign an investigator to determine if probable cause exists that a local district is not in compliance with the law. The commissioner will seek to provide a remedy for any noncompliance. Complaints may be filed even if a due process hearing is contemplated. If all administrative remedies are fruitless, a lawsuit may be filed. Frequently lawsuits are the only way to ensure legal compliance. Guardians and organizations should not be afraid to use the due process provided by law.

Role of the Advocate in Educational Due Process

The term "advocacy" means different things to different people. Usually, advocacy is thought of as interceding for someone or something, helping, or otherwise pursuing rightful claims. Advocates plead the case of another. Although guidelines for advocates vary among state agencies, some commonalities do exist. Advocates will inform people with disabilities as to their rights to admission, placement, and programming. They may participate in administrative hearings and assist in the complaint process. In some states they also assist with applications or appeals to the Social Security

Administration, negotiate with institutions, and monitor the quality of services received. Professional advocates can provide cool-headed, objective expertise and knowledge to parents caught up in emotionally charged situations.

As educators, professional advocates encourage parents to help themselves by collecting and organizing documents, making local contacts and arrangements, and sharing strategies. Advocates work with families and share responsibilities.

After due process information has been collected, advocates act as coordinators. If a due process hearing is necessary, the advocate may either represent the client or refer the case to an attorney. More and more, experts in management of PWS are called upon to testify to the need for appropriate services and funding. This may take the form of formal court testimony or a hearing before administrating agencies such as a county board of supervisors or a board of education.

Organized advocacy programs ensure that change does not happen arbitrarily. They provide continuity and direction by helping individuals with a common interest such as PWS work together. In addition to state and local advocacy and service groups, the following national organization resources may be helpful:

Center for Law and Education
Larsen 6th Floor
14 Appian Way
Cambridge, MA 02138
(617) 495-4666

Children's Defense Fund
122 C Street, NW
Washington, DC 20001
(202) 628-8787

Federation for Children with Special Needs
312 Stuart Street
Boston, MA 02116
(617) 482-2915

Mental Health Law Project
2021 L Street, NW, 8th Floor
Washington, DC 20036
(202) 467-5730

Summary

The attempts of school districts to avoid their responsibility to provide a free appropriate public education to PWS students have not gone unnoticed. Advocacy agencies now provide assistance to people with disabilities in a variety of areas in an effort to positively affect the laws, rules, and regulations that govern our lives. Advocates for people with low-incidence handicaps such as PWS can network with other groups to fight for quality services.

References

Developmental Disabilities Assistance and Bill of Rights Act of 1975, §4, 42 U.S.C. §6000–6081 (1982).

Education for All Handicapped Children Act of 1975, §601 (3)(c), 20 U.S.C. §1400–1420 (1982).

Annotated Bibliography

Alinsky, S.D. (1972). *Rules for radicals.* New York: Vintage. (This book provides the foundation for the philosophy of change. A must for anyone interested in organizing parents or system advocacy.)

Children's Defense Fund. (1984). *94-142 and 504: Numbers that add up to educational rights for handicapped children.* Washington: (This guide for parents and advocates outlines the process that can be used to assure the rights of handicapped children.)

Jones, P.R. (1981). *A practical guide to federal special education law: Understanding and implementing P.L. 94–142.* New York: Holt. (Designed for educators, but parents and advocates may find it useful.)

Turnbull, A.P., Strickland, B.B., & Brantley, J.C. (1982) *Developing and implementing individualized education programs* (2nd ed.). Columbus, OH: Charles E. Merrill. (This textbook for educators provides an inside, comprehensive view of the special education process.)

Weintraub, F.J., Abeson, A., Ballard, J., & LaVor, M.L. (Eds.) (1976) *Public policy and the education of exceptional children.* Reston, VA: Council for Exceptional Children. (This book provides the historical perspective missing in many texts and points out that the law is constantly evolving, a fact that cannot be overlooked because evolution is not always progress.)

20
Residential Programs for Individuals with Prader-Willi Syndrome

DOROTHY G. THOMPSON, LOUISE R. GREENSWAG, and RHETT ELEAZER

Provision of residential services to adolescents and adults with Prader-Willi syndrome (PWS) was not seriously addressed prior to the late 1970s, primarily because until then these individuals were not expected to live very long. Now, as a result of proper diagnosis, earlier case finding, and nutritional guidance, their life span may extend at least to middle age. However, expectations for affected persons to become socially mature and function independently are rarely met, and parents face difficult decisions about their children's future. Parental responsibility does not decrease, and out-of-home living alternatives are a primary concern.

This chapter focuses on establishment of long-term residential care facilities for individuals with PWS. Important questions arise: What is it about PWS that requires such unique residential programming? What out-of-home living options currently exist? Which settings offer the best opportunities for weight control, social interactions, work, recreation, and participation in community life? What procedural steps are required to start up and operate an appropriate facility? How should parents organize to locate potential providers and find funding? What are the optimal requirements for a physical plant, staffing, and programming? The authors hope that this discussion will be reassuring to parents and useful to residential service providers and professionals who assist in program development.

General Considerations

One of the most critical periods in the cycle of life occurs when children leave the family nest. Even when offspring are normal, "letting go" is not easy. Families of children with PWS are like those with children with other developmental disabilities; separation and out-of-home placement intensifies parental feelings of vulnerability and ambivalence. Resistance to placement has been associated with guilt about "putting their child away." Many parents feel that if their child lives in a group home, they must relinquish their traditional parenting roles. What eventually seems to happen in the families with a PWS child is that, although parents *wish* to maintain their children at home, the erratic, inappropriate behaviors intensify as the children grow older even when weight has been controlled. These unpredictable outbursts, coupled with the stress of years spent in an abnormally structured household, disrupt family life beyond tolerable limits. Residential placement becomes an attractive option for emotionally exhausted parents who want to enjoy their normal offspring and their later years and also desire to deal realistically with their own mortality.

Planning residential programs requires clearing the air about how best to serve the PWS population. Regardless of the disability, residential care should focus on normalization, that is, development of social skills, creation of work programs, community participation, and healthy recreation. Additionally, facilities for the developmentally disabled are remarkably similar in that there is usually easy access to food (both preparation and consumption) and relative freedom of movement. Unfortunately, these two elements are least appropriate for the PWS population. Poorly informed and/or trained residential staff do PWS individuals a great disservice if their facilities offer unlimited availability of food and lack the capacity for 24-hour supervision. Consideration of these two issues and that of special behavioral programming are essential to the success of any facility for PWS persons; to ignore them is to undermine opportunities for affected individuals to adapt.

Residential alternatives should be constructed on the premise that individuals have a right to live in a "least restrictive environment" that maximizes opportunities for self-fulfillment. At the same time, such settings should provide the necessary protective milieu and should be defined in terms of the needs of the client rather than the convenience of the service providers or the most inexpensive alternative (Pieper, 1985). Research and practical experience indicates that, for PWS individuals, the concept of a least restrictive environment translates into homogeneous group homes where programming meets the special needs of this population. This is *not* to say that heterogeneous programs for mentally retarded individuals that have PWS residents are ineffective, merely that such placement requires a delicate balance of specialized services and dedicated, patient, and sensitive staff who are willing to go the extra mile to make an integrated program work for both PWS and non-PWS clients.

Most children with PWS should be considered functionally retarded regardless of their IQ test scores. It is recommended that the "related conditions" classification of Mental Retardation be used as the criterion for determining eligibility for services. Documented evidence of "functional retardation" is the primary rationale for both direct and indirect services. For example, when prevocational and vocational programs are based only on standard test measures, expectations for work performance may be unrealistic.

On a larger scale, social service professionals, previously unfamiliar with PWS, now are required to be knowledgeable about the syndrome and find the methods and resources to integrate this population into residential care agencies. The issue is not *if* placement is necessary, but *which* facilities offer appropriate programs.

Currently, only a few progressive states have established and funded small homogeneous PWS group homes for their own residents. Many states still fail to recognize the special needs of this population and continue to make inappropriate placements. Existing group homes designed and staffed for PWS care have long waiting lists and are very expensive. Additional low-cost facilities are long overdue.

Current Options for Residential Services

For many years the only out-of-home placements available for the PWS population were integrated group homes, private schools for the developmentally disabled, or state institutions for the mentally retarded. Most cases placed in the state facilities had severe behaviors problems. The first PWS-specific residential program opened in the state of Washington in 1979. Since then group homes ranging in size from 4 to 16 beds have been established in California, Minnesota, Connecticut, Massachusetts, Wisconsin, Illinois, New York, New Jersey, Michigan, and North Dakota. Several larger residential schools have created separate units for those PWS children who "aged out" of their regular program. One group home, established in 1981 in Minnesota for 15 PWS residents, continues to be a model program for other facilities now providing services and for those being planned. The number of PWS group homes has notably increased during the past few years. Currently, over 100 individuals live in these special settings and others are being served in integrated facilities settings scattered throughout the country.

A generic description of programs serving the PWS population offers the reader an overview of residential options currently available and some commentary about them. With the exception of state-operated institutions, these facilities function as nonprofit or for-profit corporations.

A format that has proved to be very cost-effective and programmatically successful is a 12–15 bed permanent homogeneous residential setting for PWS clients, age 15 and older, that offers nutritional, behavioral, vocational, and social programs. It is generally state and federally funded and has a private nonprofit board as its governing body. The Minnesota group home identified previously follows this model. Several 6-bed permanent group homes for adolescents (age 12 and up) that focus on educational needs, behavioral modification, diet management, and socialization are operating, and a few 6-, 8-, and 10-units are in process. Two large private, not-for-profit residential schools for the developmentally disabled currently serve PWS children and adults with special programming. Their success is based on separate living arrangements within the facility and carefully trained staff.

As previously stated, some individuals with PWS reside in 6- or 8-bed integrated group homes. Most program directors report only limited success in controlling the weight and behaviors of the PWS residents and indicate that these problems often hinder the adjustment of both PWS and non-PWS clients. Unfortunately, in cases in which the PWS clients have not been able to adapt, they have not been allowed to remain. Several state institutions for the mentally retarded are caring for some PWS patients but rarely offer the necessary special services. Follow-up of some individuals with PWS who have been placed in foster homes reveals that they receive few programming services, they gain weight, and their behaviors continue to deteriorate.

Unfortunately, there have been several reports of nursing home placements. Sending PWS individuals to such settings is a sad commentary on the extent to which lack of knowledge about the syndrome compromises their lives. Serious medical problems and/or total lack of mobility should be the only justification for this type of placement.

It has been the experience of care providers who have worked closely with affected persons that independent living has not been successful for PWS individuals over a prolonged period of time. Certainly, there are some individuals with less severe symptoms who may be *surviving* in a less restrictive environment, but there are no reliable records of their health status. A report of 232 cases age 16 and over (Greenswag, 1984) indicated that those who lived independently (only 5 were reported in this group) or who were being served in heterogeneous residential programs weighed an average of 40–60 pounds more than those PWS people living in PWS-specific facilities.

Considering that the syndrome is underdiagnosed (Cassidy, 1984) and that over 1,000 affected individuals will need placement within the next 5 years (personal communication, Prader-Willi Syndrome Association, 1987), the need for more appropriate living facilities is obvious. It is anticipated that the number of syndrome-specific group residences will increase as efforts continue to heighten public awareness, educate professionals, promote research, and train care providers. To this end, plans are actively underway, through the concerted efforts of the Prader-Willi Syndrome Association (PWSA), to open a Crisis-Intervention and Transitional Center as a multifaceted resource for affected individuals and their families (see Chapter 21.) A listing of residential programs serving the PWS population can be found in Appendix H.

Criteria for Optimum Programming

One of the questions posed at the beginning of this chapter was "What are the components of an ideal residential facility for PWS?" Generally, establishing and administering any residential programs for the developmentally disabled is no simple task. To begin with, unrelated persons, coming together for the first time, bring diverse backgrounds of behaviors, mores, cultures, values, education, and environments. Effective placement acknowledges human diversity, cultivates individual growth, and encourages group participation. Individuals with PWS are no different; for some backgrounds will match or meld, whereas others will be in constant conflict. Responsibility for successful programs lies with individual care providers. Experience indicates that the most successful facilities are resident-effective, program-effective, staff-effective and cost-effective.

Resident-effective programs include:

1. Measurable weight reduction and maintenance protocols carried out through ongoing nutritional supervision.
2. An awareness that the physical aspects and emotional effects of PWS require continuous monitoring.
3. Structured behavioral programs that encourage psychological adaptation. Only the most bizarre, dangerous, and assaultive behaviors, if not changed after a long time, should be the basis for terminating a residential placement. In other words, "try, try again" should be the philosophy of the staff. Most people with PWS will respond favorably to *prolonged* sensitive programming even though their behaviors are not always constant or predictable.
4. Meaningful and appropriate educational and vocational services.
5. A safe, comfortable, carefully structured living environment that offers privacy as needed and opportunities for interpersonal growth.
6. Optimum opportunities for social adjustment and community participation in the world of work and recreation.

Program effectiveness is a multifaceted goal and requires services that extend beyond the boundaries of the group home into the school, work, community, and social settings. Whenever, wherever, and however PWS persons are served, they require total, consistent, 24-hour supervision with a minimum of changes and few surprises. (Most respond very poorly to change in any part of their lives.) Continuing communication between all participating agencies is essential since interdisciplinary collaboration plays a major role in how well clients adjust.

Staff effectiveness is the foundation of any successful program. Developing a qualified staff to work with individuals with PWS is similar to the process used for any program serving the developmentally disabled; personnel should be carefully screened, and education, training, and ongoing, problem-oriented in-services are essential. Staff development is discussed in detail later in this chapter.

The *cost-effectiveness* of a group home is a thorny issue. Programs must be fiscally sound. This means that primary providers in cooperation with local, state, and federal funding agencies are responsible for the financial integrity of any facility they wish to establish. Funding is almost always based on numerical mental retardation criteria and, because the mental retardation guidelines used by funding agencies tend to be so narrowly defined, many individuals with PWS fall between the cracks of the local, state, and federal funding system. Through the persistent efforts of parents, advocates, and agencies serving the disabled, screening committees now recognize that the PWS population does meet the criteria for classification in the "related symptoms" category. Procedures for obtaining federal funding to establish and operate a PWS group home are described in the following section.

Getting a Program Started

Establishing a group home is a long, arduous process. Most residential providers and parents will be working together to create the best possible facility and programming. Whereas professional service providers usually have had considerable experience with bureaucratic institutions, parents tend to find the process bewildering and need guidance and support. Programs are initiated through a series of predictable stages: planning, investigating funding and licensing, location of a site for the group home, design of the physical plant, staff development, and program development. Be advised that it can take anywhere from 6 months to 2 years from the initial planning stage to the time when the group home may open its doors.

Planning

The process begins with the formation of a planning committee. The composition of this group is critical since it will be the moving force behind all other phases of opening the residence. Members should be willing to make a long-term commitment. Ideally, the membership is a mix of parents, an attorney, a banking resource, local civic-minded individuals, a social worker, a psychologist, and a physician. Once philosophical guidelines and program goals have been established, the planning committee must study all dimensions of the start-up process, develop an overall stratety, and design a blueprint for implementation. The committee may wish to consider consulting with a professional health care planner, expert, or advocacy council. Also, the PWSA is very much in support of the development of out-of-home living options for affected individuals and is most anxious to act as a major resource. Once a residential format has been chosen, the legal, step-by-step process begins.

Funding

Once the planning committee has completed its initial investigation, the issue of "who pays" rears its ugly head. Funding resources available for use in establishing community living alternatives must be clearly defined and a continuing support system assured since individual funding, where a family assumes the total financial burden of residential care, is prohibitive. Understanding the various methods for obtaining financial assistance and licensing is vital. Each state, city, county, or region may use different guidelines. Are state, local, or federal funds able to be used to purchase land, buildings, and furnishings? Can these monies be used for staff development, for programming, and for ongoing operation? How much may parents have to assume in the way of fiscal responsibility?

Obtaining federal funding to build and support a group home is an option that should be given careful consideration. Since 1978, federal monies have been available through the Department of Housing and Urban Development (HUD) to build residential facilities for the handicapped and elderly under Section 202 of the Federal Housing Act. Until recently, this source had not been used for PWS group homes, but now these funds are available and can be applied for in any state as long as HUD requirements are met.

In order to obtain HUD funding, it is necessary to establish a corporation to borrow these funds. This "borrower" corporation would be the group home intended to be built. It must be established as a private, non-profit corporation in the state where the group home is to be located and be involved in no business other than the ownership and operation of the facility. The formation of such a non-profit corporation can be accomplished by retaining an attorney, and the costs should not exceed $500. In many areas, there are attorneys who will perform this service free of charge or for a very nominal fee.

After the nonprofit corporation has been chartered, it must receive tax exempt status from the Internal Revenue Service. An application for tax exempt status under the Internal Revenue Code, Section 501 (c)(3) should be submitted as soon as possible since this process usually takes 3–4 months. It is not difficult to complete this application and the IRS will be happy to assist and answer any questions.

The next step is for the nonprofit corporation to find a sponsor for the group home. Since the group home corporation has just been organized and has not yet received tax exempt status, more than likely it will not have the financial ability necessary to meet HUD requirements. Therefore, a sponsor who does have financial resources must be secured. This sponsor must also be chartered as a private nonprofit corporation and have tax exempt status. It must be able to show the financial capacity to repay the HUD loan and operate the home. HUD requires financial statements from the sponsor for the prior 3 years and also requires cash in the bank equal to one half of 1% of the amount of the funds being sought to build the facility. Additionally, the sponsor should have a good "track record" in providing services and sponsoring other group homes. Churches, experienced as sponsors, or existing in-state service providers who sponsor other programs for the mentally retarded or handicapped are good prospects.

It is recommended that an officially recognized state chapter of the PWSA act as co-sponsor for the group home. This co-sponsorship is impressive to HUD; it indicates that the national organization of parents and professionals is interested in establishing an appropriate facility and that the families of individuals with PWS seeking placement wish to play an active role in the design and operation of the home.

Once the borrower corporation is organized and a sponsor has been obtained, it must be demonstrated that monies will be available to operate the facility once it is built. There are several alternatives that can provide the funds needed to meet operating expenses. The first of these alternatives is use of private funds wherein the group home residents are each charged their pro-rata share of the expenses necessary by operate the home and repay the HUD loan. Although this is the easiest method, it excludes a number of people who are in need but simply do not have the financial resources to allow them to live in the home. A second alternative is to find a private service provider already in the business of operating group facilities *for profit* who has funds available to guarantee the operation of the home. Once again, this expense is passed on to the resident or his family and excludes many.

The third, and certainly the best, alternative is to apply to the state where the group home is to be located to guarantee operating funds. If it can be shown that federal funds are being sought to construct the facility, the state should agree to support it, once it is built. It is necessary to determine which state agency will be responsible for providing residential services to individuals with PWS and apply directly to it for operating monies. The state agency to be contacted may be the state's department of mental retardation, mental health, or social services, or the state housing authority.

It is a good idea to request time on the state agency's agenda to familiarize its personnel with PWS before asking for financial assistance. (Videotapes and printed educational information about PWS and the unique need for proper residential care are available from the PWSA.) Parents, families, and individuals with PWS themselves should appear at any subsequent meetings with the agency when financial assistance is requested. This tactic not only may impress the agency, but also will secure some publicity for PWS since these meetings usually have press coverage. When public support is forthcoming, the pressure to provide funds increases.

Additional monies are available for group homes through Title 19 (Medicaid). When application is made for funding, a request can also be made for grant funds under Section 8 of the Federal Housing Act to pay the debt service on the HUD loan and pay for maintenance and repairs to the project. When these monies are coupled with an agreement with the state to pay the balance of the operational costs, the group facility will be able to provide services at no cost to the residents.

Once the preliminaries have been completed (chartering the nonprofit corporation, establishment of a tax exempt status, and location of a sponsor and a source for operating expenses), application for federal funding can be made. The application period usually commences in late spring or early June of each year. Plan to visit the area HUD office prior to application time to inform the local officials of the intent to apply for funds and leave some information about PWS. Ask to be put on their mailing list and request to be notified when the application period begins. Follow up this visit and request with frequent telephone calls to the area office inquiring whether or not the Notification of Funding Availability has been received and when the application period expires.

Utilizing a local banker or mortage broker with previous experience in HUD funding projects to assist in obtaining notification and preparation of the funding application can be a great help. The fees for such services can be paid as an expense from HUD funds received and it is also possible to find a broker who will help on a contingency fee basis (i.e., being paid only if the application is approved and the loan closes).

Submission of a complete application for funding requires a number of exhibits. Financial statements from the borrower corporation, sponsor, and co-sponsor corporations are necessary to show financial ability. Where state support has been agreed upon, a letter from the appropriate state agency pledging operating funds is required. Recommendations from the governor and the state's senators and representatives that the project be funded should be included along with letters of local support. When elected officials are informed about PWS, letters recommending federal monies are more easily obtained since federal funding to specific states is politically advantageous. Letters from individuals who have political influence with the local HUD office are very desirable. Solicit as many endorsements as possible and then select the 8 or 10 most impressive to be included with the application.

HUD provides each applicant with a checklist to ensure that the application is complete. Make sure that nothing has been omitted, especially the required exhibits. Failure to include any required information or exhibits will result in rejection. Allow plenty of time to make sufficient copies, bind them neatly, and include a table of contents for ease of review.

Once the application has been filed, it will be reviewed and ranked by officials of the local HUD office along with all other organizations applying for federal monies. The applications together with their local ranking are sent to Washington for further review and final prioritization as to which projects will be funded. Once the PWS group home application arrives in Washington, exert as much political influence as possible to make sure it gets proper attention. Personal letters to congressional representatives are most important at this time.

In addition to learning the procedures for obtaining federal funds, the planning committee should form a subcommittee to investigate grants from civic organizations, clubs, and private sources and foundations. Actual donations and/or provision of temporary or long-term collateral may be an important aspect of parental commitment as co-sponsors of a group home nonprofit corporation. During the planning stage it is advantageous for committee members to investigate all available agencies, already committed to providing residential care in the community, who might be willing to assume responsibility for operation of the PWS group home as part of their services. Certainly, such agencies may serve as an excellent resource for expertise in planning.

After a thorough investigation of funding options, a residential facility may be developed through appropriate legal routes.

The Physical Facility

Size

The number of clients to be served determines the bed capacity of a group home. Size is also affected by local housing requirements and anticipated increases in referrals once the home is operating. To a certain extent, size is also based on federal, state, and local guidelines.

Determining the Locale

The location of a group residence has an impact on cost, staffing potential, and program implementation. The facility need not be in an expensive area or be new construction and may be either owned or rented. The site should be in a safe neighborhood that is accessible for families of residents, staff, and vendors. A large yard may be a liability because the cost of maintenance can be very high and, for the most part, PWS individuals are not outdoor people. Quiet residential areas need not be a primary consideration. In fact, nearby public transportation may be an incentive to obtaining good staff. Accessibility to public parks, community centers, and year-round swimming facilities is desirable as a means of encouraging social interactions through participation in community activities. Ideally, shopping areas should *not* be within walking distance of the residence. An apartment building may work if the residential project occupies the entire premises.

A one-, two-, or three-story structure may house 12–15 clients. Living areas should include space for programs, dining, food preparation, sleeping, bathing, staff offices, recreation/exercise, laundry, and storage. Except where the house is a ranch style there will be stairs. This should present no problems. In fact, walking stairs is good involuntary exercise and, with very few exceptions, PWS clients can manage very well. Where a residence has three floors, a lower level is a good place for recreation. If such space is limited, some other area should be set aside for exercise and/or exercise equipment. When a lower level is large, activities can be quite diverse (a workshop or dancing), and a tile floor is most practical.

Forget a big, beautiful living room! Two or three smaller comfortable rooms that can accommodate small group gatherings for educational projects, arts and crafts, group therapy, and socialization are ideal. Smaller rooms allow staff to work with clients in relatively quiet surroundings without too much distraction. Even though residents spend about 6 hours outside the group home each day and additional time is planned for evening activities, a fair amount of hours are consumed "at home." When they have to function in very close quarters, residents tend to stumble over one another; friction develops, followed by arguments and tantrums. Small rooms encourage the pursuit of individual interests, limit the potential for personality clashes, and provide privacy for visits with family, friends, staff, and other professionals; a more peaceful atmosphere may prevail.

The dining room needs to be large enough to seat all residents and staff with ample space to move around the table(s). This room may serve many other purposes as well: meetings, movies, and special events. Carpeting or acoustical tile is advised for noise control. Keeping the dining room floor clean rarely presents problems since PWS individuals are fully capable of good table manners and rarely spill edibles. A sink for handwashing on the same floor as the dining/activity area is advised.

Planning the kitchen is important. It should be well equipped and large enough to accommodate all food preparation, food storage, and dishwashing. If entrances to the kitchen cannot be closed/locked, then all closets, cupboards, refrigerators, and freezers must be secured and off limits to residents. Of course, the kitchen must conform to all public health standards and be regularly inspected and licensed.

Single or semi-private sleeping areas consisting of 80–100 square feet per person are recommended rather than a dormitory arrangements. If feasible, families should help furnish the client's room with familiar and pleasant items such as a favorite bed, bedding, table and chairs, and personal possessions. Small rooms also encourage the pursuit of individual interests, limit the potential for personality clashes, and provide privacy for visits with family, friends, social workers, and other professional. Single rooms eliminate the need for "time-out" rooms. (Time-out areas are an irritating reminder that unacceptable behavior is anticipated) Bedrooms should have locks, not just to ensure privacy, but because locks discourage stealing, prevent personality clashes, allow for differences in housekeeping traits, and reduce the spread of communicable diseases. Where separate bedrooms are not possible, a permanent room divider helps. Large closets, a built-in dresser, and vanity-desk are suggested. PWS clients are notorious collectors; they need space for accumulation of items. In shared rooms, locks on closets and drawers are essential.

Although private baths are ideal, they are *not* recommended. In a private bathroom, unobserved residents may be in danger of drowning. Also, residents are prone to storm out of an argumentative interaction and retaliate by stuffing the toilets, clogging sinks, or letting tubs overflow; such occurrences can be unpleasant and costly. Community bathrooms located near the bedrooms should have one sink and one toilet for every four people and one tub/shower (or a shower stall), in a separate enclosure if possible, for every six. Separate bedrooms and baths are recommended for men and women. Bath areas should be easy to keep clean and sanitary, with a minimum of space for clutter. They frequently require better care than most PWS residents are willing to give. A private bathroom with lock and key should be available for staff and visitors; in most states, these must be wheelchair accessible.

Lockable storage units about 3 feet square give residents a feeling of permanency and independence. Since "hoarding" is a problem, storage space may reduce congestion in bedrooms and provide a place for out-of-season clothing. Locked space is also needed to store cleaning supplies, equipment, and paper goods. The location of laundry facilities is not an issue beyond the need for adequate supervision of use. The size and number of machines and sinks is determined by the number of residents. Use tokens in machines together with packets of soap and softener to save clothes and wear and tear on the equipment. It seems to be particularly difficult for PWS individuals to measure efficiently.

Separate office space is required for the group home director and other staff. If the facility requires a secretary, the office area should also accommodate this person. This space is very necessary for staff breaks and safekeeping of staff property. If an area cannot be set aside as a nursing station, a special locked location will be required for storage of medicine and medical records. A private space is necessary for examination, treatment, and consultation. The staff room is best located near program areas to ensure adequate supervision.

If the staffing arrangements include house parents, a small, pleasant apartment should be provided that ensures privacy, but is close enough to the clients to provide quick access at any time.

Equipment

Entertainment, exercise, and maintenance equipment are important when planning a group home. A stereo tape unit is an asset to aerobics, dancing, and relaxation activities. A tape recorder can be an effective therapeutic tool and a videocassette recorder is an excellent device for implementing behavioral change. Unless there is plenty of space, Ping-Pong and pool tables and other larger surface games are not generally used enough to warrant the cost. If a videocassette recorder is too expensive, a movie projector is a good substitute. One lounge television set is ample because many residents may have a small one in their bedrooms. A piano/organ is fine if space and finances permit; either is handy for socialization, and some residents can play and sing very well. Exercise equipment encourages regular use, which helps in weight loss and maintenance of muscle tone. Exercycles are an excellent choice. Maintenance equipment should consist of any items usually needed to maintain a home. However, lightweight sweepers and long-handled feather dusters should be available since housekeeping is part of the responsibility of each resident.

Furnishings

With the exception of game/dance areas, carpeting the floors is best for both safety and soundproofing. Wooden furniture is most durable; it should be sturdy easy to dust, and comfortable for very short people since PWS adults usually have an average height of 5 feet. Upholstered pieces covered with heavy-duty attractive fabrics are better than most plastic or leather materials. Walls either painted or papered with white or light shades with accents of bright colors are very pleasant. Curtains with tie-backs are generally more suitable than pull drapes and window shades. It is a good safety measure to screw all pictures and decorations to the wall, avoid glass coverings, and use hanging rather than table lamps. Small tables with stain-resistant tops work best for puzzles and games. Wash-and-wear tablecloths or placemats are good for dining areas. Living plants in plastic containers add cheer. Basically, an inexpensive decor is suggested because some damage is likely to occur during emotional outbursts by some residents. Plan on loss of silverware; use cheap, open patterns.

Staffing

Too often parents and some professionals nurture the idea that a residential facility for PWS persons should be "just like home," with four to six clients interacting as a family unit. Those who understand the syndrome very well know that a small, intimate, "home-away-from home" setting is not ideal. If PWS individuals could function in this type of social unit, they could continue to live with their own families. The fact of the matter is that as this population enters adolescence and adulthood, their needs cannot be met in a normal, food-oriented environment. Moreover, staffing and staffing patterns used with other types of community residential programs for the mentally retarded will not suffice for a group home for PWS. Appropriate staffing (for a 12–15-bed facility) should include the following persons.

Director

The director follows the policies and guidelines established by the governing board of the facility. The director's credentials should include a bachelor's or master's degree in special education, psychology, social work, counseling, or a related field. A minimum of 3 years' experience as a supervisor, program planner, or resident director in a facility for the developmentally retarded is essential, along with experience working with a board of directors, parents, and local authorities. The position calls for a flexible individual with good communication skills who is open to learning about PWS, able to instruct and supervise staff, willing to work with outside consultants and ancillary service providers, and can step into any position in the facility when needed.

Program and Activities Coordinator

The program and activities coordinator works directly with staff, residents, families, and others, and provides direction for the program. This person also must be capable of taking charge when the overall director is absent. Qualifications for this position include a bachelor's degree in special education, recreation therapy, or a related field, and at least 2 years' experience in the field of developmental disabilities. The ability to understand PWS, develop individualized programs, and direct and work with staff in a supportive and supervisory role is essential.

Both the Director and Program Coordinator must be able and willing to be on duty when clients are in residence and during weekends on an exchange basis. It is absolutely necessary that one or the other is available every day during the late afternoon and evening hours.

Food Manager/Cook

The food manager/cook is responsible for developing individual diets in collaboration with a nutritional consultant, purchases all food supplies and prepares all meals for the residents. This person works closely with residents, staff, parents, and program consultants to maintain all aspects of dietary regimens. If a cook is not always on duty, a specific staff member should have primary responsibility for seeing that the food guidelines are followed.

Nurse

A nurse should be available at least part time to keep the health records of each resident accurate and current. Nursing responsibilities include assessing and monitoring health status and needs. Some psychiatric experience is helpful in addition to knowledge of nutrition.

Secretary/Bookkeeper

The secretary/bookkeeper may be a part-time employee when the group home does not function under the umbrella of a larger agency.

House Manager(s)

In a setting where there are appropriate arrangements, house manager(s) (a *mature* couple or a single person) keep the group home functioning. If a couple "lives in," their duties usually include building maintenance and transportation services as well as some staff responsibilities. Acting as security or back-up staff in case of emergency is part of their role, day or night, and in some instances house managers may handle food service. It should be pointed out that in instances where house managers are employed instead of a three-shift staffing pattern, they carry a tremendous load. Even with the help of very supportive staff, implementation and maintenance of an effective long-term program is very difficult.

Direct Care Staff

Direct care staff serve as counselors in a 3:1 or 4:1 ratio to the residents. Staff need to be carefully screened for different interests and a capacity to enhance program activities for the clients. In addition to identified weekend staff, some full-time people should rotate. This arrangement is essental for adequate supervision and program continuity. Counselors may be college graduates or individuals with fewer educational credentials. Their personal references should indicate considerable maturity, flexibility, patience, and the capacity and willingness to work with very difficult personalities. Realistically, considerable staff turnover is to be expected during the first year of a group home operation.

Where a 24-hour-a-day, three-shift staffing pattern is in place, staff duties must be carefully defined to cover all phases of the program and the physical needs of all the residents. Staff responsibilities include collaboration with the director and assistant director to establish goals and objectives and design individual programs, structure and scheduling of activities, transportation for residents (such as getting to school, work, or other activities), and supervision of all resident's personal hygience, clothing care, and money matters. Most often, the burden of interacting with the clients falls to the 3 p.m. to 11 p.m. shift where a 3:1 ratio is vital. If supervision, support, and training are ongoing, a three-shift staffing pattern can be very effective with relatively little turnover. Whereas replacement of part-time staff (nurse or secretary) usually does not influence programming, when full-time personnel to whom the clients have become attached decide to leave, programs tend to become at least temporarily disrupted. This is because PWS individuals react very poorly to change.

Direct care staff, regardless of their title or position, need to have a good sense of humor since most PWS individuals lack this trait. This is particularly important because staff temperament is reflected in the behaviors of the residents. Staff will not win every battle; they should be able to take defeat graciously and cultivate the ability to forgive and forget. Communicating clearly, slowly, and succinctly, with authority but without rancor, is important. Creativity is a must, along with enthusiasm and the ability to touch and hug easily and warmly. Perceptivity to mood changes is vital. Picking up clues of impending crisis or confrontation and learning to walk away or divert offensive behavior requires control and sensitivity. Qualified staff are good listeners and group facilitators who can show displeasure appropriately, are able to admit their own shortcomings, understand that they too must comply with all house rules, and are aware that consistency is the key to effective behavioral management.

Support Services

Outside support services and consultation (on an as-needed basis) consist of a physician, psychologist, social worker, and dentist; a hospital service contract; and a vocational training agency.

Programming

Programming consists of a total, balanced plan of structured living that incorporates diet control, behavioral management, social experiences, monitoring physical health, opportunities for work, and recreation. Optimum psychosocial adaptation in concert with weight management are the overall objectives and all activities reflect these goals. For example, it is recommended that residents be discouraged from taking part in food preparation; teaching them to function in a food-related activity is counterproductive. The temptation to eat can be overwhelming, and supervision will always be necessary. Group exercise activities should be a regular part of any program. Many residents actually prefer to participate in these activities at school or at a "Y." Aqua-aerobics are recommended becasue they are more therapeutic than just swimming or floating.

In most instances, residents will be together during the late afternoon and evening hours. Where evening activities are arranged with other non-PWS groups a staff-to-resident ratio of 3 : 1 or 4 : 1 is suggested to supervise food intake and behaviors. When the group is homogeneous, only two staff may be required. Although evening activities keep the residents busy and provide stimulation, it is important to remember that they typically lack much stamina and require ample rest. Late-hour activities make poor workers and poor dispositions the following day.

Effective programming acknowledges that most residents function emotionally like latency-age children (ages 7–10 years). Only a few reach the maturity of normal early adolescents (although their verbal skills tend to contradict this). Programming is best developed by a professional, knowledgeable about PWS, experienced in behavioral modification techniques, and able to design easily understood, reasonable, realistic protocols. The Woods Schools and Residential Treatment Center in Langhorne, Pennsylvania, is an example of a residential program within an established program for retarded people with a special setting dedicated to serving clients with PWS. Several years ago, this residential program dedicated exclusively to clients with PWS at the Woods Schools was established. Its model token economy program can be found in Appendix I.

Although PWS clients should be encouraged to improve their individual decision-making abilities, meeting group goals is the basis for improving interpersonal relationships (see Chapter 16). Programs should take into consideration the fact that people with PWS have short memory spans, mood swings, and a tendency to become depressed, and are negativistic and naively friendly. They tend to be vulnerable to abuse from peers and, in some cases, other adults. Overt behaviors consist of an unusual combination of aggressiveness, irritability, and stubbornness. Older individuals tend to become crafty, manipulative, and very possessive. Yet at other times they can be sociable, charming, affectionate, creative, and generous (see Chapter 10). Developing appropriate positive reinforcements is a real challenge; classic behavioral interventions require frequent changes in the reward system to avoid manipulation and boredom. A list of positive reinforcements/rewards may be found in Appendix C.

The responsibility for programming also extends beyond the residential facility into community agencies. Food control remains a primary issue no matter where residents happen to be; controlling calories only in the group home is simply not sufficient. Arrangements are needed for all outside activities. If a client attends a school or vocational training center, a packed lunch should be provided. When exposed to cafeterias or congregate lunch rooms, the PWS person assuredly will acquire extra food. Some have been known to steal personal belongings, sell them at a sheltered workshop program, and purchase edibles from vending machines. Other residents' lunches have disappeared during bus rides, which has precipitated emotional outbursts. Interestingly, in the adult population many behavioral problems seem to occur independently of food issues (see Chapter 10). Vocational training programs for PWS clients require considerable modification. Until answers are found for the compulsive eating and unacceptable behaviors, these individuals will not do well in the outside work world. Competitive employment does not offer enough supervision. Successful vocational/sheltered workshop programs within the framework of existing group home facilities are highly specialized. The issue of habilitation and vocational training is discussed in depth in Chapter 14.

Summary

As the life span of individuals with PWS lengthens, parents and care providers must look at long-term residential services. Specialized facilities are required.

Individuals with PWS should be evaluated as developmentally disabled based on the *Related Conditions* criterion of mental retardation. IQ testing does not indicate the degree to which PWS individuals are functionally retarded. As a rule, weight management and emotional lability are serious problems for the majority of cases, who, despite cognitive test results, lack the ability to reason and the insight to be able to function independently.

After observing the development and progress of the various group homes in operation since 1980, it is generally agreed by professionals who work with PWS and the Prader-Willi Syndrome Association that when PWS individuals can live together in 12–15 bed, homogeneous group homes, they are able to maintain a reasonable weight and improve their capacity to adapt. Although some smaller residences, both integrated and not have had some success, considerable efforts and special staff have been required.

Suggestions in this chapter for planning and development a group home are based on a typical PWS individual. Naturally, a diagnosis of PWS does not mean that all the characteristics of the syndrome are present, nor equally severe. It is believed, however, that less obvious cases are the exception.

Bibliography

Cassidy, S. (1984). Prader-Willi syndrome. *Current Problems in Pediatrics, 14*, 1–55. January. Year Book Medical Publishers, Chicago.

Greenswag, L.R. (1984). *The adult with Prader-Willi syndrome: A descriptive investigation.* Unpublished doctoral thesis, University of Iowa. (DA 0569252, University of Microfilms International, Ann Arbor, MI).

Pieper, B. (1985). *Residential issues for people with disabilities.* Chicago: Spina Bifida Association of America.

Thompson, D. (1987, June). *Resident staff and program development for Prader-Willi syndrome.* Proceedings of a Scientific Meeting held at the Prader-Willi Syndrome National Conference, Houston.

21
A National Parent Network: The Prader-Willi Syndrome Association

MARJORIE A. WETT

The Prader-Willi Syndrome Association (PWSA) is a group of parents, professionals, and interested individuals who are willing to take active, responsible roles in improving the lives of children with Prader-Willi syndrome (PWS) and their families. This national organization, founded to provide a vehicle of communication for these groups, has created and continues to maintain an international network of information, support services, and research endeavors expressly to meet the needs of affected children.

In 1975 Fausta and Gene Deterling learned that they were parents of a child with PWS. A referral to Vanja A. Holm, M.D., at the Child Development and Mental Retardation Center in Seattle, Washington brought the Deterlings together with other parents and professionals who were acquainted with the syndrome. These few individuals formed a group called "Prader-Willi Syndrome Parents and Friends," a name later changed to the Prader-Willi Syndrome Association. That same year the group officially incorporated, officers were appointed, and a board of directors was established. The first member registered on May 1, 1975. Although many people contributed to the formation of the association, Gene Deterling, the first president, provided the organizational expertise that spearheaded the group's initial growth and established the solid foundation for future development, and Vanja Holm, together with her coworkers, offered professional expertise and support.

By the end of 1976, membership in the PWSA had grown to 140; 118 were parents and relatives and 22 were professionals from 28 states, England, Australia, Canada, Norway, and Germany. Although the PWSA's goal is to serve affected children, their parents, and families, the increase in the number of professional members indicates that the organization has become an acknowledged resource for health care personnel, hospitals, medical schools, universities, state and county health departments, educational specialists, PWS clinics, residential facilities, developmental disability service providers, the Association for Retarded Citizens, and vocational training/sheltered workshop programs. Originally professionals repre-

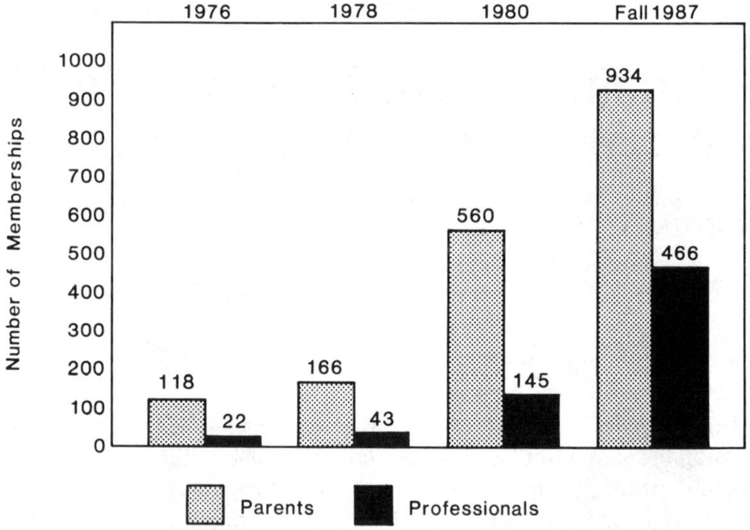

FIGURE 21.1. Growth and distribution of memberships in PWSA. From Data Report, Fall 1987, the Prader-Willi Syndrome Association, Edina, MN.

sented one fifth of the membership; this has increased to one third. The shift in the ratio of parents to professionals who are members of PWSA is indicated in Figure 21.1.

In an effort to overcome the glaring lack of information available about the syndrome, Shirley Neason created and initially edited the PWSA newsletter, *The Gathered View*. The first issue, July 1975, consisted of a three-page introduction to the association and was included with an annual membership fee of $5.00. Currently, the bimonthly issues contain 12 pages and continue to be the primary source of information. For parents and providers who do not have the opportunity to attend small group meetings or the national conferences, the publication serves as a link to those who either have children with the syndrome or serve them. *The Gathered View for the Younger Set* was first published in 1986; it is the regular newsletter with special articles for parents of children under the age of 10 years.

The PWSA's first publication, *Prader-Willi Syndrome—A Handbook for Parents*, also written by Neason, was welcomed by the membership in 1978. It incorporated pertinent facts that had been collected from parents and professionals in the Seattle clinic and reported them in concise, lay terms. Since then, many booklets, articles from newsletters, an annotated bibliography, and medical papers have been made available through the national association; some are printed in several languages (Spanish, French, German, and Dutch). Early in 1979, two conferences were held to discuss PWS. The first was a workshop at the University of Washington attended by parents and professionals. A hardcover book, *Prader-Willi Syndrome* (Holm, Sulzbacher, & Pipes, 1981) published much of what was reported at this meeting. The second conference, sponsored by the PWSA, was held in Minneapolis. Since then, a national PWSA meeting has been held annually in a variety of geographical locations, and conference attendance continues to grow. It is at these yearly gatherings that parents and individuals with PWS have an opportunity to meet, talk with one another, discuss issues with professionals, and share concerns. A general meeting of the members of the PWSA is held during the conference to discuss organizational issues, activities, and directions for future growth.

Not long after the first Minnesota conference, the Deterlings realized that they could no longer keep up with the numerous requests for help and sought assistance from the Minnesota parents' group. Shortly thereafter, an office was established as a worldwide clearinghouse for information and referral. By the summer of 1980 it was determined that the organization could best be served by appointing an Executive Director. An elected, working board of directors and officers, comprised of both parents and professionals, meets twice yearly to conduct official business.

Goals and Objectives

A broad spectrum of concerns are reflected in the PWSA's overall goals and specific objectives.

Improving Communication

PWS was generally unknown 10 years ago and is still relatively unfamiliar to many. Fortunately for people afflicted with PWS and for their families, this picture is changing. With the support of the PWSA, parents are now willing to share their experiences. Through media exposure (print, radio, and television), case-finding is increasing and parents' support groups are growing. For professionals, the PWSA is the main source for up-to-date data, and the association's national conferences, held annually, provide a forum for presentation and discussion of current research and management issues, interdisciplinary communication, and professional/parent interaction.

Lifetime Advocacy for Affected Individuals

For many years parents of individuals with PWS were the only people able to advocate for their children and, because they lacked information and had limited resources, they had a great deal of difficulty convincing professionals of their children's special problems. Many were greeted with, "Why do you feel your child's needs are any different than those of any other mentally retarded person?", "With your child's IQ, he should achieve in this program," or "Don't you know how to feed an infant?" This implies that the lack of weight gain in infancy or the tremendous weight gain by the age of 2–3 years is the parent's fault, or that behavior problems occur only because the child has been "spoiled." Advocacy is a special challenge because the potential for individuals with PWS to adapt is often restricted by unknowledgeable services providers. For example, once the diagnosis of PWS has been made, the role of the family physician tends to diminish. Individual education plans are inappropriately designed around standardized IQ scores. Social service personnel mistakenly assume that existing programs designed for all of the mentally retarded are adequate. As a result of such judgments, people with PWS tend to be managed by a few providers with very narrow points of view that overlook the needs of the "whole person." The fact of the matter is that the medical community should not abandon parents nor should educators accept cognitive capacity as their primary criterion. The psychological aspects of PWS cannot be ignored. All providers should have a clear understanding of the necessity for interdisciplinary collaboration as a basis for providing opportunities for optimum adjustment to life. Achieving the "full potential" of children with the syndrome is a major goal of PWSA. Chapter 19, which discusses the rights of individuals with PWS to services, indicates the important role the PWSA plays in the advocacy process . As recognition and understanding about PWS increases and as more information and support becomes available through the national association, parents are better prepared to advocate for the rights of their offspring.

Support for Research about PWS and the Development of a National Center for Services

Unfortunately, federal research funds are limited and rarely awarded to study low-incidence syndromes such as PWS. The PWSA has just completed a seven-part survey of over 700 cases, the data from which will be made available to qualified researchers. In a concerted effort to expand the knowledge base about PWS, the national association has established two funds of its own. The first, supported by donations from members and friends, is designated to be awarded for direct research, for seed money to enable researchers to seek larger grants, and for projects directly related to the syndrome. A Scientific Advisory Committee (SAC), formed in 1980, is responsible for overseeing these endeavors. It is comprised of PWSA members who are professionals in the fields of medicine, nutrition, and education, and who donate their time and talent to review all research fund applications. The SAC has the overall responsibility for the presentation of the Prader-Willi Scientific Session, a 1-day research symposium that is held in conjunction with the annual PWSA conference.

A second fund has been established to develop a Crisis Intervention and Transitional Center (CITC) for individuals with PWS, their families, and care providers. The center will serve as temporary placement for individuals in crisis situations where they can be kept alive and controlled until appropriate services become available in their home communities. It will offer opportunities for research, develop models for management programs, and provide training for direct care staff of facilities currently serving or planning to serve the PWS population. The PWSA recognizes that the CITC can be attained only through the collaborative efforts of the organization's membership and outside resources, since a privately supported, comprehensive facility simply cannot be funded solely by individual parent groups.

Normalization of Life for Affected Children and Their Families

Normalization of life for people with PWS and their families is very important. Affected individuals are "trapped" in a food-oriented world and deserve an environment in which they can function to the best of their ability. A recent letter to PWSA from a parent stated that "raising a child with PWS is not fair to her and not fair to the rest of the family." The organization directs considerable efforts to identifying available services to assist families to cope, and provides current information about out-of-home residential options and summer programs throughout the country (Appendix H).

Encouragement of Interdependent Relationships Between Parents and Professionals

With the national office as the hub of the wheel and local groups as the spokes, parents, professionals, and all service providers can work together on behalf of affected children. All PWSA members receive *The Gathered View*, which, in addition to updating information about PWS, reports on national and local group activities. This includes notification of times, dates, and locations of all national, regional, and state meetings. As one of the few resources for current literature about the syndrome, the PWSA provides a listing of all available publications about PWS and assists professionals interested in research and case management. The PWSA office is a place to call or write anytime questions arise; it maintains a directory of available services (diagnostic and treatment settings, service providers, and agencies), and provides information about professionals familiar with PWS who may be available for consultation and/or speaking engagements.

One of the most important roles of the PWSA is to promote parent networks in a variety of geographical areas as a means of strengthening support groups and facilitating the establishment of state chapters. The association's goal of networking parents and professionals has been met repeatedly during the annual conferences. The dialogues have found "experts" learning from the parents, and the workshop format is an effective method of interaction. Increase in the conference attendance has been attributed to the fact that the PWSA not only plans a very extensive agenda for the participants but also provides an equally impressive program for affected children and their siblings. Each year the host committee meets the tremendous challenge of organizing activities for persons with PWS ranging in age from infants of a few months to adults in their 30s, no easy task. Youth programs have included educational sessions and entertaining field trips, but the highlight of the gathering for children and parents continues to be a youth banquet followed by a dance with a live band. Dance night at the conference has been likened by parents of affected offspring to the thrill of normal teens going to a junior prom.

Organization of Chapters

In 1980, the PWSA determined that a system of official incorporated chapters would be the logical way to link the many groups of parents who had been meeting informally in different geographical areas. A group of parents in Connecticut was the first to become affiliated with the PWSA as an official chapter in July 1982; six other chapters were also formed that year. By 1983, three more joined, and by fall 1986, 19 parent groups were linked nationwide. Other chapters continue to develop and affiliate (Table 21.1).

Establishment of a chapter system enables the national office to remain a clearinghouse for dissemination of information while individual chapters are in the best position to educate families and primary care providers and increase public awareness of PWS through exposure in local media. Local chapters can initiate action to develop appropriate state and community services and schedule group support meetings. It has been noted that parents who are members of a state chapter of the PWSA may have a considerable impact on agencies who serve the developmentally disabled. Decisions about state funding and licensing are made only after close investigation of identified needs, and when services to people with PWS are requested, particularly regarding developing educational services and residential programs, the credibility of the parents' local group is enhanced when it is formally linked to a credentialed, internationally recognized organization (see Chapter 20).

The PWSA believes that a national network is the best way to serve the needs of the children, their parents, and professionals. The natural sequence of events that follows the birth of a child with PWS requires intervention from informed sources, and the PWSA serves in that vital role. As an organization, the PWSA can make a difference.

TABLE 21.1. Official chapters of PWSA.

Chapter	State/region	Number of members	Official joining date
PWSA–Connecticut Chapter, Inc.	Connecticut	25	7-31-82
PW New York Association, Inc.	New York	60–75	9-02-82
PW Kentucky Association	Kentucky	20	10-13-82
PWS Missouri Association	Missouri	20	10-26-82
PW Midlantic Association	Pennsylvania, New Jersey, Maryland, Delaware, New York	100–125	10-26-82
PWA of Minnesota	Minnesota	40	10-30-82
PW Colorado Association	Colorado	20	11-08-82
The PWS of New England, Inc.	Massachusetts, New Hampshire, Maine	20–25	2-04-83
PWS Texas Association	Texas	42	8-09-84
PWS of Michigan	Michigan	35	10-30-84
PW Frontier Regional Association	Montana, North Dakota, South Dakota, Wyoming	12–15	6-03-85
PW Utah Association	Utah	10–12	6-10-85
PW Arizona Association	Arizona	12–15	2-03-86
Illinois PW Group	Illinois	15–20	2-21-86
PWSA of South Carolina	South Carolina	10–12	4-29-86
PWSA of Virginia	Virginia	15–18	7-14-86
PW Greater Kansas City Association	Missouri, Kansas	10–12	9-01-86
PWS Southeastern Association	Alabama, Georgia, Florida	30–40	1-16-87
PWSA of Ohio	Ohio	30–35	2-06-87
PWSA of Georgia, Inc.	Georgia	12–15	6-01-87

Note: From Data Report, Fall 1987, The Prader-Willi Syndrome Association, Edina, MN.

References

Holm, V.A., Sulzbacher, S.J., & Pipes, P.L. (Eds.). (1981). *The Prader-Willi syndrome.* Baltimore: University Park Press.

Neason, S. (1978). *Prader-Willi syndrome—A handbook for parents*. Edina, MN: The Prader-Willi Syndrome Association.

Glossary

Amniocentesis: A procedure in which a small amount of the amniotic fluid surrounding the fetus is drawn off and subjected to genetic and biochemical analysis.

Chromosome: Carrier of hereditary material that appear in the nucleus of a cell. Each cell has a specific number of chromosomes; normal humans have 46.

Chromosome abnormality: Any variation from the normal chromosomal pattern. The common abnormalities found in Prader-Willi Syndrome are:

1. *Deletion:* a condition in which a piece of genetic material is lost or missing from a chromosome. Typically there is a small piece of the long arm of the 15th chromosome that is missing.
2. *Translocation:* a transfer of a fragment of one chromosome to another chromosome.

Co-contraction: The simultaneous contraction of all the muscles around a joint to stabilize it.

Cryptorchidism: Undescended testicles (testicles are not present in the scrotal sac).

Genetics counseling: Counseling that explains facts about genetics issues to parents/care providers. Emphasis is on clarification of information, possible recurrence risk, reproductive options, support to affected persons and their families, and follow-up services.

Hyperphagia: Consumption of more than an optimal quantity of food.

Hypogenitalism: The genital organs are undersized or nonexistent.

Hypogonadism: A condition of abnormal decrease in the function of the ovaries and testes, causing retardation of growth and sexual development.

Hypothalamus: The part of the brain that controls appetite, body temperature, hormones, and other vital functions.

Hypotonia: Decreased muscle tone. The muscles are soft, weak, and flabby.

Learning disabled: A term applied to low-achieving children whose performance is inconsistent with overall intelligence. These children may be part of an identifiable group who are limited in their ability to process written or spoken language, which may result in limited capacity to master some basic academic tasks.

Lability: Marked fluctuations in mood/disposition.

Mental age: A measured level of cognitive function established by a test of intelligence.

Mental retardation: A level of mental functioning identified as significantly subaverage existing concurrently with the ability to function and adapt; this level of functioning is at least two standard deviations below the mean (i.e., below an IQ of 70).

Metabolism: Pertaining to the body's process of absorbing nourishment from food and turning it into energy or stored fat.

Motor planning: The ability of the brain to conceive of, organize, and carry out a sequence of unfamiliar activities. Also known as "praxis."

Narrow bifrontal diameter: A narrow forehead.

Normalization: The effort to make available activities and patterns of everyday life that are as close as possible to the habits of normal, mainstream individuals.

Obesity: A condition in which body weight is considerably (more than two standard deviations) above the range that is normal for body height.

Praxis: The capacity of the brain to integrate and carry out unfamiliar motor activities. Also known as motor planning.

Proximal musculature: The muscles of the trunk, shoulder girdle, and hip girdle.

Rehabilitation: A dynamic process of continuing evaluation of disabled individuals in order to meet their needs and develop realistic methods of coping. This "process" acknowledges that one individual may have more than just one problem to confront and that the individual's ability to function cannot be separated from environmental concerns.

Sheltered workshop: A controlled work-oriented rehabilitation setting that utilizes work experiences and related services to assist handicapped individuals in making the maximum progress possible toward vocational productivity and normal living.

Strabismus: The condition of being "cross-eyed."

Syndrome: A term used to describe a symptom complex characterized by many medical signs. In many syndromes not all affected individuals will have every diagnostic sign.

System advocacy: Refers to actions taken by individuals or groups to influence policy making.

Suggested Readings

Alexander, R., Greenswag, L., & Nowak, A. (1987). Ruminating and vomiting in Prader-Willi syndrome. *American Journal of Medical Genetics*, *28*, 889–895.

Bray, G.A., Dahms, W.T., Swerdloff, R.S., Fisher, R.H., Atkinson, R.L., & Carrel, R.E., (1983). The Prader-Willi syndrome: A study of 42 patients and review of the literature. *Medicine*, *62*, 59–80.

Bottel, H. (1977, May). The eating disorder. *Good Housekeeping*, p. 176.

Cassidy, S.B. (1984). Prader-Willi syndrome. *Current Problems in Pediatrics*, *14*, 5–55.

Clarren, S.K., & Smith, D.W. (1977). Prader-Willi syndrome: Variable severity and recurrence risk. *American Journal of Diseases of Children*, *131*, 798–800.

Dunn, H.G., Tze, W.J., Alisharan, R.M., & Schulzer, M. (1981). Clinical experience with 23 cases of Prader-Willi syndrome. In V.A. Holm, S.J. Sulzbacher, & P.L. Pipes (Eds.), *The Prader-Willi syndrome* (pp. 69–88). Baltimore: University Park Press.

Edmonston, N.K. (1983). Management of speech and language impairment in a case of Prader-Willi syndrome. *Language, Speech and Hearing Services in Schools*, *13*, 241–245.

Greenswag, L. (1984). The adult with Prader-Willi syndrome: A descriptive investigation. Unpublished doctoral thesis, University of Iowa. (DA 056952, University Microfilms International, Ann Arbor, MI)

Greenswag, L. (1987). Adults with Prader-Willi syndrome: a survey of 232 cases. *Developmental Medicine and Child Neurology*, *29*, 145–152.

Hall, B.D., & Smith, D.W. (1972). Prader-Willi syndrome. A resume of 32 cases including an instance of affected first cousins, one of whom is of normal stature and intelligence. *The Journal of Pediatrics*, *81*, 286–293.

Hanson, J.W. (1981). A view of the etiology and pathogenesis of Prader-Willi syndrome. In V.A. Holm, S.J. Sulzbacher, & P.L. Pipes (Eds.), *The Prader-Willi syndrome* (pp. 45–53). Baltimore: University Park Press.

Herrman, J. (1981). Implications of Prader-Willi syndrome for the individual and the family. In V.A. Holm, S.J. Sulzbacher, & P.L. Pipes (Eds.), *The Prader-Willi syndrome* (pp. 229–238). Baltimore: University Park Press.

Holm, V.A., & Nugent, J.K. (1982). Growth in the Prader-Willi syndrome. *Birth Defects: Original Article Series*, *18* (No. 3 B), 93–100.

Holm, V.A., Sulzbacher, S.J., & Pipes, P.L. (Eds.). (1984). *Prader-Willi syndrome*. Baltimore: University Park Press.

Kousseff, B.G. (1982). The cytogenetic controversy in the Prader-Labhart-Willi syndrome. *American Journal of Medical Genetics*, *13*, 431–439.

LeConte, J.M. (1981). Social work intervention strategies for families with children with Prader-Willi syndrome. In V.A. Holm, S.J. Sulzbacher, & P.L. Pipes (Eds.), *Prader-Willi syndrome* (pp. 245–257). Baltimore: University Park Press.

Ledbetter, D.H., Riccardi, V.M., Airhart, S.D., Strobel, R.J., Keenan, B.S., & Crawford, J.D. (1981). Deletions of chromosome 15 as a cause of Prader-Willi syndrome. *New England Journal of Medicine*, *304*, 325–329.

Marshall, Jr., B.D., Elder, J., O'Bosky, D., Wallace, C.J., & Liberman, R.P. (1979). Behavioral treatment of Prader-Willi syndrome. *The Behavior Therapist*, *2*, 22–23.

Mitchell, L. (1981). *An overview of Prader-Willi syndrome*. Edina, MN: The Prader-Willi Syndrome Association.

Nardella, M.T., Sulzbacher, S.J., & Worthington-Roberts, B.S. (1981). Activity levels of persons with Prader-Willi syndrome. *American Journal of Mental Deficiency*, *87*, 498–505.

Neason, S. (1978). *Prader-Willi syndrome: A handbook for parents*. Edina, MN: The Prader-Willi Syndrome Association.

Prader, A., Labhart, A., & Willi, H. (1956). Ein Syndrom von Adipositas, Kleinwuchs, Kryptorchismus, und Oligophrenie nach myatonieartigem Zustand im Neugeborenenalter. *Schweizerische Medizinische Wochenschrift*, *86*, 1260–1261.

Prader, A. (1981). The Prader-Willi syndrome: An overview. *Acta Paediatrica Japonica*, *23*, 307–311.

Stephenson, J.B.P. (1980). Prader-Willi syndrome: Neonatal presentation and later development. *Developmental Medicine and Child Neurology*, *22*, 792–795.

Thompson, T., Kodluboy, S., & Heston, L. (1980). Behavioral treatment of obesity in Prader-Willi syndrome. *Behavior Therapy*, *11*, 588–593.

Wett, R.J. (1983). Prader-Willi syndrome: The disabled child. *The Journal of the American Medical Association*, *249*, 1836.

Zellweger, H., & Schneider, H.J. (1968). Syndrome of hypotonia, hypomentia, hypogonadism, obesity (HHHO) or Prader-Willi syndrome. *American Journal of Diseases of Children*, *115*, 588–598.

Appendices

Appendix A: Growth Charts for Prader-Willi Syndrome

VANJA A. HOLM

Short stature, considering genetic background, is one of the diagnostic hallmarks in the Prader-Willi syndrome (PWS) (Holm, 1981). In a previous publication, the expected linear growth in this condition has been described (Holm & Nugent, 1982). In that study we plotted growth on standard U.S. growth charts (Hamill, Drizd, Johnson, Reed, & Roche, 1977) from a mixture of cross-sectional and longitudinal data from 92 subjects, 56 males and 36 females (Figures A.1 and A.2).

From the height data obtained from age 3 years to early adulthood, growth curves were fitted for males and females that encompassed most of the data points. From these data, growth charts specific for PWS, age 3 to early adulthood, have been developed. Growth during the first 36 months of life is too unpredictable in this condition—it is characterized by a fall-off in growth—to lend itself to the development of a special growth chart for that age. The growth curves from the childhood, adolescence, and early adulthood years have been made into graphs for easy charting (Figures A.3 and A.4).

These PWS-specific growth charts can be used to clinically follow the growth of individuals with this condition. The growth of adolescents with PWS is often worrisome because their adolescent growth spurt is considerably less than expected (Holm & Nugent, 1982). Plotting the growth on these charts might be reassuring for the physician, the parents, and the adolescent. On the other hand, if a child with PWS shows a fall-off in growth during childhood, which is not typical, the physician using these syndrome-specific growth charts will easily spot this child, who needs further endocrinological workups.

Research exploring growth-promoting regimens can also benefit from these specific growth charts. They have been used in a study of the effects of oxandrolone therapy in males with this syndrome (Holm, Nugent, & Ruvalcaba, 1988). Synthetic growth hormone is now becoming widely available, and it is anticipated that growth hormone therapy soon will be used in a variety of syndromes with primordial growth deficiency, including PWS. These syndrome-specific growth charts will be useful in evaluating the effects of such future treatment in PWS.

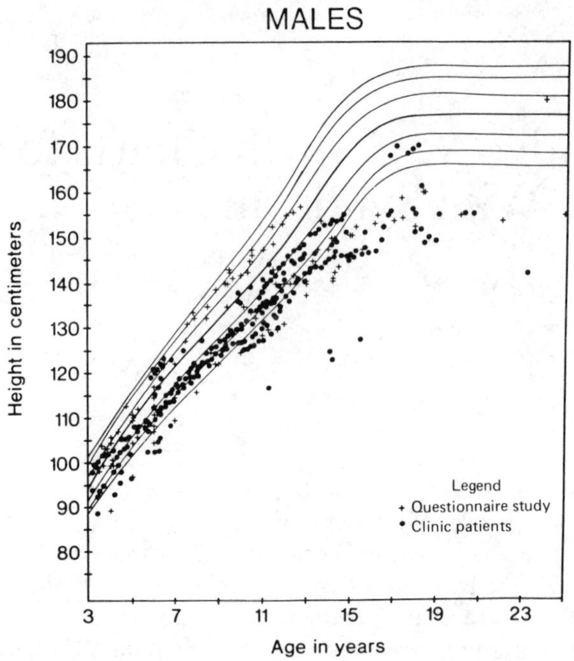

FIGURE A.1. Growth data from 56 male subjects with PWS, plotted on standard U.S. growth charts.

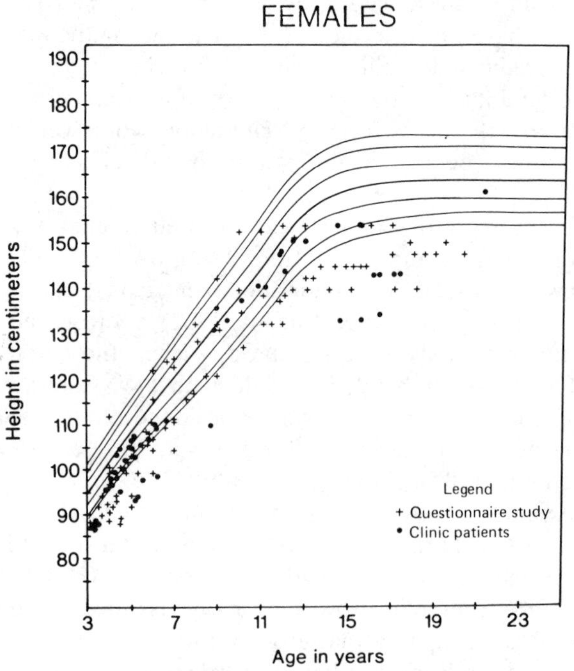

FIGURE A.2. Growth data from 36 female subjects with PWS, plotted on standard U.S. growth charts.

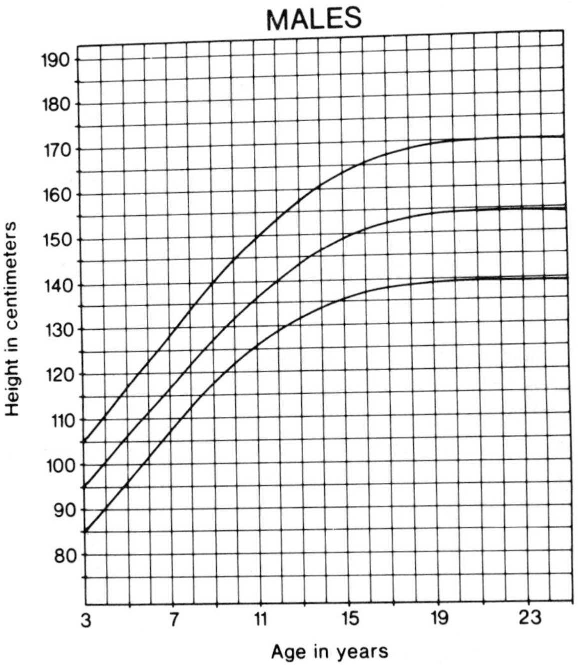

FIGURE A.3. Blank chart with growth curves for PWS males from age 3 to early adulthood.

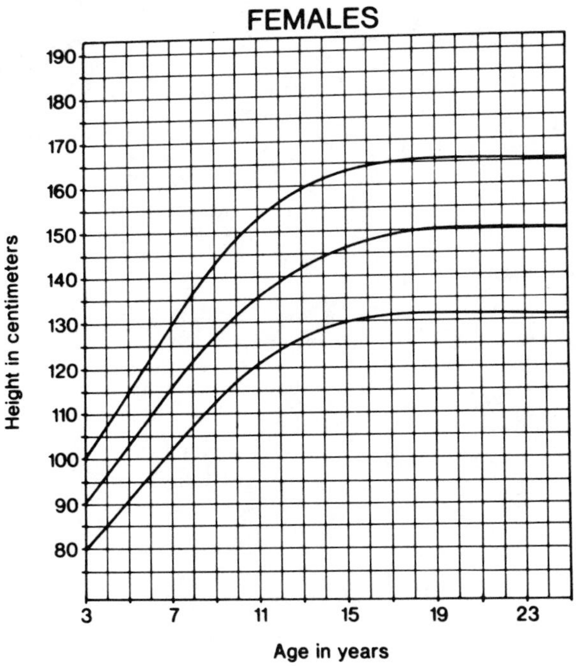

FIGURE A.4. Blank chart with growth curves for PWS females from age 3 to early adulthood.

References

Hamill, P.V., Drizd, T.A., Johnson, C.L., Reed, R., & Roche, A.F. (1977). *NCHS growth curves for children birth–18 years, United States*. Vital and Health Statistics Series 11, Number 165. U.S. Department of Health, Education, and Welfare, Pub. No (PHS) 78–1650. Washington, DC: U.S. Government Printing Office.

Holm, V.A. (1981). The diagnosis of Prader-Willi syndrome. In V.A. Holm, S.J. Sulzbacher, & P.L. Pipes (Eds.), *The Prader-Willi syndrome* (pp. 27–36). Baltimore: University Park Press.

Holm, V.A., & Nugent, J.K. (1982). Growth in the Prader-Willi syndrome. *Birth Defects: Original Article Series*, *18*, 93–100.

Holm, V.A., Nugent, J.K., & Ruvalcaba, R.H.A. (1988). *Oxandrolone therapy in males with the Prader-Willi syndrome*. Unpublished (manuscript).

Appendix B: Food Exchange Guidelines

TABLE B.1. Sample Menu

	Monday	Tuesday	Wednesday	Thursday	Friday	Saturday	Sunday
BREAKFAST	Milk, skim Pancake Diet syrup Bacon slice Peaches, sliced Orange juice Coffee Diet sweetener	Milk, skim Omelet Dry cereal Banana Tomato juice Toast Margarine Coffee Diet sweetener	Milk, skim Cottage cheese Dark toast Margarine Diet jelly Grapefruit juice Prunes Coffee Diet sweetener	Milk, skim Scrambled egg Malt-O-Meal Toast Margarine Orange juice Pears Coffee Diet sweetener	Milk, skim Cinnamon toast Dry cereal Apple juice Orange Coffee Diet sweetener	Milk, skim Boiled egg English muffin (1/2) Diet jelly Margarine Grapefruit juice Applesauce Coffee Diet sweeteneer	Milk, skim Scrambled egg Raisin toast Pineapple juice Grapefruit (1/2) Coffee Diet sweetener
LUNCH	Milk, skim Peanut butter Whole wheat bread Diet jelly Celery sticks Orange Graham cracker	Milk, skim Turkey slices Whole wheat bread Carrot coins Red apple Vanilla wafers Mayonnaise	Milk, skim Tuna salad Rye bread Radishes Seasonal fruit Crackers	Milk, skim Turkey ham Pumpernickel Cauliflower Raisins Mayonnaise Vanilla wafers	Milk, skim Sliced cheese Whole wheat bread Sliced tomato w/lettuce Mayonnaise Red apple Graham cracker	Milk, skim Cottage cheese salad Curried slaw Blueberry muffin Seasonal fruit Ice milk	Milk, skim French bread pizza Dzerta Tossed salad Seasonal fruit
	Ice water →						
DINNER	Milk, skim BBQ chicken Rice Broccoli Peas Marsh mallow crispies Tea Diet sweetener	Milk, skim Cheeseburger Dinner roll String bean salad Sauerkraut Potato salad Seasonal fruit Tea Diet sweetener	Milk, skim Baked pork chop Pasta/vegetable salad Beets/orange salad Dinner roll Margarine Seasonal fruit Tea Diet sweetener	Milk, skim Chicken Waldorf salad Dilled carrots Bread sticks Dzerta Seasonal fruit Chocolate pudding Tea Diet sweetener	Milk, skim Broiled fish w/lemon Oriental mixed vegetables Orange wheat salad Whole kernel corn Tossed salad Juice sicle Tea Diet sweetener	Milk, skim Roast beef Baked potato Mixed vegetables Spinach salad, lemon dressing Margarine Bread Peach yogurt freeze Tea Diet sweetener	Milk, skim Ham slices Sweet potatoes/ apples Seasoned rice Steamed broccoli Fruit ice Margarine Relish sticks Tea Diet sweetener
	Ice water →						
PM SNACK	Popcorn (5 c) Lemonade	Cookies (2) Apple/tea cooler	Angel food cake Frozen strawberries	Vanilla wafers (5) Applesauce	Popcorn (5 c)	Cookies (2) Grape sparkle	Graham crackers Seasonal fruit

Note: Adapted from nutritional program at Oakwood Residence, Minnetonka, MN, 1986.

TABLE B.2. Example of diet based on food exchange system

Meal	Portion/ amount	Exchange	Monday—Week 1 Calorie content of diet 900	1,000	1,200	1,500	1,800	2,000
Breakfast								
Milk, skim	1 c	1 milk	x	x	x	x	x	x
Pancake	1	1 bread/1 fat	x	x	x	2x	2x	2x
Diet syrup	—	free	x	x	x	x	x	x
Bacon	1 slice	1 fat	x	x	x	x	x	x
Peaches, sliced	1/2 c	1 fruit	0	0	0	x	x	x
Orange juice	1/2 c	1 fruit	x	x	x	x	x	x
Coffee	—	free	x	x	x	x	x	x
Diet sweetener	—	free	x	x	x	x	x	x
Lunch								
Milk, skim	1 c	1 milk	x	x	x	x	x	x
Peanut butter	2 tbsp	1 meat/1 fat	x	x	x	x	x	x
Whole wheat bread	1 slice	1 bread	x	x	x	2x	2x	2x
Diet jelly	—	free	x	x	x	x	x	x
Celery sticks	8 sticks	1 vegetable	x	x	x	x	x	x
Orange	1	1 fruit	x	x	x	x	x	2x
Graham cracker	2 squares	1 bread	0	0	0	0	0	x
Dinner								
Milk, skim	1 c	1 milk	1/2x	x	x	x	x	x
BBQ chicken	1 oz	1 meat	2 oz	2 oz	3 oz	3 oz	3 oz	5 oz
Rice	1/2 c	1 starch	x	x	x	x	x	x
Broccoli	1/2 c	1 veg	x	x	x	2x	2x	2x
Peas	1/2 c	1 starch	0	0	0	0	x	x
Marsh mallow crispies	1 square	1 fruit	x	x	x	x	x	x
Margarine	1 tsp	1 fat	0	0	x	2x	2x	2x
Tea	free	free	x	x	x	x	x	x
Diet sweetener	—	free	x	x	x	x	x	x

Note: Adapted from nutritional program at Oakwood Residence, Minnetonka, MN, 1986. X = Inclusion in diet; 2x = inclusion of twice the portion size in the daily intake; 0 = do not include in diet.

TABLE B.2. *Continued.*

Tuesday—Week 1

Meal	Portion/ amount	Exchange	Calorie content of diet 900	1,000	1,200	1,500	1,800	2,000
Breakfast								
Milk, skim	1 c	1 milk	x	x	x	x	x	x
Omelet	1 egg	1 meat	x	x	x	x	x	x
Dry cereal	3/4 c	1 bread	x	x	x	x	x	x
Banana	1/2	1 fruit	0	0	0	x	x	x
Tomato juice	6 oz	1 fruit	x	x	x	x	x	x
Toast	1 slice	1 bread	0	0	0	0	x	x
Margarine	1 tsp	1 fat	0	0	0	0	x	x
Coffee	—	free	x	x	x	x	x	x
Diet sweetener	—	free	x	x	x	x	x	x
Lunch								
Milk, skim	1 c	1 milk	x	x	x	x	x	x
Turkey slices	1 oz	1 meat	2x	2x	2x	3x	3x	3x
Whole wheat bread	1 slice	1 bread	x	x	x	2x	2x	2x
Carrot coins	1/2 c	1 veg	x	x	x	x	x	x
Red apple	1 small	1 fruit	x	x	x	x	x	2x
Vanilla wafers	5	1 bread	0	0	0	0	0	x
Mayonnaise	1 tsp	1 fat	—	x	x	x	x	2x
Dinner								
Milk, skim	1 c	1 milk	1/2x	x	x	x	x	x
Cheeseburger	1	3 oz (3 meat)	x	x	x	x	x	1 1/2x
Dinner roll	1	1 starch	0	0	0	0	x	x
String bean salad	1/2 c	1 veg	x	x	x	2x	2x	2x
Sauerkraut	1/4 c	free	x	x	x	x	x	x
Potato salad	1/2 c	1 starch	x	x	x	x	x	x
Seasonal fruit	1 or 1/2 c	1 fruit	x	x	x	x	x	x
Tea	free	free	x	x	x	x	x	x
Diet sweetener	free	free	x	x	x	x	x	x

TABLE B.2. *Continued.*

Wednesday—Week 1								
			Calorie content of diet					
Meal	Portion/ amount	Exchange	900	1,000	1,200	1,500	1,800	2,000
Breakfast								
Milk, skim	1c	1 milk	x	x	x	x	x	x
Cottage cheese	1/4 c	1 oz meat	x	x	x	x	x	x
Dark toast	1 slice	1 bread	x	x	x	x	2x	2x
Margarine	1 tsp	1 fat	x	x	x	x	x	x
Diet jelly	—	free	x	x	x	x	x	x
Grapefruit juice	1/2 c	1 fruit	x	x	x	x	x	x
Prunes	2 medium	1 fruit	0	0	0	x	x	x
Coffee	—	free	x	x	x	x	x	x
Diet sweetener	—	free	x	x	x	x	x	x
Lunch								
Milk, skim	1 c	1 milk	x	x	x	x	x	x
Tuna salad	1/4 c	1 meat/1 fat	x	x	x	2x	2x	2x
Rye bread	1 slice	1 bread	x	x	x	2x	2x	2x
Radishes	6 pieces	1 veg	x	x	x	x	x	2x
Seasonal fruit	1	1 fruit	x	x	x	x	x	x
Crackers	6	1 bread	0	0	0	0	0	x
Dinner								
Milk, skim	1 c	1 milk	1/2x	x	x	x	x	x
Baked pork chop	1 chop	3 oz	x	x	x	x	x	1 1/2x
Pasta/vegetable salad	1/2 c	1 starch	x	x	x	x	x	x
Beets/orange salad	1/2 c	1 veg	x	x	x	2x	2x	2x
Dinner roll	1	1 starch	0	0	0	0	x	x
Margarine	1 tsp	1 fat	0	0	x	x	x	x
Seasonal fruit	1 or 1/2 c	1 fruit	—	—	x	x	—	—
Tea	free	free	x	x	x	x	x	x
Diet sweetener	free	free	x	x	x	x	x	x

TABLE B.2. *Continued.*

Meal	Portion/ amount	Exchange	Calorie content of diet					
			900	1,000	1,200	1,500	1,800	2,000
Thursday—Week 1								
Breakfast								
Milk, skim	1c	1 milk	x	x	x	x	x	x
Scrambled egg	1	1 meat	x	x	x	x	x	x
Malt-O-Meal	1/2 c	1 bread	x	x	x	x	x	x
Toast	1 slice	1 bread	0	0	0	0	x	x
Margarine	1 tsp	1 fat	0	0	0	0	x	x
Orange juice	1/2 c	1 fruit	x	x	x	x	x	x
Pears	2 halves	1 fruit	0	0	0	x	x	x
Coffee	—	free	x	x	x	x	x	x
Diet sweetener	—	free	x	x	x	x	x	x
Lunch								
Milk, skim	1 c	1 milk	x	x	x	x	x	x
Turkey ham	1 oz	1 meat	x	x	2x	2x	2x	3x
Pumpernickel	1 slice	1 bread	x	x	x	2x	2x	2x
Cauliflower	1/2 c	1 veg	x	x	x	x	x	x
Raisins	1/4 c	1 fruit	x	x	x	x	x	x
Mayonnaise	1 tsp	1 fat	0	0	x	x	2x	2x
Vanilla wafers	5	1 bread	0	0	0	0	0	x
Dinner								
Milk, skim								
Chicken Waldorf salad	3/4 c	3 meat/1 fat	1/2 c	1/2 c	1/2c	x	x	1 c
Dilled carrots	1/2 oz	1 veg	—	—	x	2x	2x	2x
Bread sticks	2	1 starch	x	x	x	x	3 sticks	3 sticks
Dzerta	free	free	x	x	x	x	x	x
Seasonal fruit	1 or 1/2 c	1 fruit	x	x	x	x	x	x
Chocolate pudding	1/2 c	1 milk	x	x	x	x	x	x
Tea	free	free	x	x	x	x	x	x
Diet sweetener	free	free	x	x	x	x	x	x

TABLE B.2. *Continued.*

Friday—Week 1								
			Calorie content of diet					
Meal	Portion/ amount	Exchange	900	1,000	1,200	1,500	1,800	2,000
Breakfast								
Milk, skim	1c	1 milk	x	x	x	x	x	x
Cinnamon toast	1 slice	1 bread/1 fat	x	x	x	x	x	x
Dry cereal	3/4 c	1 bread	x	x	x	x	x	x
Apple juice	1/2 c	1 fruit	x	x	0	x	x	x
Orange	1	1 fruit	0	0	x	x	x	x
Coffee	x	free	x	x	x	x	x	x
Diet sweetener	x	free	x	x	x	x	x	x
Lunch								
Milk, skim	1 c	1 milk	x	x	x	x	x	x
Sliced cheese	1 slice	1 meat	2x	2x	2x	2x	2x	3x
Whole wheat bread	1 slice	1 bread	x	x	x	2x	2x	2x
Sliced tomato w/lettuce	1 slice	1 veg	x	x	x	x	x	x
Mayonnaise	1 tsp	1 fat	0	x	x	x	2x	2x
Red apple	1 small	1 fruit	x	x	x	x	x	x
Graham cracker	2 squares	1 bread	0	0	0	0	0	x
Dinner								
Milk, skim	1 c	1 milk	1/2x	x	x	x	x	x
Broiled fish w/ lemon	3 oz	3 meat	x	x	x	x	x	5 oz
Oriental mixed vegetables	1/2 c	1 veg	x	x	x	2x	2x	2x
Orange wheat salad	1/2 c	1 starch	x	x	x	x	x	x
Whole kernel corn	1/2 c	1 starch	0	0	0	0	x	x
Tossed salad	free	free	x	x	x	x	x	x
Juice sicle	1	1 fruit	x	x	x	x	x	x
Tea	free	free	x	x	x	x	x	x
Diet sweetener	free	free	x	x	x	x	x	x

TABLE B.2. *Continued.*

Saturday—Week 1								
			Calorie content of diet					
Meal	Portion/ amount	Exchange	900	1,000	1,200	1,500	1,800	2,000
Breakfast								
Milk, skim	1 c	1 milk	x	x	x	x	x	x
Boiled egg	1 egg	1 meat	x	x	x	x	x	x
English muffin	1/2 muffin	1 bread	x	x	x	x	2x	2x
Diet jelly	—	free	x	x	x	x	x	x
Margarine	1 tsp	1 fat	x	x	x	x	x	2x
Grapefruit juice	1/2 c	1 fruit	x	x	x	x	x	x
Applesauce	1/2 c	1 fruit	0	0	0	x	x	x
Coffee	—	free	x	x	x	x	x	x
Diet sweetener	—	free	x	x	x	x	x	x
Lunch								
Milk, skim	1 c	1 milk	x	x	x	x	x	x
Cottage cheese salad	1/2 c	2 meat	x	x	x	x	x	3/4 c
Curried slaw	1/2 c	1 veg	x	x	x	x	x	x
Blueberry muffin	1	1 starch, 1 fat	x	x	x	x	x	x
Seasonal fruit	1 or 1/2 c	1 fruit	x	x	x	x	x	x
Ice milk	1/2 c	1 starch, 1 fat	x	x	x	x	x	x
Dinner								
Milk, skim	1 c	1 milk	1/2 x	x	x	x	x	x
Roast beef	2 oz	2 meat	x	x	x	x	3 oz	4 oz
Baked potato	1 small	1 starch	x	x	x	x	x	x
Mixed vegetables	1/2 c	1 veg	x	x	x	2x	2x	2x
Spinach salad, lemon dressing	free	free	x	x	x	x	x	x
Margarine	1 tsp	1 fat	x	x	x	2x	2x	2x
Bread	1 slice	1 starch	0	0	0	x	x	x
Peach yogurt freeze	1/2 c	1 fruit	x	x	x	x	x	x
Tea	free	free	x	x	x	x	x	x
Diet sweetener	free	free	x	x	x	x	x	x

TABLE B.2. *Continued.*

Sunday—Week 1								
			Calorie content of diet					
Meal	Portion/ amount	Exchange	900	1,000	1,200	1,500	1,800	2,000
Breakfast								
Milk, skim	1 c	1 milk	x	x	x	x	x	x
Scrambled egg	—	1 meat	x	x	x	x	x	x
Raisin toast	1 slice	1 bread	x	x	x	x	2x	2x
Margarine	1 tsp	1 fat	x	x	x	x	x	2x
Pineapple juice	1/2 c	1 fruit	x	x	0	x	x	x
Grapefruit	1/2	1 fruit	0	0	x	x	x	x
Coffee	—	free	x	x	x	x	x	x
Diet sweetener	—	free	x	x	x	x	x	x
Lunch								
Milk, skim	1 c	1 milk	x	x	x	x	x	x
French bread pizza	6 inch	2 meat, 2 bread	x	x	x	x	x	x
Dzerta	free	1 veg, 1 fat	x	x	x	x	x	x
Tossed salad	free	free	x	x	x	x	x	x
Seasonal fruit	1 or 1/2 c	free 1 fruit	x	x	x	x	x	x
Dinner								
Milk, skim	1 c	1 milk	1/2x	x	x	x	x	x
Ham slices	2 oz	2 meat	x	x	x	x	3 oz	4 oz
Sweet potatoes/ apples	1/3 c	1 starch	x	x	x	x	x	x
Seasoned rice	1/2 c	1 starch	0	0	0	x	x	x
Steamed broccoli	1/2 c	1 veg	x	x	x	2x	2x	2x
Fruit ice	1/2 c	1 fruit	x	x	x	x	x	x
Margarine	1 tsp	1 fat	0	0	x	x	x	x
Relish sticks	free	free	x	x	x	x	x	x
Tea	free	free	x	x	x	x	x	x
Diet sweetener	free	free	x	x	x	x	x	x

Appendix C: Sample Positive Reinforcements for Behavioral Management

Positive reinforcement (rewards) for individuals with PWS is very effective where realistic expectations are clearly understood and consistency is maintained.

Positive reinforcement for persons with Prader-Willi syndrome should be appropriate to mental and emotional age. Rewards may need to be changed frequently and remain concrete.

Furthermore, unlike most other mentally retarded persons who tend to maintain a competency level once a task is learned, task performance of individuals with PWS tends to fluctuate broadly. They may demonstrate productivity and cooperation for a time, only to "lose it." It is practical to set rather low expectations for behavior and allow for more successful experiences than to always strive for a higher plateau. Less complicated, less stressful activities make the relearning process easier. Where possible, input from the individual with PWS should be incorporated into the decision-making process.

Behavioral charting is best done on a daily as well as a weekly basis. In addition to praise, stickers, stars, or tokens work well as long as the amount earned for a reward is relatively small and the time element short. In other words, concrete evidence of success should be available more frequently than once a week. The token/reward system should be integrated into the entire day's activities, carrying over from school to home or vocational program to group residence. Families and other primary providers appreciate specific guidelines and when all are "playing with the same set of rules" it is easier to preserve the consistency of the behavioral guidelines. For example, following directions within a set time limit may earn a token regardless of the setting.

In general, individuals with PWS have very good fine motor skills and like sedentary activities. Because they need regular exercise, any reward system should be linked to participation in specific physical programming. Also, persons with PWS, regardless of their age, seem to prefer to relate on a one-to-one with older individuals (particularly teachers and staff). They also like playing with younger children because they get to be "in charge."

1. Daily and weekly charts with age-appropriate stickers (such as stars) or tokens.
2. Puzzles, books.
3. Card games (this helps to develop interpersonal skills).
4. Workbooks: coloring (paint or crayon), "connect the numbers," or "paint by numbers."
5. Handcrafts: knitting, needlepoint (large canvas), cross-stitch, weaving, simple sewing (hand or machine), simple woodwork or leatherwork.
6. Special rewards (PWS individuals are usually very well groomed):
   brush and comb
   perfume or men's cologne
   bubble bath, bath oil, bath powder
   jewelery (bracelets, earrings, neck chains)
   fancy soaps
   makeup
   special shampoo
   towels and washcloths
   manicure sets
   small radio
7. Food items: sugarless gum, diet soda, cut-up vegetables (good for field trips).
8. Group events:
   movies
   bowling
   swimming
   roller skating
   salad bar lunch as a group with staff
   holiday party celebrations and planned picnics or camp-outs
9. Special events (PWS individuals like one-to-one interactions):
   shopping trip with a staff member
   manicure
   trip to beauty shop
   exclusive time with teacher/staff
   visit to home of staff
   extra visit with parents/family
   helping with pre-school, day care, or kindergarten activities

Appendix D: Activity Therapy Guidelines

Section 1: Annotated Bibliography of Evaluation Tools for Occupational Therapists

Evaluation

1. *Human Figure Drawing* (Florence L. Goodenough, Ph.D.). Assesses body scheme awareness in children ages 3–13.
2. *Developmental Test of Visual-Motor Integration (VMI)* (Keith E. Beery). A sequence of 24 geometric forms to be copied with pencil on paper and designed for use with students ages 3–15.
3. *The University of Kansas Fine Motor Evaluation*. An adapted instrument comprised of items selected from four standardized references, including manipulation skills in developmental sequence as well as many visual motor items and items that look at motor planning and bilateral integration. This test yields two scores, an age-equivalent score, and a score of functional level of accomplishment. Covers ages 0–72 months.
4. *Erhardt Developmental Prehension Assessment* (Rhoda Priest Erhardt). Measures prehension from the fetal and neonatal period to 15 months (which is considered the maturity level of prehension). Also measures pencil grasp and drawings for ages 1–6 years.
5. *Bruininks-Oseretsky Test of Motor Proficiency*. Fine motor component. Assesses these areas of fine motor function: 1) speed of response to a moving visual stimulus (untimed); 2) visual motor control (untimed); and 3) upper limb speed and dexterity (timed). Covers ages 4 years 11 months to 15 years 11 months. Cannot be used with children below the mild range of mental retardation.
6. *Motor Free Visual Perception Test (MVPT)*. A test of visual perception that avoids motor involvement. The five categories of visual perception assessed are visual discrimination, figure/ground, visual closure, visual memory, and spatial relationships. Covers ages 4 years to 8 years 11 months.
7. *Jebsen Test of Hand Function*. Consists of 7 subtests designed to be

representative of various hand activities and standardized for individuals ages 6–19 years.

8. *Clinical Observations* (A. Jean Ayres). A systematic nonstandardized assessment that looks at various components of sensorimotor development: muscle tone, kinesthesia, eye movements, balance and equilibrium, reflexes, motor planning, co-contractions (ability of the body to stabilize itself), and tremors.

RESOURCES

1. *Sensorimotor Integration for Developmentally Disabled Children: A Handbook*, Patricia Montgomery, M.A., R.P.T., and Eileen Richter, O.T.R. Western Psychological Services, 12031 Wilshire Boulevard, Los Angeles, California 90025.

Section 2: Sample Low-Impact Aerobic Activity Protocols for Individuals with Prader-Willi Syndrome[1]

Name:_____________ Date:_____________ Therapist:_____________

Routine low-impact aerobic exercise may contribute to weight loss in Prader-Willi syndrome (PWS) while improving general cardiovascular fitness. General fitness, including flexibility and strength, may also improve when low-impact aerobic conditioning program is performed regularly.

Aerobic conditioning is achieved by increasing the heart rate (HR) to an appropriate level for individuals with PWS 20 minutes every other day. The HR increases in response to exercise. The appropriate level of HR is called the *target heart rate*. The target heart rate is 85% of the maximum HR. The maximum HR is determined by subtracting the individual's age from 220.

Maximum HR is 220 – _____ = _____
10-second target HR is _____ = _____
Target HR is 85% of _____ = _____

Any aerobic conditioning program has three parts:

A. *Warm Up*: The warm up lasts 5 minutes. It should include two types of exercises:
   1. stretching activities appropriate to the aerobic exercise chosen to perform.
   2. exercise to gradually increase HR. This is usually the aerobic exercise performed at a slower rate.

B. *Aerobic Conditioning Exercise*: The aerobic exercise should last 20 minutes. Examples of exercises which will increase the HR to the target HR are: fast walking, stationary cycling, tricycle riding, swimming, and rowing with low resistance.

C. *Cool Down*: The cool down should last 5 minutes. This can be done using the same aerobic conditioning exercise, but at a lower intensity. Once the aerobic conditioning exercise is complete, keep moving and active, at the lower level, to allow the HR to recover and keep the blood from pooling in the arms and legs.

General Rules

1. Exercise before meals, not immediately after eating.
2. The HR should be taken immediately after the aerobic exercise phase and again 5 minutes after stopping. The HR should decline rapidly.
3. Occasionally take pulse first thing in the morning before getting out of

[1] Duesterhaus-Minor, M. (1984). University of Iowa Hospital School, Iowa City.

bed. This is called a resting heart rate. Over time, if aerobic fitness is improving, the resting heart rate will become lower.

4. The stretching exercises should help prevent injuries.
5. In the beginning it may not be possible to exercise at the target HR for 20 minutes. Gradually increase the amount of time every few days. However, keep exercising for the full 20 minutes, even if some of that is at less than target HR.
6. If there has been no exercise for a few days, reduce the level of intensity of exercise to below the level of last exercise day.
7. Do not exercise if a serious cold, flu, fever, or other illness is occurring. Wait until symptoms are gone before resuming activity.
8. Stop exercising for the day if nausea or faintness is noted. The next time, exercise at a slightly lower intensity.
9. In extreme temperatures (hot or cold) reduce the intensity of exercise.

Exercise Prescription

A. Type of aerobic exercise

_____ walking
_____ swimming
_____ stationary bike riding
_____ riding a tricycle
_____ rowing
_____ other:

B. Time

_____ as soon as home from school/work
_____ just before supper
_____ 1–2 hours after supper

C. Type of stretching

_____ hamstring
_____ gastrocnemius
_____ trunk rotators
_____ rectus femoris
_____ trunk extensors
_____ shoulder

Section 3: A Sensorimotor Program for Individuals with Prader-Willi Syndrome[2]

Purpose	Activity
Enhance tactile discrimination	*Carpet sample erase*—draw picture letter or numbers on carpet sample (or play tic-tac-toe) and have student erase with hands, feet, forearms.
Enhance tactile discrimination (good group game)	*Dried parts*—using towel or yarn ball, have child dry and name body parts.
Enhance tactile discrimination	*Inch Worm*—lying on side, have student move himself SLOWLY forward and back from one spot to another, like an inch-worm. Demonstration may be necessary.
Enhance tactile discrimination (good group game; may be adapted by having a student match the object to a picture)	*Feely-Meely*—the Feely-Meely box has a hole in the side large enough to put a hand in and remove objects. The objects are everyday items. Student reaches in, feels, names object, then brings it out. If wrong guess, object goes back in box.
Gross motor planning Bilateral motor integration	*Many Balls*—may be done in group or one-to-one. Seated on floor, child is given a utility ball that is held with both hands. Roll utility ball toward student, and student will return the ball by hitting it with the ball he or she is holding.
Reflex inhibition Bilateral motor integration Kinesthetic awareness	*Blast Off*—lying stomach down on scooter board, student places feet on wall and pushes off into a glide. He or she may need assistance with placing feet and bending knees (try it yourself to "get the idea") prior to pushing. A nice adaptation is to place a target to elicit stronger push and longer glide. It is also fun to suspend a beach or Nerf ball so the student can tag it as he or she glides past. Tag with one hand, both hands, or head.
Reflex inhibition Bilateral motor integration	*Surfing*—seated, kneeling or on stomach, lying on scooter board, student propels himself or herself simultaneously.

continued

[2]Adapted from Fink, B. (1977). *Sensory-motor integration—an activities curricula* (3rd ed.). Lowell, MI, published by the author.

Purpose	Activity
Reflex inhibition Motor planning Kinesthetic awareness	*Wheelbarrow*—using a utility ball, have student kneel over ball (4-point kneel) then "walk out" using hands (legs stay together). Ball will roll back as student moves forward. Try to get ball to ankles. Next step is to reverse the process ending in kneeling position.
Motor planning	*Obstacle Course*—stomach lying or kneeling on scooter board, student propels himself or herself through obstacle course.
Bilateral motor integration Postural adjustments Motor planning	*Body Ball*—seated on the floor, roll ball back and forth using both feet. Ask for other ideas of what body parts to use. If done in group, encourage naming the person to whom the ball is to be rolled.
Reflex inhibition	*Statue*—with student on all fours, place a beanbag or stuffed toy between right shoulder and chin. Student places right hand on hip. Student should "freeze" and hold object without dropping it while you attempt to gently push or pull student out of position. Do the same with left hand on hip. After strength is gained, downgrade items to be held (i.e., a potholder to sheet of paper)
Develop righting and equilibrium responses	*Rolling*—always roll both directions; roll with arms stretched over head (may need to hold scarf or length of rope). Encourage tucking chin down and flexing hips to initiate roll.
Encourage balance and motor planning Kinesthetic awareness	*Bean Bag Walk*—student knee-walks while balancing bean bag on head. It helps to give student a target to look at while walking (colored circle of tape on wall at eye level).
Motor planning Postural adjustments	*Stoop Tag*—tape "X"s on floor. One person is "it." He or she chases others, who must stop on X before being tagged. If tagged before stopping, that person becomes "it."
Motor planning Postural adjustments	*Kick Ball*—with a 12″ utility ball, student uses forward, backward, then sideways (to both sides) kick. Ask student to name the place or person he or she is going to kick to.
Bilateral coordination Motor planning	*Catch It*—make a catcher by cutting the bottom end out of a plastic Clorox bottle or milk carton and attach a ball on a string to it (the shorter the easier). The object is to catch the ball in the catcher with a catcher in each hand.

Section 4: Short Motor Program for Individuals with Prader-Willi Syndrome[3]

Equipment Needed: Gymnastics ball (or cage ball), scooter board, rope, two Indian clubs.
General Directions: Start with scooter board activities, then follow with ball activities. Instructor needs to try each activity before working with student.

Scooter Board Activities

1. Lie in prone position. Move to wall and push off with feet. Fly like a plane (arms outstretched).
2. Lie in prone position. Scooter stays in one spot on the floor. Student uses arms to rotate self in circle (helicopter). (Arms should cross midline and legs go out straight for good form.)
3. Sit on scooter. Teacher holds rope and student pulls hands to chest (avoid hand-over-hand patterns) moving in direction of teacher. (Teacher positions self in direct line and on either side of the student.)
4. Lie in prone position. Tie long rope to doorknob and have teacher hold free end. Have student pull self toward door, using rope and hand-over-hand pattern.
5. Lie in prone position. Move to wall and push off wall with feet (airplane). Have ball on floor several feet from wall and direct student to try to push ball with hand after "blast off."
6. Lie in prone position. Move to wall and push off with both feet. Student holds an Indian club in both hands and tries to hit ball thrown by teacher during "blast off."

Gymnastic Ball Activities

1. Lie in prone position with stomach on top of ball. Student places hands on ground and walks out using arms so knees move to top of ball and stomach is suspended in the air. Student continues walking to ankles so that knees and stomach are both suspended. Reverse procedure, so that student ends up back in prone position with stomach on top of ball.
2. Lie in prone position with stomach on top of ball. Student places hands on ground and uses legs to pull ball, so knees are positioned on top. Student then moves to balance on knees with arms out to sides like an airplane.
3. Sit on ball. Student extends legs to teacher (legs stiff). Teacher gets between student's calves and moves student to the right and left, while student shifts body weight to maintain balance.

---

[3] Carr, T. (1981). University of Iowa Hospital School, Iowa City.

4. Sit on ball. Place hands on floor. Keep hands stationary and rotate trunk around ball. Go from sitting position to stomach and back to sitting.

Small Ball Activities

1. Student on hands and knees. Teacher tosses ball and student attempts to use forehead to direct ball back to teacher.
2. Student on back with knees bent and legs in the air. Teacher tosses ball toward student and student extends legs and attempts to direct ball back to teacher.

Section 5: Sample Postural Control Exercises

These exercises have been adapted and sequenced for therapeutic purposes. It is recommended that they be demonstrated and monitored by a qualified occupational or physical therapist. Adults who carry out this program should be familiar with correct body alignment in order to avoid use of compensated postures and movement.

1

The Slide

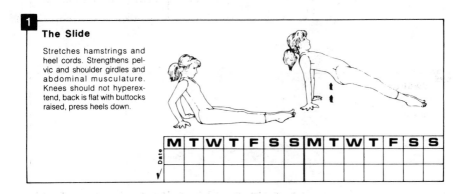

Stretches hamstrings and heel cords. Strengthens pelvic and shoulder girdles and abdominal musculature. Knees should not hyperextend, back is flat with buttocks raised, press heels down.

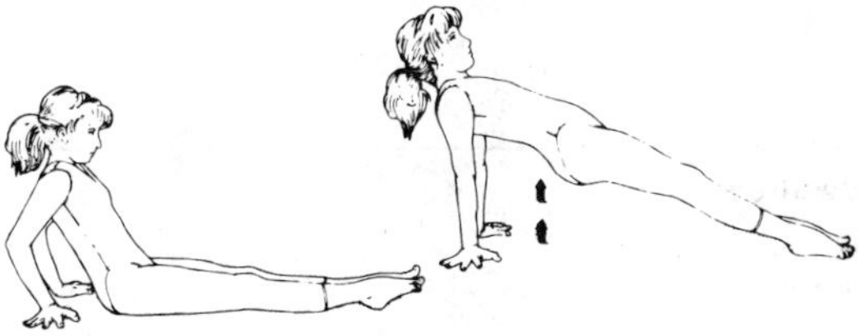

	M	T	W	T	F	S	S	M	T	W	T	F	S	S
Date														
√														

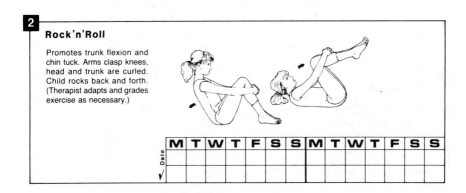

2

Rock'n'Roll

Promotes trunk flexion and chin tuck. Arms clasp knees, head and trunk are curled. Child rocks back and forth. (Therapist adapts and grades exercise as necessary.)

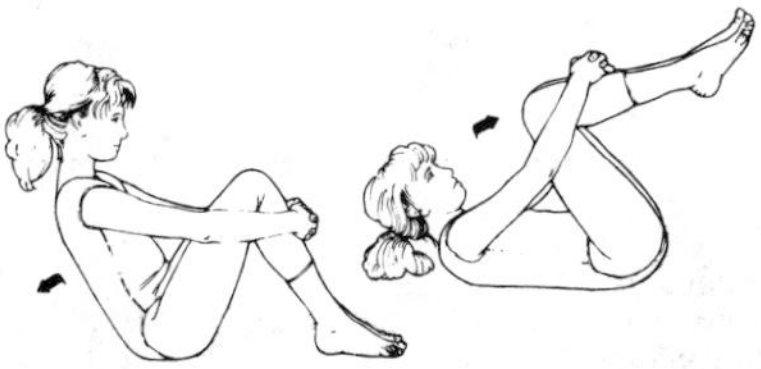

	M	T	W	T	F	S	S	M	T	W	T	F	S	S
Date														
√														

3

Side-Lying Leg Lift

Strengthens pelvic girdle musculature. Promotes co-contractions of trunk. Body is in side-lying position, legs are stacked vertically. Arm on bottom cushions head, arm on top is used for support. Leg lift is done in neutral (without hip flexion or extension.)

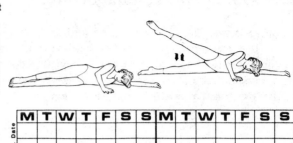

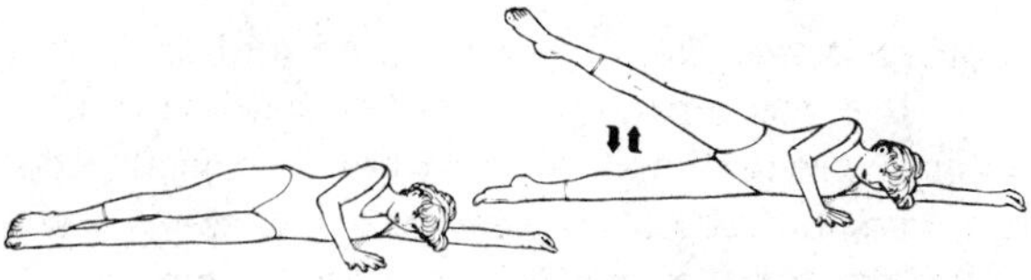

	M	T	W	T	F	S	S	M	T	W	T	F	S	S
Date														
✓														

4

Swallow

Stretches back and hip extensors.

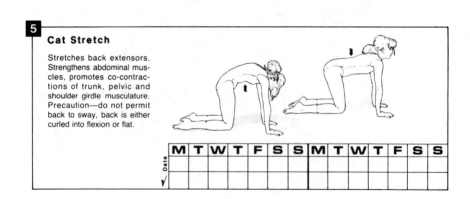

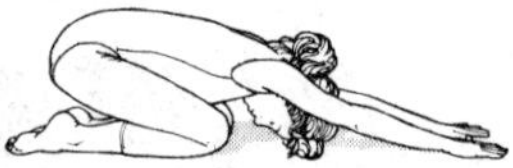

	M	T	W	T	F	S	S	M	T	W	T	F	S	S
Date														
✓														

5

Cat Stretch

Stretches back extensors. Strengthens abdominal muscles, promotes co-contractions of trunk, pelvic and shoulder girdle musculature. Precaution—do not permit back to sway, back is either curled into flexion or flat.

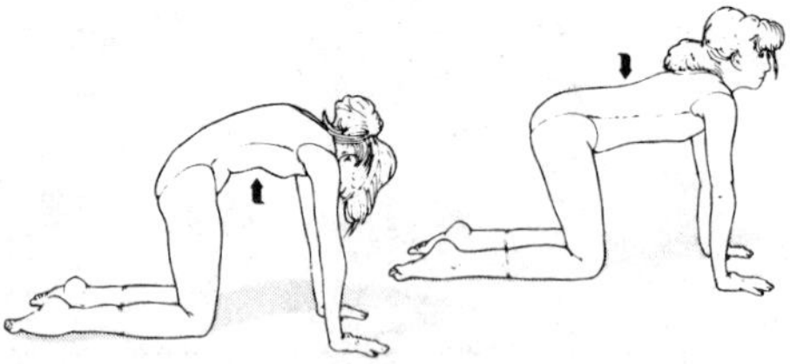

	M	T	W	T	F	S	S	M	T	W	T	F	S	S
Date														
✓														

6

Kneeling Leg Stretch

Gives total body stretch. Promotes co-contraction. Exercise begins on all fours. Curl one knee toward chest then extend the leg back. Extended leg should be at hip height. Hips should be level. Alternate right and left.

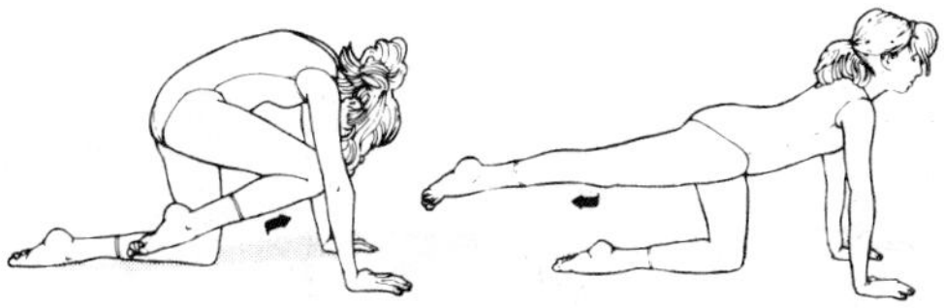

	M	T	W	T	F	S	S	M	T	W	T	F	S	S
Date														
✓														

7

Dog Stretch

Improves pelvic, trunk, and shoulder girdle stability. Chin is tucked, feet are flat on the floor, knees are straight, hands are in alignment with shoulders, elbows do not hyperextend.

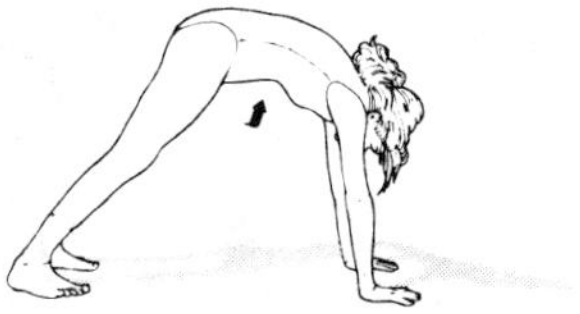

	M	T	W	T	F	S	S	M	T	W	T	F	S	S
Date														
✓														

Section 6: Sample Postural Tone Exercises[4]

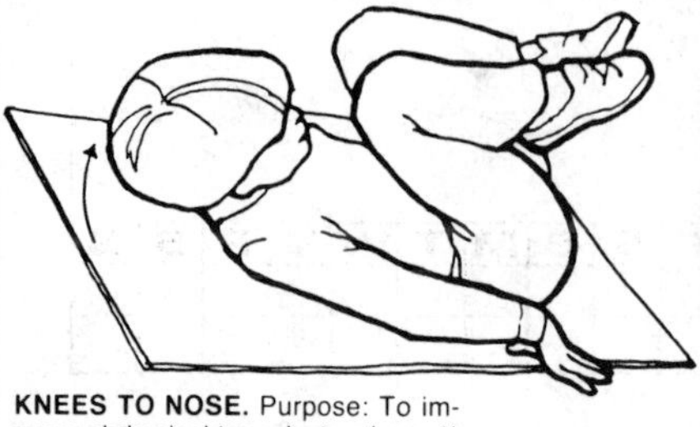

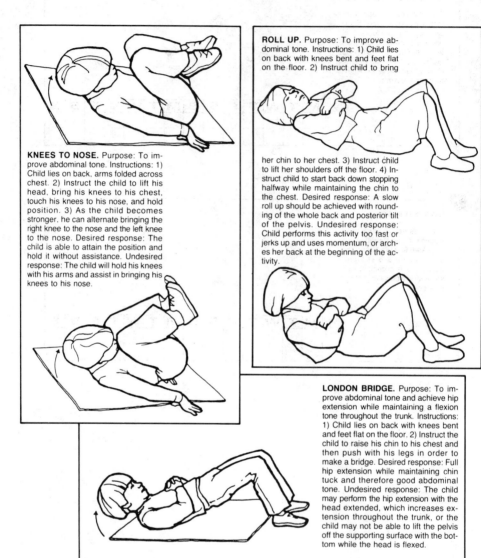

KNEES TO NOSE. Purpose: To improve abdominal tone. Instructions: 1) Child lies on back, arms folded across chest. 2) Instruct the child to lift his head, bring his knees to his chest, touch his knees to his nose, and hold position. 3) As the child becomes stronger, he can alternate bringing the right knee to the nose and the left knee to the nose. Desired response: The child is able to attain the position and hold it without assistance. Undesired response: The child will hold his knees with his arms and assist in bringing his knees to his nose.

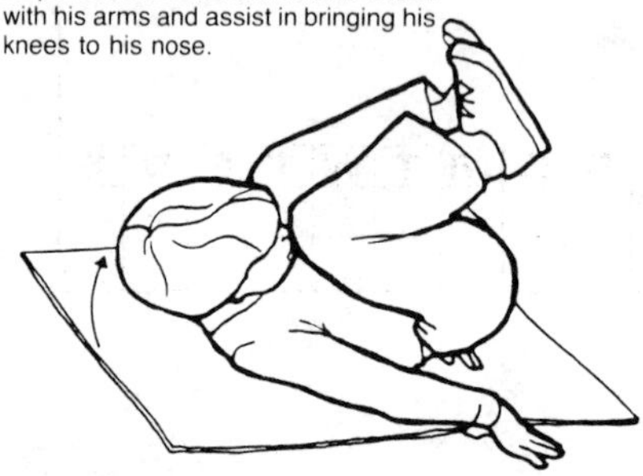

ROLL UP. Purpose: To improve abdominal tone. Instructions: 1) Child lies on back with knees bent and feet flat on the floor. 2) Instruct child to bring

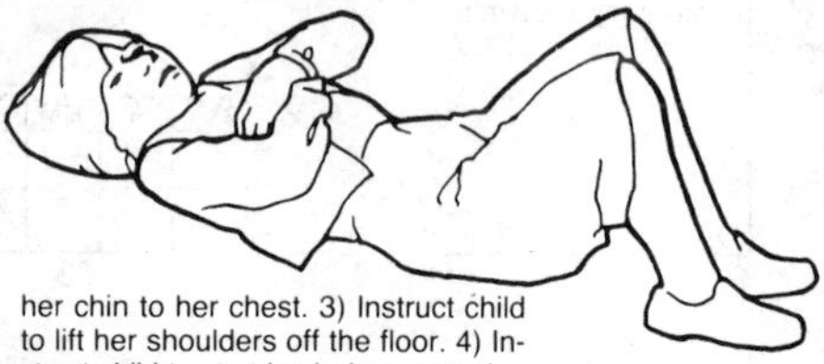

her chin to her chest. 3) Instruct child to lift her shoulders off the floor. 4) Instruct child to start back down stopping halfway while maintaining the chin to the chest. Desired response: A slow roll up should be achieved with rounding of the whole back and posterior tilt of the pelvis. Undesired response: Child performs this activity too fast or jerks up and uses momentum, or arches her back at the beginning of the activity.

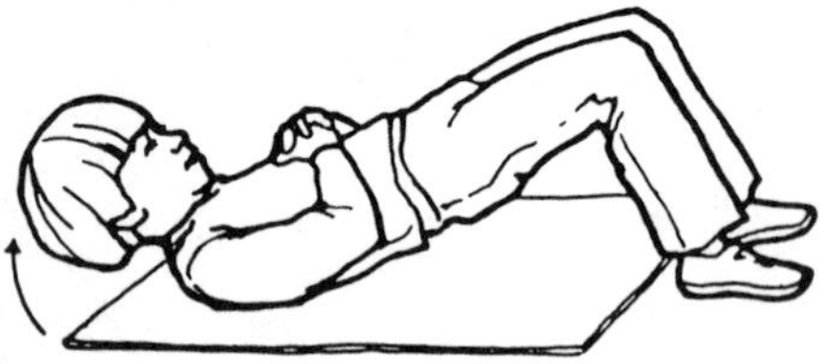

LONDON BRIDGE. Purpose: To improve abdominal tone and achieve hip extension while maintaining a flexion tone throughout the trunk. Instructions: 1) Child lies on back with knees bent and feet flat on the floor. 2) Instruct the child to raise his chin to his chest and then push with his legs in order to make a bridge. Desired response: Full hip extension while maintaining chin tuck and therefore good abdominal tone. Undesired response: The child may perform the hip extension with the head extended, which increases extension throughout the trunk, or the child may not be able to lift the pelvis off the supporting surface with the bottom while the head is flexed.

[4] Reprinted from Embrey, D., Endicott, J., Temple, G., & Jarger, D.L. (1983, Fall). Developing better postural tone in grade school children. *Clinical Management in Physical Therapy*, *3*, 6–10, by permission of the American Physical Therapy Association.

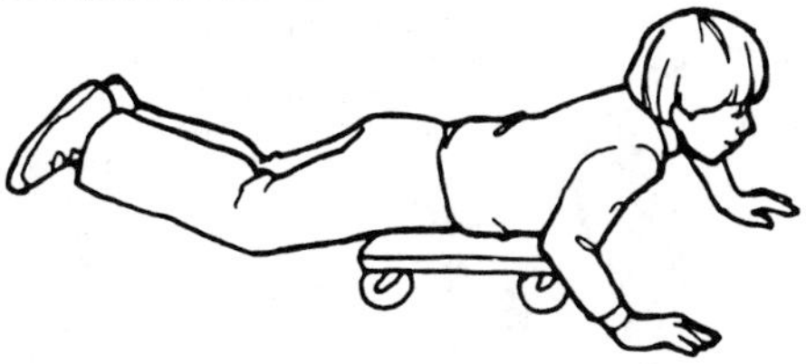

BACK-UP. Purpose: To improve shoulder stability. Instructions: 1) Child lies on stomach on a scooter board. 2) Instruct him to push with his hands on the floor to propel himself backwards while keeping his head up. Desired response: The child is able to keep the head and shoulders stable while pushing with the hands. Undesired response: The child is unable to keep the head up, or lacks the necessary shoulder stability or coordination to push backwards.

ROW YOUR BOAT. Purpose: To elongate the pectoral muscles. Instructions: 1) Two children sit erect in a ring-sitting position back to back. 2) Each pair holds a hula-hoop or dowel over their heads. 3) Instruct one child to move the hoop forward bringing the other child's arms into shoulder flexion while sitting erect. 4) Instruct the children to take turns moving the hoop. Desired response: The child whose arms are being pulled into flexion should keep the arms straight, and the pectoralis major and minor muscles should be elongated. Undesired response: The children may lean forward and backward rather than elongating the pectoral muscles.

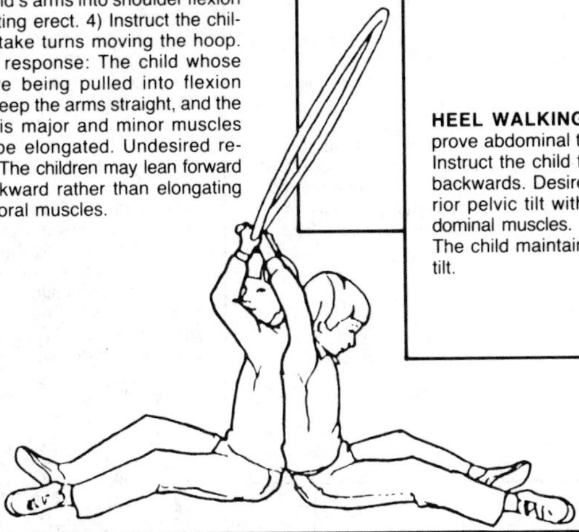

HEEL WALKING. Purpose: To improve abdominal tone. Instructions: 1) Instruct the child to walk on his heels backwards. Desired response: Posterior pelvic tilt with contraction of abdominal muscles. Undesired response: The child maintains an anterior pelvic tilt.

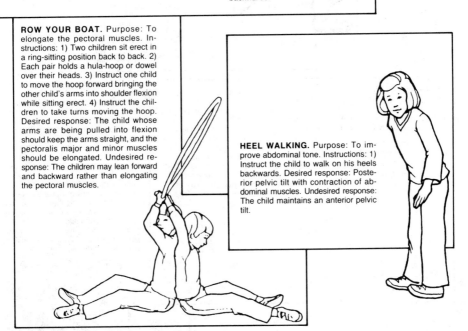

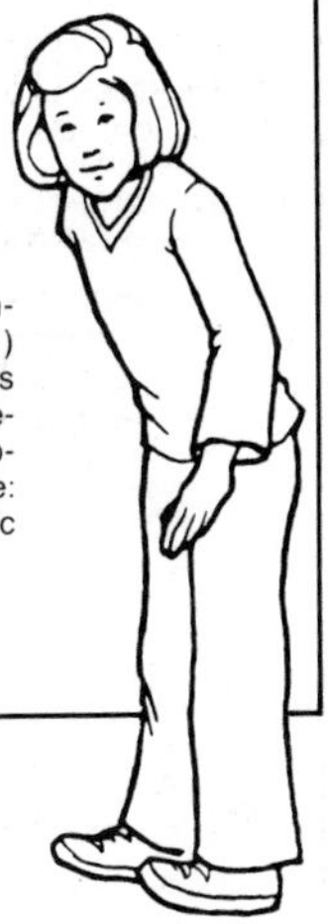

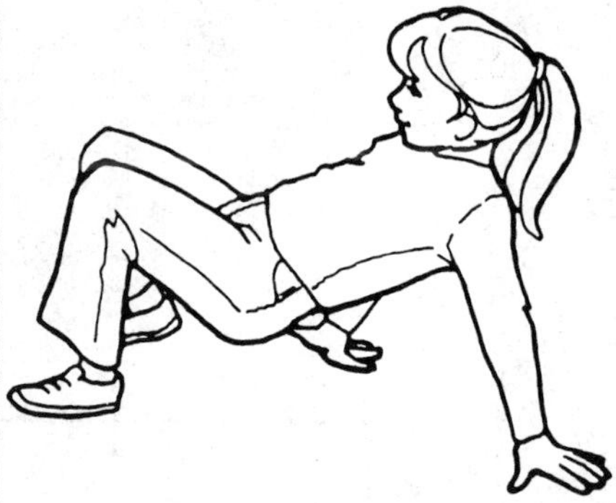

CRAB WALKING. Purpose: To improve shoulder stability and abdominal tone, and elongate the pectoral muscles. Instructions: 1) Child sits on the floor leaning back on her hands with feet flat on the floor. 2) Instruct the child to raise her bottom off the floor while her hands and feet maintain contact with the floor. 3) Instruct the child to walk backwards with the hands leading. 4) Instruct the child to walk forward with the feet leading. Desired response: The child is able to extend the shoulders sufficiently to get the pelvis off the floor and to walk in an all-fours position with only the hands and feet touching the support. Undesired response: The child drags her bottom or scoots on her bottom rather than walking with her hands and feet.

FEET OVER HEAD. Purpose: To improve abdominal tone. Instructions: 1) Child lies on back. 2) Instruct the child to bend his knees, lift his feet over his head, and touch his toes to the floor. 3) As the child returns to the starting position, instruct him to bend his knees as he slowly lowers his feet, keeping the lumbar spine flat on the floor. Desired response: The child should contract the abdominal muscles as the hips are lifted and as the feet are brought back down. Undesired response: The child may attempt to keep his knees straight and bring feet over his head without lifting the hips, or the child may arch the back as the legs are lowered.

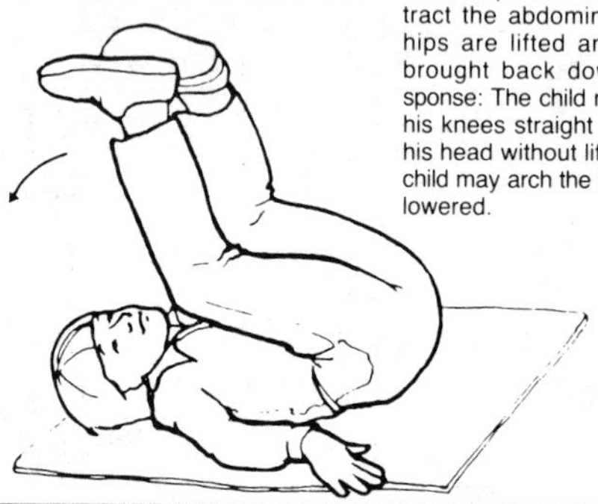

KING ON ONE KNEE. Purpose: To improve abdominal tone and balance reactions. Instructions: 1) Two children kneel facing each other, approximately two feet apart. 2) Instruct each child to raise the right knee so he is half-kneeling with the right foot forward. 3) Instruct the children to "shake hands" and try to pull each other off balance. 4) Change to the opposite foot and hand. Desired response: Children will stabilize the pelvis by bringing one leg up and maintaining a posterior pelvic tilt. This should improve balance reactions and abdominal tone. Undesired response: The children will arch the back rather than maintain a posterior pelvic tilt. Note: This activity should be done on a gymnastic mat.

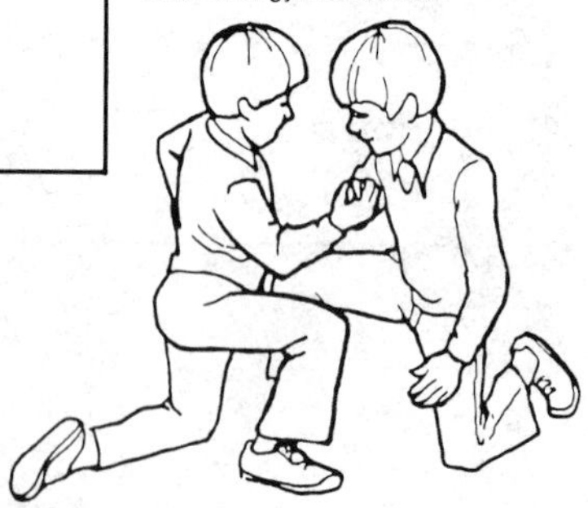

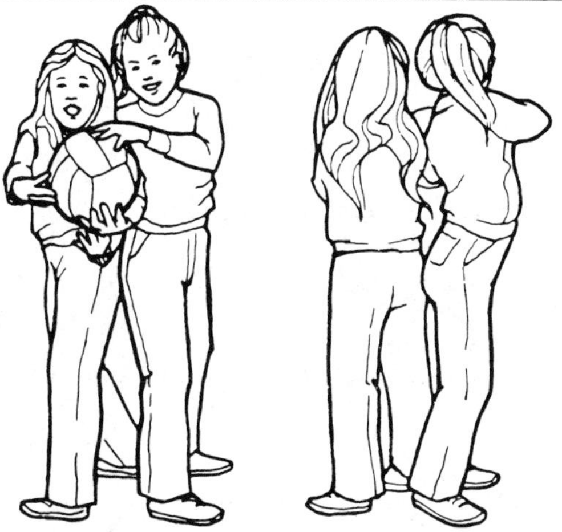

BACK-TO-BACK BALL PASS. Purpose: To improve tone of trunk musculature and range of trunk rotation. Instructions: 1) Two children stand back to back. 2) Give a ball to one child and instruct her to hand it to her partner who must then hand it back on the other side so the ball will go around in a circle. 3) Instruct the children to keep their feet stationary as they perform this activity. Desired response: The children should rotate the trunk Undesired response: Children move their feet in order to pass the ball. They lean backwards as they turn.

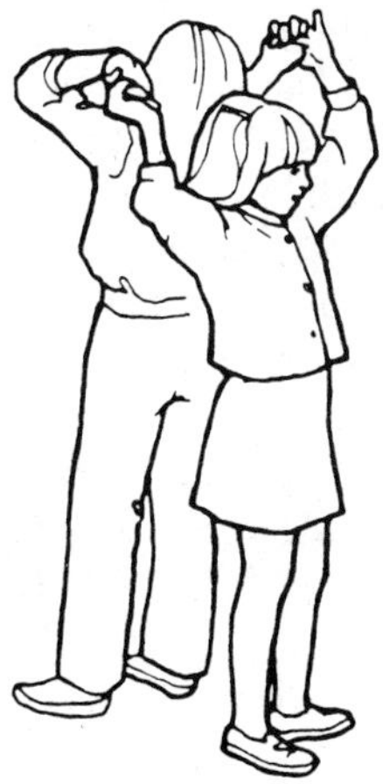

WASHING MACHINE. Purpose: To elongate the pectoral muscles. Instructions: 1) Two children face each other, holding both hands. 2) Instruct the children to turn their hands together so arms elevate as they turn. 3) Instruct the children to continue the movement until they are facing each other again. Desired response: Both children will elongate their pectoral muscles while holding hands. Undesired response: The children will not elevate their arms while they do this activity and thus will not elongate the pectoral muscles.

Section 7: Sample Occupational Therapy Evaluation and Recommendations

NAME:
B.D.:
DATE:
C.A.

CURRENT OCCUPATIONAL THERAPY EVALUATION AND RESULTS:

Feeding: Independent at age level
Undressing/Dressing: Cooperative at the 3-year level
Hand/Upper Extremity Function: Significantly delayed secondary to overall developmental delay
Adaptions/Equipment: Milwaukee brace—23 hours/day

____ was accompanied by her parents and younger sister. Tests given today were the Kansas University Fine Motor Evaluation (KUFM), the Beery Developmental Test of Visual-Motor Integration, and the Draw-a-Person. The KUFM is an adapted instrument comprised of items selected from four standardized references and including manipulation skills in a developmental sequence, as well as many visual-motor items and some items that look at motor planning and bilateral integration. This test yields a functional level of accomplishment in fine motor development that covers ages 0–72 months. ____'s age equivalent score on the KUFM was 18 1/4 months with emerging skills at 20 1/4 months. The items with which she had best results were form boards and bilateral manipulation skills. She began to experience difficulty with items that required dynamic control of the shoulder and arm and good hand stability, as well as those that required depth perception, motor planning, and perceptual acuity. The Draw-a-Person is a normed assessment that looks at the individual's awareness of body scheme. ____'s age-equivalent score on this test was 2 years. The Developmental Test of Visual-Motor Integration is a sequence of geometric forms to be copied with pencil and paper and was designed for use with students from preschool through junior high. Her age-equivalent score was below 2 years, 11 months.

By observation, ____ displays low postural tone with deficits in co-contractions (ability of the body to stabilize itself) and with antigravity holding positions. A slight tremor was observed during testing, and overflow movement was present during mild resistive activities. Grasp and release patterns used in manipulation activities at the 1 to 1 1/2 year level were good, with smooth release patterns and precise opposition being used functionally. Fingers are hypermobile, and ____ has a wavering approach to pick up or place an object that she is correcting with no difficulty or frustration at this point. Shoulder patterns are moderately immature, with excessive abduction being used to accomplish tasks. ____ has not established laterality at this point and does not have good bilateral assist when using either hand as the prime mover. For prewriting skills her pencil grasp is immature but appropriate for her developmental level (1–2 years), with the pencil being held primarily in the hand and occasionally shifting from a static tripod to a pronated grasp.

____ is able to remove and put on socks and shoes and to assist with clothing for toileting as well as to remove most clothing. Behavior during testing was cooperative and pleasant. Although she demonstrates a short attention span, ____ has a good task persistence for activities in which she is interested. She enjoys movement-based activities and follows directions well.

IMPRESSIONS: ____ has a number of subtle fine motor problems that are influencing hand/upper extremity function. In addition, she has significant perceptual deficits, including difficulties with depth perception and spatial relationships. With low postural tone and deficits in co-contractions, ____ lacks the trunk, shoulder, and head stability to form a solid physical base for moving into fine motor proficiency and dexterity. Optimal seating and appropriate level of work surface will be important in helping ____ compensate for low muscle tone and poor proximal stability.

ACTIONS TAKEN: Evaluation results and recommendations were discussed with ____'s parent. They were given a copy of *Sensorimotor Integration for Developmentally Disabled Children: A Handbook* by Patricia Montgomery, M.A., R.P.T., and Eileen Richter, O.T.R., to review for ideas for movement-based activities that they could incorporate into playtime at home.

RECOMMENDATIONS:

1. A program of movement-based activities that includes rolling, crawling, and pushing objects with weight would be good for helping ____ to develop proximal stability. These activities would also work on the areas of bilateral integration and improved motor planning (ability to organize movement).
2. Resistive activities are appropriate for improving co-contractions and joint stability. Some examples are pushing a grocery cart or a doll buggy with weight added, carrying a milk carton in from shopping, putting away canned goods, working with Play Dough.
3. Continue excellent programming at home with the "heavy work" activities that you have been providing, which include supervised climbing and swinging on playground equipment and a swim program.

4. Incorporate activities with a tactile base whenever possible to provide additional touch cues for position of hands and arms in space (examples are Play Dough, cornstarch play, fingerpaint, sand and water play).
5. Provide bilateral activities such as pushing a large ball from a seated or kneeling position, pushing a large ball with both feet from a seated position, stacking large cardboard boxes, pouring water or sand from one container to another, helping mix cookie dough.
6. Continue current excellent school program, with occupational therapist consulting to the classroom teacher regarding positioning and giving recommendations for activities that could be adapted to meet ____'s current developmental level.

____________________________ ____________________

Occupational Therapist/O.T.R./L Date

Appendix E: Vocational Training Sample Task Performance Checklists[1]

These task performance checklists are examples of task breakdowns that a Prader-Willi syndrome individual would likely be able to manage. Further breakdown in components may be needed. In some cases, focusing on just one subtask may be required.

Gardening/Outdoor Maintenance Checklist

Fertilizes plants correctly and safely:

1. Identifies need for feeding/fertilizing
2. Demonstrates proper procedure for application of fertilizer using whirly-bird type applicator
3. Demonstrates proper procedure for application of fertilizer using hose sprayer
4. Demonstrates proper procedure for application of fertilizer using spray tank
5. Follows safety precautions involved with agricultural chemicals

Plants/cultivates correctly:

1. Prepares soil properly prior to planting
2. Digs hole of proper depth
3. Places plant into hole
4. Packs dirt to proper consistency around plant
5. Uses hand shovel and cultivator properly around base of flowers, shrubs, trees, to afford better water intake

[1] From Copus, E. (1980). *The Melwood manual.* Menomonie, WI: The University of Wisconsin–Stout, Materials Development Center. Reprinted by permission.

Prunes, shapes, weeds correctly:

1. Identifies need for pruning/shaping
2. Demonstrates proper technique for pruning/shaping common flowers, trees, shrubs (roses, fuchsias, junipers, etc.)
3. Uses cutting tools safely
4. Identifies most common local weeds
5. Weeds area carefully
6. Discriminates between weeds which must be dug with tool (large root or stickers) or hand-pulled

Cleans up yard and gardening tools:

1. Determines need to sweep sidewalk, driveway, etc.
2. Selects proper broom for use
3. Sweeps sidewalk, walkway, driveway
4. Identifies properly swept sidewalk, walkway, etc.
5. Uses hose, if necessary, to wash away lawn clippings
6. Washes and wipes hand tools
7. Changes mower spark plugs monthly
8. Changes oil on mower monthly

Rakes lawn correctly:

1. Determines need to rake
2. Rakes lawn entirely free of debris
3. Removes and disposes of debris

Uses/maintains power mower correctly:

1. Determines need to mow lawn
2. Adjusts cutting height of mower properly
3. Checks gas in mower
4. Fills mower with gas
5. Checks oil in mower
6. Changes oil monthly
7. Transports mower to cutting area
8. Starts mower
9. Cuts lawn in straight line whenever possible, without missing spots
10. Recognizes completion of properly mown lawn
11. Shuts off mower
12. Follows safety procedures in use of lawn mower

Waters yard correctly:

1. Determines location to outside faucet
2. Attaches hose to outside faucet
3. Waters lawn correctly
4. Waters flowers correctly

5. Waters vegetables correctly
6. Waters trees/shrubs correctly
7. Identifies root feeder
8. Demonstrates proper use of root feeder
9. Demonstrates proper use of aerator

Identifies and demonstrates proper use/care of gardening tools:

1. Identifies and demonstrates proper use of rotary mower
2. Identifies and demonstrates proper use of gas can
3. Identifies and demonstrates proper use of spading fork
4. Identifies and demonstrates proper use of spade or shovel
5. Identifies and demonstrates proper use of hand shovel
6. Identifies and demonstrates proper use of Swedish tree saw
7. Identifies and demonstrates proper use of clippers
8. Identifies and demonstrates proper use of hoe
9. Identifies and demonstrates proper use of lawn edger
10. Identifies and demonstrates proper use of topping shears
11. Identifies and demonstrates proper use of pruning shears
12. Identifies and demonstrates proper use of broadcaster
13. Identifies and demonstrates proper use of hedge trimmer
14. Identifies and demonstrates proper use of spray atomizer
15. Identifies and demonstrates proper use of dustpan
16. Identifies and demonstrates proper use of cultivator
17. Identifies and demonstrates proper use of lawn rake
18. Identifies and demonstrates proper use of yard rake
19. Identifies and demonstrates proper use of pole pruner
20. Identifies and demonstrates proper use of mattock
21. Identifies and demonstrates proper use of wheelbarrow
22. Identifies and demonstrates proper use of soil test kit
23. Identifies and demonstrates proper use of folding tree saw
24. Identifies and demonstrates proper use of spray tank
25. Knows where tools are kept
26. Places tools in proper storage area
27. Discriminates between dull and sharp tools
28. Sharpens tools safely

Carpentry Procedures Checklist

Follows correct carpentry procedures:

1. Drives nail
2. Pulls nail
3. Identifies and demonstrates proper use of sandpaper
4. Sands with grain of wood

5. Uses correct grade of sandpaper for each job
6. Identifies need to replace sandpaper
7. Recognizes acceptably completed sanding procedure
8. Waxes wood following proper procedure
9. Stains items
10. Uses proper steps when gluing items
11. Returns items to proper storage place

Uses ladder correctly and safely:

1. Identifies and demonstrates proper use of ladder
2. Stores ladder correctly
3. Lifts ladder correctly

Identifies and demonstrates proper use of hand tools:

1. Identifies and demonstrates proper use of hammer
2. Returns hammer to proper storage place
3. Identifies and demonstrates proper use of saw
4. Returns saw to proper storage place
5. Identifies and demonstrates proper use of measure
6. Returns measure to proper storage place
7. Identifies and demonstrates proper use of screwdriver
8. Returns screwdriver to proper storage place
9. Identifies and demonstrates proper use of plane
10. Returns plane to proper storage place
11. Identifies and demonstrates proper use of pliers
12. Returns pliers to proper storage place
13. Identifies and demonstrates proper use of clamp
14. Returns clamp to proper storage place
15. Identifies and demonstrates proper use of vise
16. Returns vise to proper storage place
17. Identifies and demonstrates proper use of chisel
18. Returns chisel to proper storage place
19. Identifies and demonstrates proper use of file
20. Returns file to proper storage place

Uses power saw correctly and safely:

1. Verbalizes safety procedure for power saw
2. Identifies and demonstrates proper use of power saw under supervision
3. Feeds material to be sawed
4. Sets material to be sawed at desired point
5. Saws material accurately
6. Sets power saw to make special cut (i.e., halfway cut)
7. Identifies and demonstrates proper use of power saw independently
8. Disconnects plug when job is completed
9. Cleans area

Uses hand drill correctly and safely:

1. Identifies and demonstrates proper use of hand drill with supervision
2. Verbalizes safety procedure for using drill
3. Uses drill safely
4. Uses correct size drill bit for specific job
5. Changes drill bit
6. Recognizes dull drill bit
7. Drills to specific depth
8. Identifies and demonstrates proper use of hand drill independently
9. Stores drill properly

Uses drill press correctly and safely:

1. Follows safety measures for drill press
2. Loads material
3. Unloads material
4. Checks power switches and plugs in cord
5. Properly sets drill and table
6. Identifies and demonstrates proper use of jigs
7. Knows how to set a jig properly
8. Knows speed for separate drilling
9. Can adjust machine to separate speeds
10. Can identify drill bit
11. Uses correct size drill bit for specific job
12. Recognizes dull drill bit

Appendix F: Social Skills Training[1]

Section 1: Social Skills Training for Staff—Agenda for Format I, Session 1

I. Introduction/Agenda: Have each person give his or her name, duties, and describe the client with whom he or she feels most engaged
II. Pretest
III. Give Out Staff Questionnaires
IV. Definitions and Techniques
   A. Social skills
   B. Modeling
   C. Role playing
   D. Coaching
   E. Labeling
   F. Relaxation
V. Some Basic Concepts
   A. Mature/immature dichotomy
   B. Assertive/aggressive/passive behavior
VI. Body Language—Introduction
   A. Demonstration
   B. 80% of communication is nonverbal
VII. Planning Next Steps: Look at curricula

---

[1] Mitchell, W., & Cook, K. (1987). The Developmental Evaluation Clinic, Children's Hospital, Boston.

Section 2: Format I, Session 2

I. Go Over Agenda
II. Collect Staff Questionnaires
III. Individual Prioritizing of Goals
IV. Discussion
  A. Past week
  B. Ideas about training
  C. Review:
    1. Concepts and definitions from definitions from last week
    2. Other materials:
      a. Duso
      b. Transitions
      c. TAD (Towards Affective Development)
      d. Social Skills Training for Elementary Age Children
V. Group Prioritizing of Goals
VI. Body Language
  A. Facial expressions: video and discussions
  B. Voice and speech (volume, tone, speed): discussion
  C. Mannerisms (nervous/calm)
    1. Videotape model
    2. Model with successive approximations:
      a. Give situation to volunteers
      b. Have them demonstrate it
      c. Have group give feedback
      d. Redo demonstration
      e. Give praise for performance (specific positive feedback)
  D. Appropriate distance (arms length away)
    1. Model (live)
    2. Model with successive approximations:
      a. Give situation to volunteers
      b. Have them demonstrate it
      c. Have group give feedback
      d. Redo demonstration
      e. Give praise (specific positive feedback)
  E. Wrap up body language
    1. Set goals
    2. Discuss barriers to goals
    3. Brainstorm ways to meet goals
    4. Decide on client activities

Section 3: Format I, Session 3

I. Agenda
II. Discussion
   1. Past week
   2. Review priorities (conversational skills, inappropriate behaviors, assertiveness)
III. Review Body Language
   1. Pictures for transitions
   2. Timing game
IV. Conversational Skills
   1. Introduce *UNGAME®*
   2. Initiating conversation
      a. Joining (videotape)
      b. Joining exercise
      c. Open vs. closed questions (game)
V. Plans for Next Week

Section 4: Format I, Session 4

I. Present ABC Principles: Discuss past week in light of these principles.

II. Review of Goals from Last Session

   A. *UNGAME®*

   B. Timing, open/closed games

   C. Ending conversations

IV. Relaxation Tape

V. Sandwich Technique (© Arlyn Roffman):

VI. Plans for Next Week

Section 5: Ranking of Training Priorities

Rank the following skills in order of importance, within each category. Which one is highest training priority with this population? Give this a rank of 1. Please rank all skills in each category, from 1 to number of skills.

I. Conversational Skills. Staff should teach clients to:
_____ Initiate conversation appropriately.
_____ Maintain conversation appropriately.
_____ Express interest in other person.
_____ Express liking for others appropriately.
_____ Take turns in conversation.
_____ Listen to others.
_____ Terminate conversation appropriately.
_____ Look at the person who is talking.

II. Nonverbal Skills. Staff should teach clients to:
_____ Maintain appropriate distance.
_____ Maintain appropriate eye contact.
_____ Keep facial expressions congruent with affect or mood.

III. Assertiveness. Staff should teach clients to:
_____ Refuse requests appropriately.
_____ Make requests from others.
_____ Express annoyance and irritation appropriately.
_____ Give criticism constructively.

IV. Inappropriate Behavior of Clients. Staff should:
_____ Reduce frequency of emotional outbursts.
_____ Reduce incidents of physical assaultiveness.
_____ Reduce incidents of verbal assaultiveness.
_____ Reduce frequency of stealing or damage to another's property.
_____ Reduce food stealing
_____ Reduce noncompliance.
_____ Reduce frequency of stereotypes.

Section 6: Rating of Client Social Skill Deficits

Client Name ______________________________
Age ____
Sex ____
Weight _____ Height _____
Length of Time in Program __________
Functional Level (if known) __________

I. Below are listed some common social skills. Circle the number you think best describes this client's skills.

	Always inappropriate	Usually inappropriate	Somewhat inappropriate	More appropriate than inappropriate	Usually appropriate	Always appropriate
Conversation Skills						
1. Initiates conversation appropriately:						
with peers	1	2	3	4	5	6
with staff	1	2	3	4	5	6
2. Maintains conversation appropriately:						
with peers	1	2	3	4	5	6
with staff	1	2	3	4	5	6
3. Expresses interest in the other person (ask questions) appropriately:						
with peers	1	2	3	4	5	6
with staff	1	2	3	4	5	6
4. Expresses liking another person appropriately:						
with peers	1	2	3	4	5	6
with staff	1	2	3	4	5	6
5. Takes turns in conversation appropriately:						
with peers	1	2	3	4	5	6
with staff	1	2	3	4	5	6
6. Listens to others appropriately:						
with peers	1	2	3	4	5	6
with staff	1	2	3	4	5	6
7. Terminates conversation appropriately:						
with peers	1	2	3	4	5	6
with staff	1	2	3	4	5	6
8. Looks at the person who is talking:						
with peers	1	2	3	4	5	6
with staff	1	2	3	4	5	6

I. *Continued*

	Always inappro-priate	Usually inappro-priate	Somewhat inappro-priate	More appropriate than inappropriate	Usually appro-priate	Always appro-priate
"Body language" or nonverbal skills						
1. Maintains appropriate distance:						
with peers	1	2	3	4	5	6
with staff	1	2	3	4	5	6
2. Maintains appropriate eye contact:						
with peers	1	2	3	4	5	6
with staff	1	2	3	4	5	6
3. Keeps facial expressions congruent with affect or mood (e.g., smiles when pleased or happy; frowns when unhappy):						
with peers	1	2	3	4	5	6
with staff	1	2	3	4	5	6
Assertiveness						
1. Refuses requests appropriately:						
with peers	1	2	3	4	5	6
with staff	1	2	3	4	5	6
2. Makes requests from others appropriately:						
with peers	1	2	3	4	5	6
with staff	1	2	3	4	5	6
3. Expresses annoyance and irritation appropriately (assertively, not agressively):						
with peers	1	2	3	4	5	6
with staff	1	2	3	4	5	6
4. Gives criticism constructively:						
with peers	1	2	3	4	5	6
with staff	1	2	3	4	5	6

II. Below are listed some inappropriate behaviors. Circle the number you think best describes this client's characteristics.

1. Emotional outbursts (e.g., "tantrums")							
a. Frequency	1/mo	1–2/mo	1/wk	3/wk	1/day	2–4/day	>4/day
	1	2	3	4	5	6	7
b. Duration	1–5 mins	5–10 mins	10–15 mins	15–30 mins	30–60 mins	1–2 hrs	>2 hrs
	1	2	3	4	5	6	7
c. Intensity	Extremely mild intensity						Extremely intense
	1	2	3	4	5	6	7
2. Physical assaultiveness							
a. Frequency	1/mo	1–2/mo	1/wk	3/wk	1/day	2–4/day	>4/day
	1	2	3	4	5	6	7
b. Duration	1–5 mins	5–10 mins	10–15 mins	15–30 mins	30–60 mins	1–2 hrs	>2 hrs
	1	2	3	4	5	6	7
c. Intensity	Extremely mild intensity						Extremely intense
	1	2	3	4	5	6	7
3. Verbal assaultiveness							
a. Frequency	1/mo	1–2/mo	1/wk	3/wk	1/day	2–4/day	>4/day
	1	2	3	4	5	6	7
b. Duration	1–5 mins	5–10 mins	10–15 mins	15–30 mins	30–60 mins	1–2 hrs	>2 hrs
	1	2	3	4	5	6	7
c. Intensity	Extremely mild intensity						Extremely intense
	1	2	3	4	5	6	7
4. Taking possessions belonging to others: frequency	1/mo	1–2/mo	1/wk	3/wk	1/day	2–4/day	>4/day
	1	2	3	4	5	6	7
5. Taking food inappropriately (foraging, stealing, etc.): frequency	1/mo	1–2/mo	1/wk	3/wk	1/day	2–4/day	>4/day
	1	2	3	4	5	6	7
6. Noncompliance: frequency	1/mo	1–2/mo	1/wk	3/wk	1/day	2–4/day	>4/day
	1	2	3	4	5	6	7
7. Stereotypies (e.g., jiggling legs, biting nails, pulling hair, picking skin): frequency	1/mo	1–2/mo	1/wk	3/wk	1/day	2–4/day	>4/day
	1	2	3	4	5	6	7

Section 7: Prader-Willi Syndrome Social Skills Training Program/Staff Questionnaire

Name ____________________

Date ____________________

We would like to help you in your work with Prader-Willi clients, but we need your help. Please answer the following questions and give us any other information you think helpful. Thank you!

I. Background

1. Your job title ____________________
   Brief description of duties ____________________
   ____
2. How many hours a week are you in your present job? ____ hours.
   How many hours a week do you work with Prader-Willi clients? ____ hours.
3. How long have you been in your present job? ____ years ____ months.
   How long have you worked with Prader-Willi clients? ____ years ____ months.
   How long have you worked with other MR clients? ____ years ____ months.
4. In your work with Prader-Willi clients,
   What do you find most rewarding? ____________________
   ____
   What do you find most frustrating? ____________________
   ____
5. What is your highest degree? Degree: ____ Date: ____
   School: __________ Other degrees (if any): __________

II. In-service training

1. Have you participated in any in-service training in the last 2 years?
   ____ Yes ____ No If yes, topic(s): ____________________
   ____
2. Have you participated in a social skills training program before?
   ____ Yes ____ No If yes, briefly describe: ____________________
   ____
3. Have you participated in a training program for Prader-Willi clients?
   ____ Yes ____ No If yes, briefly describe: ____________________
   ____
4. What would you like to know about Prader-Willi syndrome?
   ____ a. Better description of disorder
   ____ b. Better understanding of behavior management
   ____ c. Other techniques for working with clients
5. Any other comments: ____________________
   ____

Section 8: Social Skills Training Curriculum Test

Name ______________________________

I. Basic Social Skills

1. Briefly define the terms:
   a. social skills
   b. modeling
   c. role-playing

In the following two questions, mark the appropriate point on the continuum.

2. In conversation, good eye contact consists of looking at the speaker:

   Never Rarely Some of the time Most of the time Always

   |——|————|——————|————|

3. Nonverbal communication should be consistent with words:

   Never Rarely Some of the time Most of the time Always

   |——|————|——————|————|

For the following three questions, write the letter of the phrase that best completes the statement in the blank to the left of the number.

_____ 4. When giving criticism, it is helpful to begin by:
  (a) telling the other person what's bothering you.
  (b) telling them how it makes you feel.
  (c) giving a positive statement.
  (d) giving guidelines for change.

_____ 5. When initiating conversation with someone you do not know, it is helpful to:
  (a) tell them something about yourself.
  (b) ask a question about them.
  (c) ask them a question about sports.
  (d) tell them something that you will be doing later today.

_____ 6. When receiving criticism, it is helpful to:
  (a) paraphrase the criticism.
  (b) tell them how you feel.
  (c) make an excuse.
  (d) say nothing.

II. Techniques: Fill in the blank before each training context with the appropriate technique or techniques to use in that context. You may not need to use each technique.

Key to social skills training techniques:

Modeling (MO)

Role play (RP)
Labeling (LA)
Coaching (CO)
Timing (TI)
Biofeedback (BI)
Relaxation (RE)

_____ 1. The person needs to know when a skill is appropriate.
_____ 2. The person needs to become aware of the emotions behind an acton.
_____ 3. The person needs to practice a new skill.
_____ 4. The person has a high level of anxiety in social situations.
_____ 5. The person has not learned the skill.
_____ 6. The person's skill needs refining.

III. Assertiveness: In the two sections below, fill in the blanks with the appropriate term:

Key to Behaviors:
Assertive (AS)
Aggressive (AG)
Passive (PA)

A. Behaviors
_____ 1. Uses apologetic tone of voice.
_____ 2. Expresses own needs.
_____ 3. Makes "I" statements.
_____ 4. Bossy.
_____ 5. Talks seldom and quietly.
_____ 6. Makes too much eye contact.

B. Situations.
_____ 1. You'd like to take a break from work. You say to your boss, "Do you think, uh, by any chance, you might give me a break?"
_____ 2. Someone you work with interrupts you whenever you try to talk with her. You say, "Stop interrupting me."
_____ 3. At dinner, someone grabs a roll off your plate. You say, "Keep your hands off my food."
_____ 4. A friend borrows your shoes and does not return them. The next time this friend asks to use your clothes, you say, "Gee, it's my favorite shirt, but ok."
_____ 5. A coworker keeps asking you out. You say, "I'd rather be your friend, not your date."

Section 9: Social Skills Training for Staff—Agenda for Workshop Format II

I. Introduction
II. Questionnaires
  A. Client questionnaires
  B. Staff questionnaires
  C. Curriculum test (prestest)
  D. Rating of client social skills deficits
III. Definitions
  A. Organizing concepts
    1. Mature/immature
    2. Aggressive/assertive/passive
  B. Social skills
    1. Nonverbal skills
      a. facial expressions
      b. voice/speech
      c. nervous/calm mannerisms
      d. keeping an appropriate distance
    2. Verbal skills
      a. initiating conversations—open and closed questions
      b. maintaining conversation
      c. ending conversations
      d. "sandwich technique" by Roffman for giving criticism
IV. Techniques
  A. Reward
  B. Modeling
  C. Role Play
  D. Labeling
  E. Coaching
  F. Timing
  G. Biofeedback
  H. Relaxation
V. Activities (Premack Principle)
  A. *UNGAME®*
  B. Assertiveness game
  C. Timing game
  D. Open/closed question game
  E. Sandwich technique activity
VI. Assessment
  A. Curriculum test (Posttest)
  B. Rating of effective activities and techniques

Appendix G: State Protection and Advocacy Agencies[1]

ALABAMA
Suellen R. Galbraith, Program Director
Alabama DD Advocacy Program
P.O. Drawer 2847
The University of Alabama
Tuscaloosa, AL 35487-2847
(205) 348-4928

ALASKA
David Maltman, Director
Protection and Advocacy for the Developmentally Disabled, Inc.
325 E. 3rd Avenue, 2nd Floor
Anchorage, AK 99501
(907) 274-3658

AMERICAN SAMOA
Minareta Thompson, Director
Client Assistance and Protection and Advocacy Program
P.O. Box 3407
Pago Pago, American Samoa 96799
(684) 633-2418

ARIZONA
Amy Gittler, Executive Director
Patricia Brown, Director, P&A
Arizona Center for Law in the Public Interest
112 N. Central Avenue, Suite 400
Phoenix, AZ 85004
(602) 252-4904

ARKANSAS
Nan Ellen East, Executive Director
Advocacy Services, Inc.
12th & Marshall Streets, Suite 504
Little Rock, AR 72202
(501) 371-2171

CALIFORNIA
Albert Zonca, Executive Director
California Protection & Advocacy, Inc.
2131 Capitol Avenue
Sacramento, CA 95816
(916) 447-3331
(800) 952-5746

COLORADO
Mary Anne Harvey, Executive Director
The Legal Center
455 Sherman Street, Suite 130
Denver, CO 80203
(303) 722-0300

COMMONWEALTH OF NORTHERN MARIANA
John Castro, Director
Protection and Advocacy Agency
Catholic Social Services
P.O. Box 745
Saipan, CNMI 96950

[1] As of Summer 1987.

Connecticut
Eliot J. Dober, Executive Director
Office of P&A for Handicapped & DD Persons
90 Washington Street, Lower Level
Hartford, CT 06105
(203) 566-7616
(203) 566-2102 (Teletype)
(800) 842-7303 (Statewide toll-free)

Delaware
Christine Long, Program Administrator
Disabilities Law Project
144 E. Market Street
Georgetown, DE 19947
(302) 856-0038

District of Columbia
Yetta W. Galiber, Executive Director
Information, Protection and Advocacy Center for Handicapped Individuals (IPACHI)
300 I Street, N.E., Suite 202
Washington, DC 20002
(202) 347-4986

Florida
Jonathan P. Rossman, Executive Director
Governor's Commission on Advocacy for Persons with Disabilities
Office of the Governor, Capitol
Tallahassee, FL 32301
(904) 488-9070

Georgia
Donald G. Trites, Executive Director
Georgia Advocacy Office, Inc.
1447 Peachtree Street, N.E., Suite 811
Atlanta, GA 30309
(404) 885-1447
(800) 282-4538

Guam
Tomas G. Basa
Acting Client Assistance Program Administrator
Marianas Association for Retarded Citizens
P.O. Box 8830
Tamuning, Guam 96911
(671) 646-9026/9027

Hawaii
Patty Henderson, Executive Director
Protection and Advocacy Agency
1580 Makaloa Street, Suite 860
Honolulu, HI 96814
(808) 949-2922

Idaho
Brent Marchbanks, Director
Idaho's Coalition of Advocates for the Disabled, Inc.
1510 W. Washington
Boise, ID 83702
(208) 336-5353

Illinois
Zena Naiditch, Director
Illinois DD P&A Board
175 W. Jackson, Suite 2103
Chicago, IL 60604
(312) 341-0022

INDIANA
Ramesh K. Joshi, Executive Director
Indiana P&A Service Commission for the Developmentally Disabled
850 N. Meridian Street, Suite 2-C
Indianapolis, IN 46204
(317) 232-1150
(800) 622-4845

IOWA
Mervin L. Roth, Executive Director
Iowa Protection and Advocacy Service, Inc.
3015 Merle Hay Road, Suite 6
Des Moines, IA 50310
(515) 278-2502

KANSAS
Joan Strickler, Executive Director
Kansas Advocacy & Protective Services
Suite 2, 513 Leavenworth Street
Manhattan, KS 66502
(913) 776-1541
(800) 432-8276

KENTUCKY
Gayla O. Peach, Director
Division for Protection & Advocacy
Department of Public Advocacy
151 Elkhorn Court
Frankfort, KY 40601
(502) 564-2967
(800) 372-2988

LOUISIANA
Lois V. Simpson, Executive Director
Advocacy Center for the Elderly & Disabled
1001 Howard Avenue, Suite 300A
New Orleans, LA 70113
(504) 522-2337
(800) 662-7705

MAINE
Advocates for the DD
2 Mulliken Court
P.O. Box 5341
Augusta, ME 04330
(297) 289-5755
(800) 452-1948

MARYLAND
David Chavkin, Director
Maryland Disability Law Center, Inc.
2510 St. Paul Street
Baltimore, MD 21218
(301) 383-3400

MASSACHUSETTS
Richard Howard, Executive Director
DD Law Center for Massachusetts
11 Beacon Street, Suite 925
Boston, MA 02108
(617) 723-8455

MICHIGAN
Elizabeth W. Bauer, Executive Director
Michigan P&A Service
109 W. Michigan, Suite 900
Lansing, MI 48933
(517) 487-1755

MINNESOTA
Luther Granquist, Director
Legal Aid Society of Minneapolis
222 Grain Exchange Building
323 Fourth Avenue, S.
Minneapolis, MN 55415
(612) 332-7301

MISSISSIPPI
Rebecca Floyd, Executive Director
Mississippi P&A System for DD, Inc.
4793-B McWillie Drive
Jackson, MS 39206
(601) 981-8207

Missouri
Carol D. Larkin, Director
Missouri DD P&A Service, Inc.
211 B Metro Drive
Jefferson City, MO 65101
(314) 893-3333
(800) 392-8667

Montana
Kris Bakula, Executive Director
DD/ Montana Advocacy Program, Inc.
1219 E. 8th Avenue
Helena, MT 59601
(406) 444-3889
(800) 332-6149

Nebraska
Timothy Show, Executive Director
Nebraska Advocacy Services for DD Citizens, Inc.
422 Lincoln Center Building
215 Centennial Mall S., Room 422
Lincoln, NE 68508
(402) 474-3183

Nevada
Holli Elder, Project Director
DD Advocate's Office
2105 Capurro Way, Suite B, 1st Floor
Sparks, NV 89431
(702) 789-0233
(800) 992-5715

New Hampshire
Donna Woodfin, Director
DD Advocacy Center, Inc.
6 White Street
P.O. Box 19
Concord, NH 03301
(603) 228-0432

New Jersey
Sarah W. Mitchell, Director
Division of Advocacy for the Developmentally Disabled
N.J. Dept. of Public Advocate
Division of Advocacy for the DD
Hughes Justice Complex CN 850
Trenton, NJ 08625
(609) 292-9742
(800) 792-8600

New Mexico
James Jackson, Executive Director
P&A System for New Mexicans with DD
San Pedro N.E., Building 4, Suite 140
Albuquerque, NM 87110
(505) 888-0111

New York
Clarence J. Sundram, Commissioner
NY Commission on Quality of Care for the Mentally Disabled
99 Washington Avenue, Suite 1002
Albany, NY 12210
(518) 473-4057

North Carolina
Lockhart Follin-Mace, Director
Governor's Advocacy Council for Persons with Disabilities
116 W. Jones Street
Raleigh, NC 27611
(919) 733-9250

North Dakota
Barbara C. Braun, Director
P&A Project for the DD
Governor's Council on Human Resources
13th Floor, State Capitol
Bismarck, ND 58505
(701) 224-2972
(800) 472-2670

Northern Mariana Islands
Felicidaed Ogamuro, Executive Director
Remedio R. Sablan, Administrator
Catholic Social Services, Box 745
Saipan, Commonwealth of the Northern Mariana Islands 96950
9-011-670-6981

Ohio
Carolyn Knight, Executive Director
Ohio Legal Rights Service
8 E. Long Street, 5th Floor
Columbus, OH 43266-0523
(614) 466-7264
(800) 282-9181

Oklahoma
Bob M. VanOsdol, Ph.D., Director
Protection and Advocacy Agency for DD
9726 E. 42nd
Osage Building, Room 133
Tulsa, OK 74146
(918) 664-5883

Oregon
Elam Lantz, Jr., Director
Oregon Advocacy Center
Advocacy Center
310 S.W. 4th Avenue, Suite 625
Portland, OR 97204
(503) 243-2081

Pennsylvania
Elmer L. Cerano, Executive Director
Pennsylvania Protection and Advocacy, Inc.
3540 N. Progress Avenue
Harrisburg, PA 17110-9659
(717) 657-3320
(800) 692-7443

Puerto Rico
Luis Ramos Milian
Ombudsman for Disabled Persons
Chardon Avenue, 916 Hato Rey
San Juan, PR 00916
(809) 766-2372/2388/2415

Rhode Island
Elizabeth Morancy, Executive Director
Rhode Island P&A System (RIPAS), Inc.
86 Weybosset Street, Suite 508
Providence, RI 02903
(401) 831-3150

South Carolina
Louise Ravenel, Executive Director
S. C. P&A System for the Handicapped, Inc.
2360-A Two Notch Road
Columbia, SC 29204
(803) 254-1600

South Dakota
Robert J. Kean, Executive Director
South Dakota Advocacy Project, Inc.
221 S. Central Avenue
Pierre, SD 57501
(605) 224-8294
(800) 742-8108

Tennessee
Marriette J. Derryberry, Executive Director
EACH., Inc.
P.O. Box 121257
Nashville, TN 37212
(615) 298-1080
(800) 342-1660

TEXAS
Dayle Bebee, Executive Director
Advocacy, Incorporated
7700 Chevy Chase Drive, Suite 300
Austin, TX 78752
(512) 454-4816
(800) 252-9108

UTAH
Phyllis Geldzahler, Executive Director
Legal Center for the Handicapped
455 East 400 S., Suite 201
Salt Lake City, UT 84111
(801) 363-1347
(800) 662-9080

VERMONT
William J. Reedy, Esq., Director
Vermont DD P&A
P.O. Box 1367
Burlington, VT 05402
(802) 863-2881

VIRGINIA
Carolyn White Hodgins, Director
Department for the Rights of the Disabled
James Monroe Bldg., 17th Floor
101 N. 14th Street
Richmond, VA 23219
(804) 225-2042
(800) 552-3962 (TDD and voice)

VIRGIN ISLANDS
Russell Richards, Director
Committee on Advocacy for the Developmentally Disabled, Inc.
31-A New Street, Apartment 2
Frederiksted, St Croix
U.S. Virgin Islands 00840
(809) 772-1200

WASHINGTON
Katie Dolan, Executive Director
The Troubleshooters Office
50 W. Armory Way, Suite 204
Seattle, WA 98119
(206) 284-1037

WEST VIRGINIA
Nancy Mattox, Executive Director
West Virginia Advocates for the Developmentally Disabled, Inc.
1200 Brooks Medical Bldg.
Quarrier Street, Suite 27
Charleston, WV 25301
(304) 346-0847
(800) 642-9205

WISCONSIN
Lynn Breedlove, Executive Director
Wisconsin Coalition for Advocacy, Inc.
16 N. Carroll, Suite 400
Madison, WI 53703
(608) 251-9600
(800) 328-1110

WYOMING
Jeanne A. Kawcak, Executive Director
P&A System, Inc.
2424 Pioneer Avenue, # 101
Cheyenne, WY 82001
(307) 632-3496
(800) 328-1110

Appendix H: Residential Facilities and Summer Camps

Section 1: Residential Facilities

Two types of residential facilities currently serve the Prader-Willi syndrome (PWS) population: those that are designed specifically for PWS individuals, and integrated facilities that serve both PWS and non-PWS individuals. The following list is provided by the Prader-Willi Syndrome Association. This association makes no specific recommendations about any of the listed facilities nor is it an official accrediting agency. Inspection and review of any residential program is the responsibility of those seeking placement.

Facilities Specifically Designed for PWS Clients

Bedford and Brookhaven Homes
Carolyn Champlin, Director
12461 N.E. 173rd Avenue
Woodinville, WA 98072
(206) 488-3534
Duplex, capacity: 8 each, ages 18+

Corte Maria
Friends of Handicapped Children
George Lawler
P.O. Box 97, 7733 Palm Street, # 201
Lemon Grove, CA 92045
(619) 466-9981
Capacity: 6, ages 18+

Devine House IV
Irene Otteman, Director
1801 Lynnwood
Mt. Pleasant, MI 48858
Capacity: 6, ages 18+

Dorothy Group Home
American Institute at Vineland
Kathleen Costello, Director
15th & NJ Avenues
Dorothy, NJ 08317
(609) 476-4399

Gatehouse
Oconomowoc Developmental Training Center
Debbie Frisk, Director
36100 Genesee Lake Road
Oconomowoc, WI 53066
(414) 567-5515

Gilbough Center
Residential Rehabilitation Center
P.O. Box G, Route 6A
Brewster, MA 02631
(617) 896-5776
Capacity: 8, ages 16+

Glenview
Glenkirk, Inc.
3675 Commercial Avenue
Northbrook, IL 60062
(312) 657-7727
Capacity: 8, ages 20+

Granada Hills Home
Dubnoff Center
Gil Freitag, Ph.D., Director
10527 Victory Place
N. Hollywood, CA 91606
(213) 877-5678
Capacity: 6, ages 14+

Lee Street House
Linda Hamilton, Owner, Operator
25401 Lee Street
Los Molinos, CA 96055
(916) 384-1488
Capacity: 6, ages 18+

McArthur Group Home
Meredith Green Director
349 E. McArthur Street
Sun Prairie, WI 53590
(608) 837-2499
Capacity: 3, ages 18+

Oakwood Residence, Inc.
Sandra Singer, Director
13403 McGinty Road
Minnetonka, MN 55343
(612) 938-8130
Capacity: 12, ages 18+

Othmer House
State of New York
McAlpin Avenue
Mahopac, NY 10541
Capacity: 11, ages 18+

Southern Road Group Home
14101 Southern Road
Grandview, MO 64030
c/o Jackson Country Board of Services for Developmental Disabilities
8508 Hillcrest
Kansas City, MO 64138
(816) 363-2000
Capacity: 12, ages 18+

Waltham Group Home
Human Service Options, Inc.
The Adams Office Park
Quincy, MA 02169
(617) 770-1405
Capacity: 4, ages 18+

Integrated Facilities for PWS and Non-PWS Clients

Adriel School
Box 188
West Liberty, OH 43357
(513) 465-5010

Area Residential Care
2909 Kaufman Avenue
Dubuque, IA 52001
(319) 556-7560

Arlington Community Residences
5015 10th Street, North
Arlington, VA 22205
(703) 522-8719

ATCO Enterprises
P.O. Box 1030
Watertown, SD 57201
(605) 886-7601

Benedictine School for Exceptional Children
Ridgely, MD 21660
(301) 634-2112

Bethshan
12927 South Monitor Avenue
Palos Heights, IL 60463
(312) 371-0800

Caswell Center
State of North Carolina
2415 W. Vernon Avenue
Kinston, NC 28501
(919) 522-1261

Charles River A.R.C.
P.O. Box 169

Needham, MA 01292
(617) 444-4347

Childeda Habilitation Institute
P.O. Box 2799
LaCrosse, WI 54602
(608) 782-6480

Children's Haven & Adult Center
4405 Desoto Road
Sarasota, FL 33580
(813) 355-8808

Cole County Residential Services
220 E. Dunklin
Jefferson City, MO 65101
(314) 634-4555

Community Options, Inc.
P.O. Box 1944
Montrose, CO 81404
(303) 249-1412

Curtis Home Children's Program
380 Crown Street
Meriden, CT 06450
(203) 237-9526

Deepwood Center
8121 Deepwood Boulevard
Mentor, OH 44060
(216) 255-7411

Ellington Community Residence
12 Westview Terrace
Vernon, CT 06066
(203) 646-4446

Exceptional Persons, Inc.
2530 University
Waterloo, IA 50701
(319) 232-6671

Fraser Hall
711 S. University
Fargo, ND 58103
(701) 293-8458

Francis X. Gallagher Services
2520 Pot Spring Road
Timonium, MD 21093
(301) 252-4005

Gateways to Better Living
130 Javit Court
Youngstown, OH 44515
(216) 792-2854

Glenwood State School
Glenwood, IA 51534
(712) 527-4811

Good Shepherd Manor
P.O. Box 387
Wakefield, OH 45687
(614) 289-2861

Guild School
W. 2118 Garland
Spokane, WA 99205
(509) 326-1651

Hillcrest Educational Centers, Inc.
Housatonic Street, P.O. Box 794
Lenox, MA 01240
(413) 528-0080

Hope Haven
1800 19th Street
Rock Valley, IA 51247
(712) 476-2737

Hull House
Farmington Hills, MI
(313) 858-1225

Johnson County Mental Retardation Center
9090 Nieman
Overland Park, KS 66214
(913) 492-6161

Keystone City Residence
406 N. Washington Avenue
Scranton, PA 18503
(717) 346-7561

Lakemary Center
100 Lakemary Drive
Paola, KS 66071
(913) 294-4361

Laura Baker School
P.O. Box 611
Northfield, MN 55057
(507) 645-8866

Linnhaven, Inc.
360 Seventh Avenue
Marion, IA 52302
(319) 377-9788

Little Keswick School, Inc.
P.O. Box 24
Keswick, VA 22947
(804) 295-0457

J. Clifford MacDonald Center
4304 Boy Scout Boulevard
Tampa, FL 33607
(813) 870-1300

Maryhaven Center of Hope
450 Myrtle Avenue
Port Jefferson, NY 11777
(516) 473-8300

Monroe Developmental Center
750 Latta Road
Rochester, NY 14612
(716) 461-8500

New Hope of Indiana
8450 N. Payne Road
Indianapolis, IN 46268
(317) 872-421

New Hampton Group Home
841 W. Main
New Hampton, IA 50659
(515) 394-2670

Northern RI ARC
80 Fabien Street
Woonsocket, RI 02895
(401) 769-9720

NYALD Community Residence
232 Gay Street
Delmar, NY 12054

Oak Hill School
120 Holcomb Street
Hartford, CT 06112
(203) 242-2274

Redford Opportunity House
17360 Beech Daly
Redford, MI 48240
(313) 531-3411

REM-Mankato
210 Thomas Drive
Mankato, MN 56001
(507) 387-3181

Residential Support Services
Panner Place Group Home
1320 Panner Place
Billings, MT 59105
(406) 248-4211

The Rhinebeck Country School
P.O. Box 191
Rhinebeck, NY 12572
(914) 876-7061

RICA Regional Institute for
Children and Adolescents
150004 Broschart Road
Catonsville, MD 21228
(301) 455-6000

Riverbrook School
Ice Glen Road
Stockbridge, MA 01262
(413) 298-4626

School of Hope
819 S. Laurel
Hope, AR 71801
(501) 777-4501

Shepherds Baptist Ministries
P.O. Box 400
Union Grove, WI 53182
(414) 878-2451

Sikeston Regional Center for MR/DD
Box 966, Plaza Drive
Sikeston, MO 63801
(314) 417-9455

Society for Handicapped Citizens
4283 Paradise Road
Seville, OH 44273
(216) 722-1900

Southern Concepts
826 N. Thorp Spring Road
Granbury, TX 76048
(817) 573-3821

Straight Talk, Inc.
3350 Olive Avenue
Signal Hill, CA 90807
(213) 424-5557

Summer House, Inc.
206 5th Street
Woodland, CA 95695
(916) 662-8493

Sunflower Training Center
P.O. Box 838
Great Bend, KS 67530
(316) 792-1321

Sunny Acres Homes
810 College Hill Drive
Paradise, CA 95969
(916) 877-5389

Utah State Training School
American Fork, UT 84003
(801) 756-6022

Vasa Lutheran Home for Children
5225 W. Highway 61
Red Wing, MN 55066
(612) 388-8845

Village Northwest Unlimited
330 Village Circle
Sheldon, IA 51201
(712) 324-4873

Woodward State School
Woodward, IA 50276
(515) 438-2600

The Woods School
354-5 Roebling Drive Langhorne, PA 19047
(215) 750-4054

Section 2: Summer Camp Programs for Individuals with PWS

This list of summer programs is provided by the Prader-Willi Syndrome Association. It was compiled on the basis of recommendations from members of the organization. Camp directors and staff frequently change, and anyone interested in a summer program is advised to conduct a thorough investigation.

Camp Blue Sky
St. Louis A.R.C.
P.O. Box 27809
St. Louis, MO 63146
(314) 569-2211

Camp Huntington
Bruceville Road
High Falls, NY 12440
Camp (914) 687-7840
Office (914) 462-0991

Camp Keystone
406 N. Washington Avenue
Scranton, PA 18503
(717) 346-7561

Camp Lee Mar
Lackawaxen, PA 18435
(717) 685-7188
Office (212) 988-7260

Camp New Horizons
P.O. Box 98
Shawnee-on-Delaware, PA 18356
Office (518) 761-4690

Camp Wonderland
Lake of the Ozarks
Rocky Mount, MO 65072
Camp (314) 392-8886
Office (314) 634-2321

Eagle Springs
RD # 2, Box 427
Pine Grove, PA 17963
Office (215) 849-2744
Camp (717) 345-9984

Meteor Ranch Bible Conference
2255 E. Highway 20
Upper Lake, CA 95485
(707) 275-2170

The Rehabilitation Institute of Pittsburgh
6301 Northumberland Street
Pittsburg, PA 15217
(412) 521-9000

Rock Creek Farm
RD # 1
Thompson, PA 18465
(717) 756-2706

Rosemont
RD # 3
Honesdale, PA 18431
(717) 253-3770
Office (516) 764-5021

Shady Brook Camp (Learning Disabled and Mental Retardation)
Route 151, P.O. Box 365
Moodus, CT 06469

Trade Lake Camp
Grantsburg, WI 54840
Office (612) 776-6945

Appendix I: A Sample Token Economy Behavioral Program for Individuals with Prader-Willi Syndrome[1]

JERI J. GOLDMAN and WILLIAM D. BLEVINS

As the residential placement of (PWS) clients has become refined, so too have the programs to address the particular needs of this population. An integral part of the behavior management plan for these clients is a token economy. Although this system is very similar to other token economies, it has been specially modified and tailored to meet the particular needs of the PWS client.

Within five privilege levels categorized from "A" to "E," with Level A being the least restrictive and Level E being the most restrictive, clients are able to earn "+" marks for the absence of maladaptative behaviors. The client can then "buy" his or her way into the next privilege level. Those clients on Level A may use their accumulated tokens to make purchases at the "token store," such as stamps, stationery, pencils, pens, and notebooks. Although available on a very limited and restricted basis at the token store, food items are not generally used as reinforcers, and the token system is not directly tied to the loss or maintenance of weight.

Maladaptive behaviors are weighted as to the seriousness and/or the potential for injury to others. (As an example, theft, property destruction, or failure to follow program each results in a drop of one privilege level, while an assault upon another person will result in an immediate demotion to Level E.) A drop to Level E results in the loss of all accumulated tokens and requires 3 days to move to the next level. A drop to any other level does not mean a loss of all tokens but does not permit the cashing in of tokens for 24 hours.

Residents are not required to comply with the token economy, instead being offered the opportunity to earn tokens through compliance. The emphasis is placed on teaching the residents that appropriate choices have

[1] Reprinted with the permission of The Woods Schools and Residential Treatment Center, Langhorne, PA 19047. Principal program planners: P.T. Barnes, W.D. Blevins, M. Cornell, J.F. Downing, J.J. Goldman, C. Kombacher, W. Lundahl, W.R. Martys, M. Oswald, R. Schall, and H. Turner, working in an ongoing IDT process (1984 to present).

positive effects and that each is responsible for his or her own choices. Thus compliance with the token system results in attainment of greater independence and more privileges, and failure to comply means that the resident has chosen to relinquish the opportunity to earn these rewards. Additionally, of course, the utilization of a token system provides an objective measurement of the overall effectiveness of the program.

The most indispensable part of any token economy is that of the reinforcement. This sample system consists of the immediate reinforcer of the "+" for compliance, the privilege level system, and the token store. Each "+" mark represents one token, which is later utilized at the daily opening of the token store to purchase higher privilege levels or more material objects. Purchasing ability is correlated with one's privilege level, which is directly related to compliance with rules and manifestation of appropriate social behavior. The privileges assigned to each level are listed below.

Level A

1. Unrestricted use of all west-campus activity areas without direct staff supervision. Residents are required to check in with their staff every 10 minutes.
2. Full access to all areas of the residence without direct staff supervision with the exception of the kitchen.
3. Privilege of inviting guests to the residence with prior supervisory permission.
4. Opportunity to purchase a "Weight Watchers" dinner each Friday.
5. Full participation in the token store.
6. Participation in all on-campus and off-campus activities.
7. In-room curfew at 11:00 p.m. Sunday through Thursday, with no established time for Friday and Saturday.

Level B

1. Use of west-campus activity areas with line of sight supervision only.
2. Full access to all public areas of the residence without direct staff supervision with the exception of the kitchen.
3. Participation in the token store limited to purchasing Level A or extended curfew.
4. Participation in all on-campus and off-campus activities.
5. In-room curfew at 10:30 p.m. Sunday through Thursday and 11:00 p.m. Friday and Saturday.

Level C

1. Full access to all public areas of the residence without supervision with the exception of the kitchen.
2. Use of the token store limited to purchasing Level B or extended curfew.
3. Participation in all on-campus and off-campus activities.
4. In-room curfew at 10:00 p.m. Sunday through Thursday and 11:30 p.m. Friday and Saturday.

Level D
1. Full access to all public areas of the residence with the exception of the kitchen.
2. Requirement for staff permission to be in the bedroom areas of the residence.
3. Participation in all on-campus activities.
4. Participation in the token store limited to purchasing Level C.
5. In-room curfew at 9:30 p.m.

Level E
1. Participation in residence-based activities only.
2. Access to public areas in the residence other than the dining/activity area requires direct staff supervision.
3. Participation in the token store limited to the purchase of Level D.
4. In-room curfew at 9:30 p.m.

Token System Guidelines

1. Once earned, tokens may not be taken away except in the event of an aggression or assault.
2. Clients are to be informed immediately if they have failed to earn a token or have experienced a level drop.
3. All clients are to be warned prior to taking any action that may result in their failure to earn a token or be dropped a level.
4. Level assignments are made daily.
5. Behaviors resulting in a level demotion and/or other consequences are as follows:
    a. Aggression/assault: immediate assignment to Level E and loss of all accumulated tokens.
    b. Program refusal: demotion of one privilege level and the failure to earn tokens during the time the program was scheduled.
    c. Noncompliance: inability to earn tokens for the period of noncompliance.
    d. Destruction of personal property: demotion of one privilege level.
    e. Destruction of other person's property: demotion of one privilege level and restitution required.
    f. Stealing: demotion of one privilege level with required restitution.
    g. Unauthorized absence from program area: drop of one privilege level and failure to earn tokens during the time of absence.
    h. Unauthorized absence and observed off-campus: demotion of two privilege levels and the failure to earn tokens for the period absent.
    i. Failure to follow house/work rules: failure to earn tokens.
6. A resident may only be demoted one level per day except in the case of an unauthorized absence off-campus or an aggression or assault.

Token Store Inventory

Item	Cost in tokens	Limit
Decaffeinated coffee[a]	20	1
Diet gum[a]	5	5
Diet candy[a]	5	3
One-half hour curfew extension	10	1
Uptown trip[a]	70	1
Allowance $.50[a]	50	1
Stationery[a]	2 per sheet	—
Envelopes[a]	10	5
Stamps[a]	25	5
Pencil[a]	5	1
Pen[a]	10	1
Notebook[a]	50	1
Next Level D through B	85% for 1 day	1
Move from Level E	90% for 3 days	1

[a] Level A only.

Index

R